A Special Notation of thanks to my dear friends:

George Barnett for taking the cover photograph.

Larry Quinn for taking the author photograph.

I appreciate your kindness in bringing this project to the public.

Patient Empowerment Guide and Journal

The Thirty-Day Planner, Organizer, and Journal for Your Inpatient Visit

A Powerful Tool To Inform You of How To Protect Yourself From:

- Neglect
- Inflated Billing
- Hospital-Acquired Infections
- Possible Wrongful Death

In Layman's Terms This Guide Will Assist You In Understanding The Following:

- Lab Tests
- Medical Imaging
- Medical Procedures
- Medical Language and Terminology

This Is A Must Have For Anyone Entering The Healthcare Setting

Johnilynn Wunderlich, RN, CLNC

iUniverse, Inc.
New York Bloomington

Patient Empowerment Guide and Journal
The Thirty-Day Planner, Organizer, and Journal for Your In-patient Visit

iUniverse books may be ordered through booksellers or by contacting:

iUniverse
1663 Liberty Drive
Bloomington, IN 47403
www.iuniverse.com
1-800-Authors (1-800-288-4677)

ISBN: 978-1-4401-7169-7 (sc)
ISBN: 978-1-4401-7170-3 (ebk)

Printed in the United States of America

iUniverse rev. date: 10/21/2009

Dedicated to:

My Lord and Savior, Jesus Christ. May all I do be pleasing to you.

My mother, Gail Sandefur, for encouraging me to write this journal to help others. Mom, you are my best friend and my rock. Thank you for everything. I love you.

My children: Jessica, thank you for your assistance. Eric and Graisen, thank you for your patience and understanding.

My granddaughter Ireland, you are a blessing.

I love you all.

To the memory of L ____ and C ____:

May the circumstances of your tragic suffering and deaths never be repeated.

I pray that now you may rest in peace.

INTRODUCTION

First, I would like to apologize if my grammar is not perfect. At the present time I do not have the extra finances to afford a professional edit. I feel it important enough to publish this book "as is" for your protection. When finances improve, I may in the future restructure this journal. I am not a professional writer, I am nurse. I am a nurse that has a great deal of compassion for people. I believe in treating people with dignity and respect. I feel this so strongly that I left my position in the Intensive Care Unit to write this book after often witnessing criminal negligence brought on by corporate greed. I have been told to falsify charting and strongly cautioned to watch what I say if I wanted to keep my job. I am not the only nurse that has been told this; I am just someone who believes in taking a stand when it comes to providing quality care to those in need.

This guide and journal is designed to empower you and your loved ones while in the hospital or an inpatient facility. I created this guide and journal for you in hopes that it will inform and protect you. The public needs to realize that healthcare is big business and with any big business the bottom line is money and not the patient's well-being. Many people think that hospitals are there to make them well and in many cases that is what happens, in many cases it is not what happens. I have often witnessed unfortunate patients suffer and die needlessly. This is due to greedy administrators wanting to make their bonuses by keeping staffing below a substandard level. This is a major contributor to patients lying in their own waste, patient falls, injuries, pressure ulcers, pneumonia, hospital acquired infections, and even deaths.

I noticed while providing care for patients over the last thirteen years as a Registered Nurse that patients and their loved ones typically do not question the physician or healthcare provider. Most patients shake their heads in agreement to anything since they think that physicians and healthcare providers know best. When the physician or the healthcare provider leave the room the patient is then left in a state of confusion wondering what happens next. I suggest that you do not agree to anything you do not thoroughly understand! Unfortunately patients and their families agree to tests and procedures that are not necessary because they are not educated in medicine. If you do not thoroughly understand something ask your healthcare provider to repeat everything in terms you understand. I suggest that you question everything because you may be surprised to find that some of the people taking care of you may not know the answers themselves. I have had conversations with healthcare providers that knew very little about the condition of their patient. I suggest that you question everyone that provides care for you about your condition and why you are there. This will empower you and force the healthcare industry to be accountable.

The agency that accredits hospitals typically informs facilities that they are coming for a visit in advance. This allows administrators to have time to staff the units appropriately and clean the areas for inspection. It has been my observation that this agency rarely makes surprise visits. Hospitals spend billions of dollars lobbying our government to keep healthcare from being regulated. This means no one is watching how they take care of you or your loved one. This guide will help inform you of how to protect yourself from negligence, hospital-acquired infections, inflated billing, and possible wrongful death. It will assist you in understanding various tests, scans, procedures, and medical language.

You need to protect yourself by always asking questions and documenting everything. Take charge of your healthcare. Remember that without you, they would be out of business. You do have choices. If you do not approve of the care that is being provided inform the chief nursing officer, case manager, and social worker. Do not settle for substandard care.

Johnilynn Wunderlich, RN, CLNC

Contents

MY HOSPITAL JOURNAL

This journal belongs to: ______________________________

I stayed at ______________________________ hospital.

Dates of my stay: ______________________________

My reason for coming to hospital: ______________________________

My diagnosis: ______________________________

My physician's names: ______________________________

My day shift nurses names: ______________________________

My night shift nurses names: ______________________________

My patient care technician's names: ______________________________

Names of charge nurses: ______________________________

Name of case manager: ______________________________

Name of social worker: ______________________________

Name of nurse manager: ______________________________

Names of nursing supervisors: ______________________________

Name of inpatient service director: ______________________________

Name of chief nursing officer: ______________________________

Name of CEO at hospital: ______________________________

This hospital is owned by ______________________________ Corporation.

Is this a for profit hospital: _____ yes, _____ no.

MY INSURANCE INFORMATION

My primary insurance company is: ______________________________

My policy number is: ________________ Group number: ______________

My ID number is: ______________ Insurance phone number: ______________

Mailing address of insurance company: ______________________________

____

I am the primary/secondary (circle) policy holder.

If secondary policy holder, name of primary: ______________________

My co-pays are: ______________________________

Do all my physicians take my insurance that see me during my

hospital stay: _____ yes, ____ no. This is important to ask.

My secondary insurance company is: ______________________________

My policy number is: ________________ Group number: ______________

My ID number is: ______________ Insurance phone number: ______________

Mailing address of insurance company: ______________________________

____

I am the primary/secondary (circle) policy holder.

If secondary policy holder, name of primary: ______________________

My co-pays are: ______________________________

Notes: ____

____

____

____

____

____

____

____

____

MAKING DECISIONS

There are times when we need to make our decisions known in advance. Spending time in the hospital setting is one of those times. I have witnessed all too often patients suffer needlessly due to not having made these important wishes clarified in writing.

If you do not currently have these in place, I strongly urge you to complete them before you come into the hospital. If this is not possible, the hospital can assist you with them. Do not hesitate to ask!

I have a Living Will: ____ yes, ____ no.
Copy given to the hospital: _____ yes, _____ no.
Is a copy on the chart (ask)! ____ yes, ____ no.
I would like information regarding a Living Will: _____ yes, _____ no.

I have a Healthcare Surrogate: ________ yes, ______ no.
If yes, name of person: ____

If no, I wish to initiate __________________________ as my Healthcare Surrogate if I am unable to become unable to make my own decisions.

Copy given to hospital: _____ yes, _____ no.

Is a copy on the chart (ask)! _____ yes, _____ no.

I would like information regarding the responsibilities of my Healthcare Surrogate: ____ yes, _____ no.

If yes, ask for the form from the hospital and have your healthcare provider explain it to you.

I have a Medical Power Of Attorney: _____ yes, _____ no.
My medical power of attorney is: ______________________________
Their contact information is: ______________________________
____
Copy given to the hospital: _____ yes, _____ no.
Is a copy on the chart (ask)! _____ yes, _____ no.
I would like information regarding the responsibilities of my Power Of Attorney: _____ yes, _____ no.
If yes, ask for the form from the hospital and have your healthcare provider explain it to you.

TERMS TO KNOW

Full Code: This is where every attempt is made to save a patient during cardiopulmonary arrest. This includes but not limited to: medications, chest compressions, electrical shocks to the heart, intubation and line insertions.

DNR or Do Not Resuscitate: You will be cared for as any other patient. If your heart or lungs fail, then we allow nature to take its course and provide comfort to the patient.

CMO or Comfort Measures Only: This is when it has been determined that the end of life is inevitable. IV fluids, nutrition, and medications are stopped. Pain medications are allowed.

PRIVACY CODE

There are federal laws that protect your privacy. The Health Insurance Portability and Accountability Act of 1996 is known as HIPAA. It is important to understand that in accordance with the law healthcare professionals are not allowed to discuss your condition or that you are patient with anyone that does not have your privacy code.

Note: It is strongly suggested that one main contact person be named and that everyone else contact that individual for updates. Nursing staff are very busy giving patient care and too many updates take time away from the patients.

My privacy code: ____________ Name of primary contact: ____________

The following persons are allowed to have my privacy code and information regarding my condition:

Name: ____________ Home phone: ____________

Work: ____________ Cell: ____________

Name: ____________ Home phone: ____________

Work: ____________ Cell: ____________

Name: ____________ Home phone: ____________

Work: ____________ Cell: ____________

Name: ____________ Home phone: ____________

Work: ____________ Cell: ____________

Name: ____________ Home phone: ____________

Work: ____________ Cell: ____________

Name: ____________ Home phone: ____________

Work: ____________ Cell: ____________

Name: ____________ Home phone: ____________

Work: ____________ Cell: ____________

MEDICATION LIST

I take (medication name) ________________, dosage amount ______________
How many times per day ______________ at what times ______________________
Purpose for medication ____

I take (medication name) ________________, dosage amount ______________
How many times per day ______________ at what times ______________________
Purpose for medication ____

I take (medication name) ________________, dosage amount ______________
How many times per day ______________ at what times ______________________
Purpose for medication ____

I take (medication name) ________________, dosage amount ______________
How many times per day ______________ at what times ______________________
Purpose for medication ____

I take (medication name) ________________, dosage amount ______________
How many times per day ______________ at what times ______________________
Purpose for medication ____

I take (medication name) ________________, dosage amount ______________
How many times per day ______________ at what times ______________________
Purpose for medication ____

I take (medication name) ________________, dosage amount ______________
How many times per day ______________ at what times ______________________
Purpose for medication ____

I take (medication name) ________________, dosage amount ______________
How many times per day ______________ at what times ______________________
Purpose for medication ____

I take (medication name) ________________, dosage amount ______________
How many times per day ______________ at what times ______________________
Purpose for medication ____

I take (medication name) ________________, dosage amount ______________
How many times per day ______________, at what times ______________________
Purpose for medication ____

I take (medication name) ________________, dosage amount ______________
How many times per day ______________, at what times ______________________
Purpose for medication ____

I take (medication name) ________________, dosage amount ______________
How many times per day ______________, at what times ______________________
Purpose for medication ____

I take (medication name) ________________, dosage amount ______________
How many times per day ______________, at what times ______________________
Purpose for medication ____

I take (medication name) ________________, dosage amount ______________
How many times per day ______________, at what times ______________________
Purpose for medication ____

MEDICATION LIST

I take (medication name) ____________, dosage amount ____________
How many times per day ____________ at what times ____________
Purpose for medication ____________

I take (medication name) ____________, dosage amount ____________
How many times per day ____________ at what times ____________
Purpose for medication ____________

I take (medication name) ____________, dosage amount ____________
How many times per day ____________ at what times ____________
Purpose for medication ____________

I take (medication name) ____________, dosage amount ____________
How many times per day ____________ at what times ____________
Purpose for medication ____________

I take (medication name) ____________, dosage amount ____________
How many times per day ____________ at what times ____________
Purpose for medication ____________

I take (medication name) ____________, dosage amount ____________
How many times per day ____________ at what times ____________
Purpose for medication ____________

I take (medication name) ____________, dosage amount ____________
How many times per day ____________ at what times ____________
Purpose for medication ____________

I take (medication name) ____________, dosage amount ____________
How many times per day ____________ at what times ____________
Purpose for medication ____________

I take (medication name) ____________, dosage amount ____________
How many times per day ____________ at what times ____________
Purpose for medication ____________

I take (medication name) ____________, dosage amount ____________
How many times per day ____________, at what times ____________
Purpose for medication ____________

I take (medication name) ____________, dosage amount ____________
How many times per day ____________, at what times ____________
Purpose for medication ____________

I take (medication name) ____________, dosage amount ____________
How many times per day ____________, at what times ____________
Purpose for medication ____________

I take (medication name) ____________, dosage amount ____________
How many times per day ____________, at what times ____________
Purpose for medication ____________

I take (medication name) ____________, dosage amount ____________
How many times per day ____________, at what times ____________
Purpose for medication ____________

LIST OF SURGERIES AND PROCEDURES

I had ______________________________ (Surgery/Procedure)
Reason: ______________________________
Year: ______________, Physician: ______________

I had ______________________________ (Surgery/Procedure)
Reason: ______________________________
Year: ______________, Physician: ______________

I had ______________________________ (Surgery/Procedure)
Reason: ______________________________
Year: ______________, Physician: ______________

I had ______________________________ (Surgery/Procedure)
Reason: ______________________________
Year: ______________, Physician: ______________

I had ______________________________ (Surgery/Procedure)
Reason: ______________________________
Year: ______________, Physician: ______________

I had ______________________________ (Surgery/Procedure)
Reason: ______________________________
Year: ______________, Physician: ______________

I had ______________________________ (Surgery/Procedure)
Reason: ______________________________
Year: ______________, Physician: ______________

I had ______________________________ (Surgery/Procedure)
Reason: ______________________________
Year: ______________, Physician: ______________

I had ______________________________ (Surgery/Procedure)
Reason: ______________________________
Year: ______________, Physician: ______________

I had ______________________________ (Surgery/Procedure)
Reason: ______________________________
Year: ______________, Physician: ______________

I had ______________________________ (Surgery/Procedure)
Reason: ______________________________
Year: ______________, Physician: ______________

I had ______________________________ (Surgery/Procedure)
Reason: ______________________________
Year: ______________, Physician: ______________

I had ______________________________ (Surgery/Procedure)
Reason: ______________________________
Year: ______________, Physician: ______________

I had ______________________________ (Surgery/Procedure)
Reason: ______________________________
Year: ______________, Physician: ______________

LIST OF PHYSICIANS AND THEIR SPECIALTY

This is a list of the different types of physicians that may see you during your hospital stay:

You will always have a Primary Physician (also called Attending Physician, this is the doctor in charge of your care.)

Check and list names of the physicians that apply to you during your hospitalization.

__Primary: Dr.________________________________

__Allergist (allergies): Dr.________________________________

__Anesthesiologist (pain control, puts you to sleep and monitors during procedures):

Dr: ________________________________

__Cardiologist (heart): Dr.________________________________

__Dermatologist (skin conditions): Dr. ________________________________

__Endocrinologist (hormones, diabetes, thyroid): Dr. ________________________________

__ENT (ear, nose, throat): Dr.________________________________

__Gastroenterologist (stomach, intestines, liver): Dr. ________________________________

__Gynecologist (female reproductive system): Dr. ________________________________

__Hematologist (blood disorders): Dr.________________________________

__Infectious Disease: Dr.________________________________

__Internal Medicine: Dr.________________________________

__Neonatologist (premature infants): Dr: ________________________________

__Nephrologist (kidneys and urinary tract): Dr. ________________________________

__Obstetrician (pregnancy, childbirth, and post partum): Dr: ________________________________

__Oncologist (cancer): Dr. ________________________________

__Ophthalmologist (diseases of the eye): Dr. ________________________________

__Optometrist (eyes, vision correction): Dr. ________________________________

__Orthopedist (bones, joints): Dr.________________________________

__Pediatrician (children): Dr. ________________________________

__Proctologist (disorders of the rectum or anus): Dr. ________________________________

__Psychiatrist/psychologist (mental health): Dr. ________________________________

__Pulmonologist: (lungs and ventilator management): Dr. ________________________________

LIST OF PHYSICIANS AND THEIR SPECIALTY

__Radiologist (X-rays and various scans): Dr. ____________

__Rheumatologist (treat arthritis, diseases of the joints, connective tissues, muscles and bones): Dr. ____________

__Surgeon (surgical procedures): Dr(s). ____________

__Urologist (urinary system): Dr. ____________

__Dr(s). ____________

ITEMIZED BILLING

In this journal you will have the ability to keep a complete record of physician visits, nursing visits, therapies, medications, and supplies you receive.

You need to understand that you will be billed for any visit from the doctor or their assistant. The fee will be charged as a physician visit even if it is from the assistant, resident, intern, or medical student that visited the patient and not the actual physician. The assistant talks with the physician about the condition of the patient and may not even actually visit or examine the patient but will sign the progress report or orders. Unfortunately some physicians will not see the patient at all but ask the nurse about the patient while filling out the progress notes and orders. The patient is still being charged for that visit since there are notes and orders as if they were actually seen by the physician. This is why there is a section about which physicians visited and if you were actually examined. You should compare this to your bill.

Look at the section of your bill that addresses various types of therapies. Physical and Occupational Therapy typically bill in unit time. A unit of time is usually a few minutes. A patient may be billed for therapy including range of motion exercises lasting a few minutes for the entire day or getting them in a chair and leaving them until the nursing staff puts the patient to bed. Look at how you are being billed for these services.

You should ask about medications you are receiving and record them if possible. Ask for a daily record of medications administered. Take a recording device and say what medications you are receiving and the times administered. Record the medications in your journal. Ask about the medications you are receiving. You will notice that occasionally the staff administering the medications have no idea why they are giving the medication to the patient due to the nurse having too many patients and not enough time to think about what is happening with each of the patients. This is usually the result of understaffing caused by corporate greed and the frustration of the nursing staff that filters down to the patient.

Keep a record of all things brought into your room. Ask why you are receiving the items. Do not allow yourself to be billed for any unused supplies. It is not uncommon for items to be brought into a patient's room and left not opened. The end result is you are being billed for items that end up in the trash.

Keep a separate folder for test results, X-rays, scans, and discs for your records. Ask the physician and anyone acting on their behalf for a business card. If you cannot obtain a card, write their title in your journal under the physician section.

OBTAINING MEDICAL RECORDS

It is a wise decision to obtain a copy of your medical records. This will require you to sign a release form. You should ask for the release form while you are still in the hospital. You may get the necessary release forms in the medical records department if your healthcare provider does not provide a form to you. You or a person having legal rights to your health information may contact the facility if you have left the facility and are unable to return to sign the form. The healthcare facility should be able to mail, fax, or e mail the request form to you to sign and return. You may obtain specific information or the entire record.

Types of information in a medical record are: Emergency room record, physician notes and orders, progress notes, nurses notes, admission record, medication record, lab test results, X-ray and scan reports, pathology reports, history and physical, therapy notes, surgical report, anesthesia report, cardiology reports, radiology reports, respiratory therapy notes, dialysis record, blood products record, patient care duties performed including oral care, bathing, how often a patient is repositioned, wound care management, code blue record, social services reports, case management reports, and discharge record. Ask the medical records department of the cost of your records. Typically there is a per page fee in addition to an hourly fee for someone to copy the records. This can become extremely expensive. If you have the records sent to your Primary Care Physician instead of you there may not be a charge.

If you are not the patient but have the legal right to the health information you must provide the legal document as proof before records will be released.

The availability of obtaining your medical records differs from state to state. Typically records are available for approximately five to six years after discharge from the facility. There is an exception with children's records. Children's records are accessible for three to ten years beyond the age of eighteen to twenty one depending upon the facility.

KEEP YOUR EYES OPEN

Make sure your room has been terminally cleaned. You should insist on it! The term terminally cleaned means that every surface has been wiped down with a disinfectant to help kill bacteria. It also means that a new privacy curtain has been hung. Healthcare providers open and close these curtains with dirty gloves after cleaning blood, urine, and feces from patients. Wound dressings that are saturated with life threatening bacteria are changed and then the curtains are opened with contaminated gloves. The curtains are not changed on a routine basis after every patient.

Please ask your healthcare providers and guests to wash their hands for at least twenty seconds with soap and water. Do not retouch the handle with bare hands. This is the best way to prevent the spread of viruses and bacteria.

Have your healthcare provider or anyone assisting with your care change gloves between cleaning wounds, urine and feces, bathing, trach care, and ventilator care. This is a source of bacterial cross contamination.

Gowns, gloves, and masks: This is extremely important when someone is on isolation precautions. Make sure the physicians are putting on protective gear - don't be afraid, they know to do this. Do not be afraid to ask them to gown up, wash hands, and wear gloves. Make sure your healthcare provider cleans their stethoscope or covers it before touching you.

Look at your healthcare providers hands. Do they have overlays on their fingernails? Acrylic and gel nails can harbor bacteria, fungus, and some viruses between the natural nail and overlay. There have been instances where a link between the death of premature babies and the bacteria from healthcare providers acrylic nails. Most hospitals do not allow their employees to have fake nails due to the risk of harboring infection which could be transmitted to patients.

If the healthcare provider is wearing excessive or dangling jewelry, ask them to remove or cover it. Jewelry is a host for bacteria like MRSA. This also includes badge holders that hang around the neck.

You should request at the beginning of each shift that the nurse clean the computers and scanners with a disinfectant. This is especially important if the computers are portable and enter other patient's rooms.

Ask your healthcare provider to label your IV lines with insertion dates to reduce risk of infection. A peripheral IV site is to last three to four days. A central line may last a week to ten days depending upon protocol at each facility. Request a new bandage if the dressing gets wet, soiled, or edges begin to lift.

Ask your surgeon about antibiotics before having surgery. Make sure your antibiotics are given on time. Prophylactic antibiotics are to be given one hour prior to surgery. Frequently understaffing can cause a delay in correct timing of your medications. Do not hesitate to speak up when it comes to your health.

A checklist is to be completed for any procedure or surgery. This checklist identifies that it is the correct patient, procedure, and site. This is to be done at the bedside immediately before the procedure. Many times physicians are in a rush and this checklist is not completed until after the procedure is over and the nurse is chasing them down for a signature. Insist that the checklist be completed, the correct site is marked, and you are having the correct procedure before any sedation is administered.

Make sure your healthcare provider are turning, suctioning, checking for incontinence, and cleaning the patient's mouth every two hours. This will help reduce infection and decrease the risk of pressure ulcers.

KEEP YOUR EYES OPEN

Ask about one time use or disposable blood pressure cuffs and oxygen saturation probes. These are recycled and should not be reused, these are single use items. They are often used several times by for profit hospitals! This is totally disgusting and should not be tolerated. Ask how you are being charged for disposable equipment others have used. You are being charged for new equipment, you should demand the equipment provided for you not be recycled possibly giving inaccurate information and having terrible consequences. This is a way for the facility to cut cost and charge you for something that should be discarded. If your heart is being monitored look at the connections. These are often not cleaned from patient to patient.

Ask if you are in a semi-private room and if your roommate is on isolation precautions. If your roommate is on isolation precautions, request a different room. Hospitals can place you in a room with other patients that have life threatening illnesses as long as they follow hospital protocol. Hospital protocol could mean only a three foot barrier between you and being compromised, leaving you at risk! From experience I can tell you this is at times compromised.

Ask about the medications you are receiving. Take notes of the medications you decide to refuse. If the medications have already been scanned and charted as given, you will be charged for those medications unless you have a record of refusing them. Your healthcare provider should unchart that the medications were given and note them as refused. Take notes of the healthcare providers name, date, time, and type of the medications refused. Keep your own records and compare to your itemized bill.

Activities that compromise patients well being: ______________________________

____

____

____

____

____

____

____

____

____

____

____

____

____

____

NOSOCOMIAL INFECTIONS

Nosocomial infections are infections acquired during your hospital stay or at a nursing home. Most people have the perception that hospitals are sterile and clean. In reality, most hospitals are not clean or sterile. Approximately two million nosocomial infections are reported in the United States annually. Approximately ninety thousand deaths are related to hospital acquired infections annually. Medicaid no longer reimburses hospitals for nosocomial infections, remember this when you get your bill. You should not be held responsible to pay for extra care due to a hospital acquired infection. Take good notes of when or if you acquire a nosocomial. Obtain an itemized statement. Look for what you are being charged for after the date of infection. You and your loved ones must be the guardians of your own healthcare. Good hand washing, wearing gloves, cleaning the stethoscope, and cleaning the IV ports with alcohol before accessing will decrease the risk of you becoming a statistic. A list of the most common nosocomial infections is listed below.

Acinetobacter: This is one of the most common infections in the hospital. This type of bacteria can be life threatening in compromised patients. This bacterium can affect the lungs causing a nosocomial pneumonia or ventilator acquired pneumonia. It can cause infections of the skin, wound, and blood. Acinetobacter can cause Meningitis. This type of bacteria is resistant to many types of antibiotics.

Candida: This is more commonly known as a yeast or fungal infection. This infection can be acquired when a patient is on long term antibiotics or is immunocompromised. Candida can be found on the skin and reproductive organs and in the gastrointestinal tract and mouth. Oral Candida is commonly known as thrush. Treatment for Candida is oral and intravenous antifungals.

Clostridium Difficile or C Diff: This bacterium is found in the gastrointestinal tract. It can cause diarrhea and colitis. The elderly and people on long term antibiotics are at a higher risk of acquiring this disease. This type of bacteria can be easily transferred from patient to patient if healthcare professionals are not washing hands between patients. It can also be acquired if the patient is not allowed to wash their hands after using the bedside commode or bedpan.

Escherichia Coli: This bacterium is found in the gastrointestinal tract. It is associated with urinary tract infections. If you are to have a urinary catheter placed in the hospital you may want to ask for a urine culture to be done prior to insertion. This will inform you if you acquire an infection prior to or after insertion. Ask what hospital policy is regarding securing the catheter and how long it may be remain. Have the person inserting the catheter date the drainage bag upon insertion.

Influenza: This commonly referred to as the flu. This infection can lead to pneumonia, cardiac or respiratory failure. The very young and elderly are at highest risk. Annual vaccinations are recommended as prevention.

Klebsiella: This bacterium is found in the intestinal tract. Klebsiella can affect the blood, lungs, urinary tract, and wounds. This is a very serious infection and is becoming more common in the hospital environment. Have your healthcare provider take all precautions to prevent transmission.

Methacillin-Resistant Staphylococcus Aureus or MRSA: This is a common nosocomial infection. This infection affects the lungs, blood, wounds, eyes, ears, nose, mouth, and urinary tract. Surgical wounds and soft tissues are especially at risk. Central and peripheral IV sites at susceptible. This infection can be fatal. Good hand washing, gloves, mask, gown, cleaning the stethoscope, and cleaning the IV sites with alcohol before accessing will help decrease the risk of infection.

NOSOCOMIAL INFECTIONS

Pseudomonas Aeruginosa: This bacterium affects the lungs, blood, wound, and urinary tract. This infection is resistant to many antibiotics and is characterized by a fruity odor especially in wounds. This infection can be fatal if acquired.

Staphylococcus Aureus: This infection is related to approximately twelve thousand hospital deaths annually. This bacterium is responsible for many hospital-acquired respiratory infections, nosocomial pneumonia, blood stream infections, and post surgical site infections. This infection increases the risk of mortality.

Streptococcus Group A: This infection is not limited to a particular site. This infection is associated with Necrotizing Fasciitis and Sepsis. This infection can lead to multi system organ failure, shock, and even death.

Streptococcus Pneumoniae: This infection is associated with ear infections, Pneumonia, Cellulitis, Endocarditis, Peritonitis, Oseomyelitis, Meningitis, and abscesses of the brain. This infection is spread from person to person. Good hand washing, gown, mask, and gloves should be worn.

Vancomycin-Resistant Enterococcus or VRE: Persons at risk for acquiring VRE are patients that have received Vancomycin, Penicillin, or Gentamycin in the past, and persons that have been on long term antibiotic therapy. Elderly, critically ill patients, cancer, and post surgical patients are at risk. Patients with central IV catheters and urinary catheters are at an increased risk. This is a very serious infection due to it is resistant to most antibiotics.

Note: Always ask your healthcare provider to wash hands, wear gloves, clean and cover stethoscope. If the patient is on isolation precautions, gown, gloves, and mask should be worn. Have your visitors wear protective gear as well. If at all possible keep small children from visiting. If they must visit, do not allow them to touch anything including the privacy curtain. Wash the child's hands thoroughly for at least thirty seconds with soap and water. If they are brought in by stroller, wash the surfaces on the stroller including the wheels. There are highly infectious bacteria everywhere!!

If you acquire a nosocomial infection list type, date, and treatment:

Infection: ______________________________

Date: ____________ treatment: ____________________

Infection: ______________________________

Date: ____________ treatment: ____________________

Infection: ______________________________

Date: ____________ treatment: ____________________

Infection: ______________________________

Date: ____________ treatment: ____________________

INFORMATION REGARDING ADMINISTERING BLOOD PRODUCTS

The following information is designed to help aid you in your decision to either accept or decline blood products. You should discuss this subject further with your physician and anyone that may make decisions for you in the event you cannot make decisions. This is meant to be a basic overview and not an actual consent. An actual consent must be signed and witnessed prior to the administration of blood products.

The purpose of transfusing blood components is to help improve the oxygen-carrying capacity to the circulatory system and tissues. Depending on the type of component it may also aid in replacing circulating volume, clotting factors and platelets.

Types of Blood Components:

Packed Red Blood Cells: This is indicated for correcting the oxygen carrying capacity in patients with low Hemoglobin/Hematocrit levels. This is indicated for patients that have severe blood loss.

Platelets: Indicated for patients with low platelet counts of 100,000/ul

FFP or Fresh Frozen Plasma: Indicated for patients with coagulation deficiencies, Coumadin overdose, Thrombotic Thrombocytopenic Purpura (TTP) or a patient with active bleeding and is receiving massive blood transfusions.

Cryoprecipitate: It is used in the treatment of Hypofibrinogenemia that is associated with Disseminated Intravascular Coagulation. DIC is basically when your body produces small clots all over your body and you also have abnormal bleeding at the same time. It is also used when a patient has massive blood loss.

Albumin: Used as a volume expander. Used in emergent treatment of shock, managing burn victims, and Hypovolemia (low circulatory volume).

Blood types and compatibility:

Recipient type	donor type	Rhesus factor or commonly named RH factor
A	A , O	Positive or Negative: this is an antibody
B	B , O	that is attached to the surface of the blood
AB	AB , A , B , O	cell. Example: A positive or A negative.
O	O (only)	

My blood type is: _________ positive / negative.

What to expect: (take notice if this is done correctly-steps are often skipped)

Blood sample taken: _____yes, _____ no.
Blood band on patient: _____ yes, _____ no.
Identified patient by two identifiers: _____ yes, _____ no.
When blood product administered, two nurses (administering nurse must be RN) at bedside checking blood together using two identifiers: _____ yes, _____ no.
Vital signs taken prior to receiving product: _____ yes, _____ no.
Vital signs taken in 15 minutes: _____ yes, _____ no. One hour: _____yes, _____ no.
Vital signs taken at completion: _____ yes, _____ no. Reaction: _____yes, _____ no.

RECORD OF BLOOD PRODUCTS

This is a record of blood products given to: ______________________________.
Attach one sticker from each band placed on your arm and write down the information in case the sticker is misplaced.

My blood band number(s): __________, __________, __________, __________, __________.

Place blood band stickers here:

On the back of the blood product you should find stickers attached. This contains all the information regarding the product. You may want to keep a label for your future records. You will also find a donor number on the bag. This is the number assigned to the individual(s) that donated the blood product that you are receiving.

Donor numbers: __________, __________, __________, __________, __________,

__________, __________, __________, __________, __________, __________, __________,

__________, __________, __________, __________, __________, __________, __________,

__________, __________, __________, __________, __________, __________, __________.

Attach donor stickers here:

Reactions to blood products: fever, chills, hives, itching, severe headache, shortness of breath, back and muscle ache, chest pain, blood in the urine, and anaphylaxis.

Any reactions to blood products: ____ yes, ____ no.

List reaction: ______________________________

Donor number associated with reaction: ______________________________

List treatment: ______________________________

Note: it is very important to inform your healthcare provider if you have previously received blood products and had a reaction. Medications may be given to prevent minor reactions.

MEDICAL IMAGING

There are many types of scans offered that are used as tools to detect abnormalities in the body. Listed below are the main types of X-rays and scans. There are various tests within each category.

Cat Scan or Computerized Axial Tomography Scan: This type of scan takes a series of two dimensional X-rays and creates a three dimensional picture. This type of scan can view internal structures of the body including bone, soft tissues including brain, organs, blood vessels, abnormal collection of fluid and air, certain cancers, and tumors. This test is not reliable for screening the heart, due to the heart is in constant motion. This scan may be performed with or without contrast depending on the structures to be identified. You not be allowed to eat for several hours depending on the structures being scanned.

Doppler Studies: This test is performed using a Doppler Ultrasound. This is a painless test. It is used to detect blood flow through a vessel using sound waves. It can show narrowing of a vessel and blocked blood flow. Doppler studies evaluate the risk of Deep Vein Thrombosis or DVT, Pulmonary Embolus or P.E., embolus, Stroke, and blood flow in an unborn fetus.

EBCT or Electron Beam Computed Tomography: This is a very fast form of x-ray imaging. It measures the amount of calcium deposits in the coronary arteries, evaluates the patency of bi-pass grafts, various cardiac lesions, measure cardiac output, cardiac ejection fractions, cardiac muscle mass, and the amount of blood volumes in the chambers. This is ordered as a tool to predict heart attacks and the need for invasive testing or cardiac surgery.

MRA or Magnetic Resonance Angiography: This test is used to view the blood vessels in heart, lungs, brain, liver, kidneys, neck, abdomen, pelvis, arms, and legs. This test detects aneurysms, Atherosclerosis, and Arteriovenous Malformations. This test also views blood flow to tumors and masses. Contrast media may or may not be ordered. Patients with metal clips, screws, metallic implants, pacemakers or defibrillators, artificial heart valves, implanted nerve stimulators, implanted medication pumps, metallic artificial limbs and prostheses, and cochlear implants are prohibited from this test.

MRI or Magnetic Resonance Imaging: This test uses a magnetic field to view internal structures of the body. This type of imaging is used when a greater contrast between the soft tissues is needed. Contrast media may or may not be ordered. Patients with metal clips, screws, metallic implants, pacemakers or defibrillators, artificial heart valves, implanted nerve stimulators, implanted medication pumps, metallic artificial limbs and prostheses, and cochlear implants are prohibited from this test.

Pet Scan or Positron Emission Tomography: This test uses a small amount of radioactive material that can be injected, swallowed, or inhaled. The radioactive material collects in the area that is to be scanned. This scan assists in the how well the organs and tissues are functioning. Pet scans are used to detect cancer and evaluate effectiveness of treatment. It is used to evaluate heart function and blood flow. It is used to evaluate central nervous system disorders, brain mapping and abnormalities. You will not be allowed to eat several hours before the test. Remove all metal objects including glasses, jewelry, dentures, hearing aids, and metallic hair accessories. If you are breastfeeding pump breast milk and store until the radioactive contrast material is eliminated from your body. Inform your physician of what medications you are taking and your allergies.

MEDICAL IMAGING

Ultrasound: This type of scan uses sound waves to visualize various body structures. It is used in pregnancy to view the unborn fetus and placenta. The test typically involves conducting gel to be placed over the site that is viewed and a wand is placed on the skin. Depending on the structures that are being scanned it may require an ultrasound probe be inserted into the body.

X-Ray or Radiography: This type of imaging visualizes the bones, joints, organs, certain cancers and tumors if present in a two dimensional view. Dentists use this type of imaging to evaluate the condition of your teeth. Images may be with or without contrast. The types of contrast media used in x-rays are iodine based or barium. The iodine based contrast medium is injected and used to image typically vascular structures and types of cancers and masses in the body if present. Barium contrast is administered orally or rectally. Barium contrast is given to enhance images of the abdomen and pelvis.

INFORMATION REGARDING CONTRAST MEDIA

Iodine based contrast media is given intravenously or through a vein, Intrathecally or in the spine, Intrabdominally or in the abdomen, Intraarterially or through an artery, or Intraosseous or through an insertion made in the bone for IV access. A warm sensation may be felt if iodine based contrast is used. Warning: Contrast media may cause reactions in some patients: A mild reaction includes hot flushed feeling and vomiting. Skin reactions such as itching, swelling, and hives may occur. Breathing difficulties such as a tightening of the lungs, throat, and face may occur. A systemic reaction can occur leading to a drop in blood pressure leading to shock, respiratory, and cardiac arrest. A delayed reaction to iodine based contrast may occur up to forty-eight hours after administration. Delayed symptoms include flu-like symptoms, headaches and muscle pain. If you have experienced a mild reaction in the past tell your healthcare professional. Medications including steroids and Benadryl can be ordered to reduce the risk of a reaction. Contrast media can be toxic to the kidneys. A blood test may be ordered to evaluate your kidney function prior to the scan.

Barium contrast media is given orally or rectally. It used to view the digestive system. Oral contrast is given to view the esophagus, stomach, and small bowel. A barium enema is given to view the distal small intestine and large intestine. Barium should not be used if there is a known or suspected obstruction of the colon or a perforation of the bowel. Increased risks include impaction, perforation leading to Peritonitis, granulomas, adhesions, Anaphylaxis and death.

Note: If you take the medication Metformin, it should be stopped if possible for two days prior to the scan and until after the administration of intravenous contrast media is completely excreted from the body and renal function is normal. Metformin is excreted by the kidneys. Not allowing the allotted time may increase the risk of lactic acidosis.

ROUTES OF OXYGENATION

There are several types of devices that deliver supplemental oxygen. It is important to understand what type of device your physician has prescribed. If you have any questions regarding these devices ask your healthcare provider to explain further

Note: Room air is about 21%

Nasal Cannula: This device is a thin tube that loops over the ears and has two prongs that are placed in the nostrils that deliver oxygen. The prongs are to face downward. Oxygen is delivered by liters (0.25 to 6) and may even be humidified for comfort. Do not use a petroleum based product to lubricate the nose. It is not wise to mix concentrated oxygen with petroleum based products or any type of fire causing agents. Oxygen and smoking are a dangerous combination.

LOW FLOW DEVICES

Simple Face Mask: This device is a mask that fits over the nose and mouth. It delivers oxygen by liters (6 to 10) and mixes with room air. Oxygen concentration delivered is about 35 to 60%.

Partial Rebreather: This device is a mask that fits over the nose and mouth. This device has a reservoir bag. Oxygen is delivered at 5 to 15 liters per minute. At 6 to 10 liters oxygen delivered is about 40 to 70%.

HIGH FLOW DEVICES

Non-rebreather: Looks similar to a Rebreather mask but it incorporates a series of one way valves that prevent exhaled air returning to the patient. Minimum oxygen delivery is at 10 liters. Oxygen delivered is between 60 and 80%, this is dependent on the patients breathing pattern.

Venturi mask: This device delivers oxygen up to 40%. Tracheostomy collars, t-tube adapters, aerosol masks and face tents can be used with this system. This system is not intended for a patient in respiratory distress.

FACTS REGARDING MECHANICAL VENTILATION

A Pulmonologist (lung doctor) is the physician that will manage the ventilator. A Respiratory Therapist is the person that will assist in managing the ventilator and administers respiratory treatments. The Critical Care Nurse will help assist in monitoring the ventilator and provide care to the patient.

Mechanical ventilation requires the person to be intubated with an Endotracheal Tube that is inserted into the trachea and held there by a balloon that is inflated with air to hold it in place. This tube will be held in place by either a stabilization device or tape. Frequent oral care including oral suctioning and endotracheal suctioning should be performed at least every two hours. Ask the healthcare provider to adjust the tube side to side every two days to help prevent tissue breakdown in the mouth and lips.

A Closed Ballard is the device that is used for suctioning out secretions from the lungs. This should be done at least every two hours or more frequently. Ask about your hospital protocol. This should also be labeled with the date on it indicating time to be changed.

Make sure the healthcare professional has washed hands and is wearing gloves. This will aid in decreasing the possibility of contaminating the lungs with foreign bacteria. It has been reported all too often of patients acquiring lung infections due to providers not following proper technique. I have known of patients even acquiring E. Coli (found in feces) in the lungs. This happens when a patient is being cleaned and the healthcare provider doesn't change gloves before suctioning the patient or providing oral care. This is not an uncommon event!

VAP or Ventilator Acquired Pneumonia: This peaks at or around day 5 on the ventilator. The risk can be reduced by having the patient positioned in no less than a 30 degree angle with the head up. This helps reduce the risk of aspiration. Antibiotics, frequent suctioning and good hand washing are also important to reduce the risk of VAP.

Arterial Blood Gases are often done on a daily basis to determine patient oxygenation status and if a patient is ready to be weaned from ventilator.

MECHANICAL VENTILATION SETTINGS (IN BASIC TERMS)

CMV or Controlled Mandatory Ventilation: This setting is where the machine does the breathing for you if you are unable to take a breath on your own. Every breath is a full ventilation breath. The ventilator is set to a minimum number of breaths per minute and the amount of volume that is placed in the lungs. The patient never receives less.

ACV or Assist Control Ventilation: The patient assists in the initiation of each breath. Typically the patient is breathing over the set rate of ventilation. The patient cannot breathe less than the set rate. The amount of volume is always the same with each ventilated breath. The patient also takes spontaneous breaths and the volume is measured.

IMV or Intermittent Mechanical Ventilation: Mechanical breaths are delivered intermittently with the patient's breathing. This is used sometimes in the weaning process. The patient also has to have an intact breathing process.

CPAP or Continuous Positive Airway Pressure: Delivers a prescribed amount of oxygen that is at a compressed pressure and given to the patient via a full face mask or nose mask that is strapped to the patients face. This can be delivered while on the ventilator and is used as a weaning process. CPAP can also be used while not being on the ventilator for conditions including obstructive sleep apnea.

Bi-pap or VPAP: Bi-level or Variable Positive Airway Pressure provides two levels of pressure. First level is IPAP or Inspiratory Positive Airway Pressure which helps decrease the work of breathing by supplementing the Inspiratory Airway Pressure and helps decrease the work on the inspiratory muscles. The second level is Expiratory Positive Airway Pressure which helps aid in keeping the lungs from collapsing.

MY VENTILATOR SETTINGS

Setting: ______________, Rate: _______, O2%: ______, Tidal Volume: ________,

Spontaneous Tidal Volume: _______, Peep: _______, Pressure Support: ________,

Peak Pressure: ________ Suctioned at least every two hours? ____ yes, _____ no

Date intubated: ______________________, Date extubated: ______________________

Did I acquire an infection related to the ventilator: ______ yes, _______ no

If yes, what is the name of the infection: ______________________________

What was the treatment: ____

____

Did I require a Bronchoscopy: _______ yes, _______ no.

Did I acquire an infection from the Bronchoscopy: ______ yes, _____ no.

Type of infection: ____

Treatment: ____

REHABILITATION THERAPIES

The types of therapies offered vary from each institution. There are four main types of therapy: Physical Therapy, Occupational Therapy, Respiratory Therapy, and Speech-Language Therapy. Each therapy specializes in a specific scope of practice. There are additional types of therapies offered at varying facilities. These types of therapies are massage therapy, alternative therapy which includes acupuncture, light or healing touch, and music therapy. Ask your facility what types of services they provide and most importantly…how they bill for their services. Some facilities bill in as little as eight minute increments for Physical and Occupational Therapy (this is called a unit of time), meaning your therapy session is only eight minutes in length. You can be billed for physical therapy even if it is only getting the patient up in a chair and then leaving them for the nursing staff to put them back to bed - when the nurse finds the time. The therapist may not come back to assist the patient back to bed due to they do not get paid to put patients back to bed.

Note: It is important to get therapy started as soon as possible (as long as it is more than a few minutes per day, which does very little to benefit the patient.) Family members or friends should assist the patient with exercises as long as the physician agrees it is safe.

Physical Therapy: Assist with functional capacity evaluations to determine the ability to perform activities of daily living. Services include restoring muscle, joint and range of motion function, improve mobility, and help relieve pain. Therapists help restore, maintain, and promote fitness and overall health. Therapy includes testing and measuring patients' strength, flexibility, mobility, range of motion, balance, endurance, coordination, posture, muscle, and motor function. They assist the physician with a treatment plan for the best possible physical outcome.

Occupational Therapy: Aid the patient in returning to the best possible level of function. Assist in helping the patient problem-solve to improve the quality of life. Types of therapies include improving mobility, memory, and thinking skills. Teach patients how to feed and dress themselves. Train patients in how to use adaptive equipment such as wheelchairs, walkers, and prosthetics.

Respiratory Therapy: Aids the patient with respiratory treatments. The Respiratory Therapist assists the physician with respiratory procedures, treatments, intubation, and mechanical ventilation management.

Speech-Language Therapy: Assess, diagnose, treat, and help prevent disorders related to swallowing, speech, and language. Assist patients that are unable to swallow due to stroke, brain injury, and cleft palate. Assist patients with learning disabilities and hearing loss to improve communication more effectively.

My Physical Therapist name(s): ______________________________

My Occupational Therapist name(s): ______________________________

My Respiratory Therapist name (s): ______________________________

My Speech-Language Therapist name(s): ______________________________

Other Therapist (list type) name(s): ______________________________

____

____

THERAPY SCHEDULE CONTINUED FROM ________ TO ________

Therapist: ______________, Performed: P.T./O.T./R.T./Speech/Other (circle) Therapy
On ______________ at __________ am/pm. Length of visit: ___________ minutes.
Activities performed: ____.

Therapist: ______________, Performed: P.T./O.T./R.T./Speech/Other (circle) Therapy
On ______________ at __________ am/pm. Length of visit: ___________ minutes.
Activities performed: ____.

Therapist: ______________, Performed: P.T./O.T./R.T./Speech/Other (circle) Therapy
On ______________ at __________ am/pm. Length of visit: ___________ minutes.
Activities performed: ____.

Therapist: ______________, Performed: P.T./O.T./R.T./Speech/Other (circle) Therapy
On ______________ at __________ am/pm. Length of visit: ___________ minutes.
Activities performed: ____.

Therapist: ______________, Performed: P.T./O.T./R.T./Speech/Other (circle) Therapy
On ______________ at __________ am/pm. Length of visit: ___________ minutes.
Activities performed: ____.

Therapist: ______________, Performed: P.T./O.T./R.T./Speech/Other (circle) Therapy
On ______________ at __________ am/pm. Length of visit: ___________ minutes.
Activities performed: ____.

Therapist: ______________, Performed: P.T./O.T./R.T./Speech/Other (circle) Therapy
On ______________ at __________ am/pm. Length of visit: ___________ minutes.
Activities performed: ____.

Therapist: ______________, Performed: P.T./O.T./R.T./Speech/Other (circle) Therapy
On ______________ at __________ am/pm. Length of visit: ___________ minutes.
Activities performed: ____.

Therapist: ______________, Performed: P.T./O.T./R.T./Speech/Other (circle) Therapy
On ______________ at __________ am/pm. Length of visit: ___________ minutes.
Activities performed: ____.

Therapist: ______________, Performed: P.T./O.T./R.T./Speech/Other (circle) Therapy
On ______________ at __________ am/pm. Length of visit: ___________ minutes.
Activities performed: ____.

Therapist: ______________, Performed: P.T./O.T./R.T./Speech/Other (circle) Therapy
On ______________ at __________ am/pm. Length of visit: ___________ minutes.
Activities performed: ____.

Therapist: ______________, Performed: P.T./O.T./R.T./Speech/Other (circle) Therapy
On ______________ at __________ am/pm. Length of visit: ___________ minutes.
Activities performed: ____.

Therapist: ______________, Performed: P.T./O.T./R.T./Speech/Other (circle) Therapy
On ______________ at __________ am/pm. Length of visit: ___________ minutes.
Activities performed: ____.

Therapist: ______________, Performed: P.T./O.T./R.T./Speech/Other (circle) Therapy
On ______________ at __________ am/pm. Length of visit: ___________ minutes.
Activities performed: ____.

THERAPY SCHEDULE CONTINUED FROM __________ TO __________

Therapist: ________________, Performed: P.T./O.T./R.T./Speech/Other (circle) Therapy
On __________ at __________ am/pm. Length Of visit: __________ minutes.
Activities performed: ____.

Therapist: ________________, Performed: P.T./O.T./R.T./Speech/Other (circle) Therapy
On __________ at __________ am/pm. Length Of visit: __________ minutes.
Activities performed: ____.

Therapist: ________________, Performed: P.T./O.T./R.T./Speech/Other (circle) Therapy
On __________ at __________ am/pm. Length Of visit: __________ minutes.
Activities performed: ____.

Therapist: ________________, Performed: P.T./O.T./R.T./Speech/Other (circle) Therapy
On __________ at __________ am/pm. Length Of visit: __________ minutes.
Activities performed: ____.

Therapist: ________________, Performed: P.T./O.T./R.T./Speech/Other (circle) Therapy
On __________ at __________ am/pm. Length Of visit: __________ minutes.
Activities performed: ____.

Therapist: ________________, Performed: P.T./O.T./R.T./Speech/Other (circle) Therapy
On __________ at __________ am/pm. Length Of visit: __________ minutes.
Activities performed: ____.

Therapist: ________________, Performed: P.T./O.T./R.T./Speech/Other (circle) Therapy
On __________ at __________ am/pm. Length Of visit: __________ minutes.
Activities performed: ____.

Therapist: ________________, Performed: P.T./O.T./R.T./Speech/Other (circle) Therapy
On __________ at __________ am/pm. Length Of visit: __________ minutes.
Activities performed: ____.

Therapist: ________________, Performed: P.T./O.T./R.T./Speech/Other (circle) Therapy
On __________ at __________ am/pm. Length Of visit: __________ minutes.
Activities performed: ____.

Therapist: ________________, Performed: P.T./O.T./R.T./Speech/Other (circle) Therapy
On __________ at __________ am/pm. Length Of visit: __________ minutes.
Activities performed: ____.

Therapist: ________________, Performed: P.T./O.T./R.T./Speech/Other (circle) Therapy
On __________ at __________ am/pm. Length Of visit: __________ minutes.
Activities performed: ____.

Therapist: ________________, Performed: P.T./O.T./R.T./Speech/Other (circle) Therapy
On __________ at __________ am/pm. Length Of visit: __________ minutes.
Activities performed: ____.

Therapist: ________________, Performed: P.T./O.T./R.T./Speech/Other (circle) Therapy
On __________ at __________ am/pm. Length Of visit: __________ minutes.
Activities performed: ____.

Therapist: ________________, Performed: P.T./O.T./R.T./Speech/Other (circle) Therapy
On __________ at __________ am/pm. Length Of visit: __________ minutes.
Activities performed: ____.

DIALYSIS

There are four types of dialysis: Hemodialysis, Peritoneal Dialysis, Continuous Renal Replacement Therapy or more commonly known as CRRT, and Intestinal Dialysis. All share the same common goal of filtering toxins, regulating electrolytes, correcting ph balance, and maintaining fluid balances in the body when a patient is in either acute or chronic renal failure. A patient on dialysis will have a Nephrologist monitoring their dialysis. A nurse or technician certified in dialysis will administer and monitor the patient during the process.

Hemodialysis: This route of filtration is through the circulatory system. A minor surgical procedure will be required to create a fistula or graft between a vein and artery. Patients requiring immediate access will have a temporary venous catheter placed in the neck, chest, or groin.

There are three types of access for Hemodialysis. The first is Arteriovenous Fistula or AV Fistula. This requires a surgeon to connect an artery to a vein. Typically the site preferred is the lower forearm. This site may take several months to heal properly and is used for planned dialysis. This site usually last the longest amount of time and has the least risk of blood clots or infection. The second type of access is the Arteriovenous Graft. This type of graft is used when the patient's veins are too small to create a fistula. A synthetic graft or tube is implanted under the skin. The most common site for this is the upper forearm. This type has a slightly higher risk of blood clots and infection. This type may take a couple of weeks to heal and is not intended for emergent dialysis. The third type of access is a venous catheter that is inserted into a main vein in your neck, chest, or groin. This is used for immediate access. This type of catheter can be used for several weeks to months in patients that plan to have a more permanent type of access placed. Complications from this type of access include blood clots, narrowing of the vessel after removal, and infection.

Peritoneal Dialysis: A soft catheter tube is placed in your abdominal cavity usually by your belly button allowing the dialysis fluid to enter the abdomen and filter toxins and pull off extra fluid. This may be either by Continuous Ambulatory Peritoneal Dialysis (CAPD) or Continuous Cycler-Assisted Peritoneal Dialysis (CCPD). CAPD allows the patient to fill the abdomen with the dialysis solution and have a dwell time of four to six hours before emptying. This step must be repeated after each emptying. CCPD performs the exchange while you sleep. A machine cycles during sleep allowing for only one exchange during the time the patient is awake. Complications associated with peritoneal dialysis include infection of the peritoneum. Signs of infection include fever, nausea, vomiting, redness or pain at site, bulging at catheter site, and cloudiness from dialysis solution.

Continuous Renal Replacement Therapy: This type of dialysis is used for patients that cannot tolerate conventional dialysis sessions due to complications such as hypotension. This type of dialysis is used until the patient is stable enough to tolerate shorter four hour sessions. There are four different types of CRRT: Continuous Veno-Venous Hemofiltration or CVVH. Continuous Veno-Venous Hemodialysis or CVVHD. Continuous Veno-Venous Hemodiafiltration or CVVHDF. Slow Continuous Ultrafiltration or SCUF. All have a maximum fluid removal rate of 1000ml/hour except for SCUF that has a 2000ml/hour rate during ultra filtration and does not replace fluids.

Intestinal dialysis: This type of dialysis uses activated charcoal to remove poisons and toxins from the gastrointestinal tract. Used mainly in the removal of drugs and poisons. Electrolytes should be monitored. This will cause diarrhea.

DIALYSIS

How to care for your Fistula or Graft: Do not allow blood pressures in that arm, check your pulse, don't lay on the arm with the fistula or graft, keep your site clean, and make sure the professional administering your dialysis cleans and checks the site before accessing. After leaving the hospital do not wear anything that constricts the site. If your site is in the lower forearm by the wrist, do not wear jewelry as this increases your risk of infection. Do not place heavy objects or lift heavy objects with the arm that has the fistula or graft.

How to care for your Peritoneal Dialysis Catheter: Wash your hands thoroughly with soap and water for at least twenty seconds making sure to vigorously rub hands together before handling your catheter every time. Wear a surgical mask when accessing site. Thoroughly "scrub the hub" or clean the catheter site with prescribed antiseptic for at least ten seconds before access. Inspect the dialysis solution for signs of cloudiness which means the solution may be contaminated. Always perform in a well lighted area. Store supplies in a cool, dry place.

My Nephrologist is Dr. ____________________.

I go to ________________ facility for dialysis.

I have chronic renal failure: ________ yes, _________ no.

I have acute renal failure: __________ yes, _________ no.

I receive ______________________ dialysis.

My fistula or graft site is located: _______________.

My dialysis schedule is every _________________, _________________, _______________,

_________________, ________________, ________________, _______________.

My dialysis last for: _______________ hours.

Notes: ____

____

____

____

____

____

____

____

____

____

MY DIALYSIS SCHEDULE

I received ________________ dialysis on ______________. Run time is _______hours.
Amount of fluid removed ______________. Nurse or Tech name ______________________.
Current weight ________________________.

I received ________________ dialysis on ______________. Run time is _______hours.
Amount of fluid removed ______________. Nurse or Tech name ______________________.
Current weight ________________________.

I received ________________ dialysis on ______________. Run time is _______hours.
Amount of fluid removed ______________. Nurse or Tech name ______________________.
Current weight ________________________.

I received ________________ dialysis on ______________. Run time is _______hours.
Amount of fluid removed ______________. Nurse or Tech name ______________________.
Current weight ________________________.

I received ________________ dialysis on ______________. Run time is _______hours.
Amount of fluid removed ______________. Nurse or Tech name ______________________.
Current weight ________________________.

I received ________________ dialysis on ______________. Run time is _______hours.
Amount of fluid removed ______________. Nurse or Tech name ______________________.
Current weight ________________________.

I received ________________ dialysis on ______________. Run time is _______hours.
Amount of fluid removed ______________. Nurse or Tech name ______________________.
Current weight ________________________.

I received ________________ dialysis on ______________. Run time is _______hours.
Amount of fluid removed ______________. Nurse or Tech name ______________________.
Current weight ________________________.

I received ________________ dialysis on ______________. Run time is _______hours.
Amount of fluid removed ______________. Nurse or Tech name ______________________.
Current weight ________________________.

I received ________________ dialysis on ______________. Run time is _______hours.
Amount of fluid removed ______________. Nurse or Tech name ______________________.
Current weight ________________________.

I received ________________ dialysis on ______________. Run time is _______hours.
Amount of fluid removed ______________. Nurse or Tech name ______________________.
Current weight ________________________.

I received ________________ dialysis on ______________. Run time is _______hours.
Amount of fluid removed ______________. Nurse or Tech name ______________________.
Current weight ________________________.

I received ________________ dialysis on ______________. Run time is _______hours.
Amount of fluid removed ______________. Nurse or Tech name ______________________.
Current weight ________________________.

I received ________________ dialysis on ______________. Run time is _______hours.
Amount of fluid removed ______________. Nurse or Tech name ______________________.
Current weight ________________________.

MY DIALYSIS SCHEDULE CONTINUED

I received ________________ dialysis on ______________. Run time is _______hours.
Amount of fluid removed ______________. Nurse or Tech name _____________________.
Current weight _______________________.

I received ________________ dialysis on ______________. Run time is _______hours.
Amount of fluid removed ______________. Nurse or Tech name _____________________.
Current weight _______________________.

I received ________________ dialysis on ______________. Run time is _______hours.
Amount of fluid removed ______________. Nurse or Tech name _____________________.
Current weight _______________________.

I received ________________ dialysis on ______________. Run time is _______hours.
Amount of fluid removed ______________. Nurse or Tech name _____________________.
Current weight _______________________.

I received ________________ dialysis on ______________. Run time is _______hours.
Amount of fluid removed ______________. Nurse or Tech name _____________________.
Current weight _______________________.

I received ________________ dialysis on ______________. Run time is _______hours.
Amount of fluid removed ______________. Nurse or Tech name _____________________.
Current weight _______________________.

I received ________________ dialysis on ______________. Run time is _______hours.
Amount of fluid removed ______________. Nurse or Tech name _____________________.
Current weight _______________________.

I received ________________ dialysis on ______________. Run time is _______hours.
Amount of fluid removed ______________. Nurse or Tech name _____________________.
Current weight _______________________.

I received ________________ dialysis on ______________. Run time is _______hours.
Amount of fluid removed ______________. Nurse or Tech name _____________________.
Current weight _______________________.

I received ________________ dialysis on ______________. Run time is _______hours.
Amount of fluid removed ______________. Nurse or Tech name _____________________.
Current weight _______________________.

I received ________________ dialysis on ______________. Run time is _______hours.
Amount of fluid removed ______________. Nurse or Tech name _____________________.
Current weight _______________________.

I received ________________ dialysis on ______________. Run time is _______hours.
Amount of fluid removed ______________. Nurse or Tech name _____________________.
Current weight _______________________.

I received ________________ dialysis on ______________. Run time is _______hours.
Amount of fluid removed ______________. Nurse or Tech name _____________________.
Current weight _______________________.

I received ________________ dialysis on ______________. Run time is _______hours.
Amount of fluid removed ______________. Nurse or Tech name _____________________.
Current weight _______________________.

TYPES OF NUTRITION

You may notice that your diet has changed from what you regularly have at home depending on your diagnosis, surgical procedures, and current health. Diets will range from a regular diet to tube feedings to parenteral nutrition which is nutrition that is administered intravenously. This guide of some of the more frequently ordered diets. There are many variations to the ones listed below. This will help you better understand your diet plan.

Bland diet: This diet is ordered when a patient has Reflux Esophagitis, Dyspepsia, Peptic Ulcer Disease, and Chronic Gastritis. It may also be ordered in patients with Hiatal Hernia. The diet ordered will have foods that are soft, lightly seasoned and easily digestible.

Clear liquids: Ordered when your gastrointestinal tract needs to rest. This may be the first nutrition you receive after surgery. Patients on this diet will be offered clear juice, broth, popsicles, gelatin, and tea. Occasionally coffee will be allowed.

Full liquids: Used as a transition between clear liquids and either a soft diet or regular diet. All liquids included from the clear liquid diet with the addition of milk, pudding, custard, yogurt, and smooth cream soups.

Nothing by mouth or NPO: This is what is ordered for patients that are scheduled for surgery. Nutrition may be held for some post surgical patients and for patients that have gastrointestinal disorders that have stopped functioning or require rest.

Pureed diet: Ordered when a patient is having pain or difficulty swallowing. Specified diet ordered from physician blended to consistency of baby food.

Regular diet: This diet is similar to what you would have at home.

Soft diet: Eases the difficulty of chewing and swallowing. It may be ordered for patients that have gastrointestinal disorders. Used as transition from clear liquids to regular diet. This diet restricts certain “gas producing” foods. It also restricts spicy, greasy, or fried foods.

Soft mechanical diet: This is a soft diet with the exception of allowing fat, spices, and fiber.

TYPES OF NUTRITION

A therapeutic diet may be ordered to treat disease or metabolic disorders depending upon your diagnosis and nutritional needs.

Cardiac Diet: This diet is low in saturated fat, cholesterol, and salt. This is ordered for patients that have elevated cholesterol and blood pressure.

Diabetic Diet: This diet is ordered to keep your glucose levels within a desired range. This diet is low in sugars and fat. Calories will be restricted according to your dietary needs. Glucose monitoring tests will be ordered.

Fiber High or Low: A high fiber diet aids in digestion by promoting peristalsis or the wavelike contractions in your intestines to remove wastes. A low fiber diet may be ordered for patients having flare ups of Diverticulitis, Crohns, or Ulcerative Colitis. It may also be ordered as a pre or post surgical diet to reduce volume in the bowel. If the patient is on a low residual diet long term, a vitamin and mineral supplement may be ordered.

Gluten Free: Ordered for the treatment of Celiac Sprue disease. These patients have intolerance to wheat, rye, and barley.

Gout Diet: Gout is a form of arthritis. These patients will have elevated levels of Uric Acid. The Uric Acid forms crystals in the joints and surrounding tissues. Foods high in purines will be avoided.

Lactose Intolerant: Patients with lactose intolerance are unable to digest and absorb lactose or the sugars found in milk. This condition causes pain and abdominal distress. These patients will have lactose free or reduced lactose milk products. Soy may be substituted.

Low Protein: A low protein diet is ordered for patients diagnosed with liver or kidney disease. Along with a low protein diet, lower salt intake will also be ordered to decrease fluid retention.

Low Residual Diet: Same diet as the low fiber diet except it excludes milk and milk products, and prune juice. A vitamin and mineral supplement may be ordered.

Low Sodium Diet: This diet is ordered for patients that have high blood pressure, kidney disease, Pneumonia, or patients retaining fluid. Herbs are used in the place of salt.

Neutropenic Diet: This diet is ordered for patients with cancer, chemotherapy, weakened immune systems, organ transplant, HIV, and will have or has had a stem cell transplant. This diet is typically reserved for patients that have an Absolute Neutrophil Count (ANC) of five hundred or less. It limits the exposure to harmful bacteria and organisms found in certain foods. No fresh fruits or vegetables. No raw or undercooked meats including eggs. All dairy products must be pasteurized. No yogurt with active cultures. No raw nuts (acceptable if in baked goods). Wash hands before eating.

Phenylalanine Diet: This diet is ordered for patients with Phenylketonuria or PKU. Foods that will be avoided are high in protein such as steak, fish, eggs, nuts, beans, milk, milk products and ice cream.

Renal Diet: This diet is ordered for patients having difficulty removing fluid from the body or kidney disease. You will be placed on fluid restrictions. The nutrition plan will include foods lower in Protein, Sodium, Phosphorus, Potassium, and Calcium. Lab tests will be ordered to monitor your kidney function.

TYPES OF NUTRITION

ENTERAL FEEDINGS

Enteral Tube feedings may be ordered when a patient is unable to take fluids, food, and medication by mouth. Nutrition and medications may be delivered by a Nasogastric, Dobhoff Tube, Orogastric Tube, or Percutaneous Endoscopic Gastrostomy (PEG) Tube. The Nasogastric Tube is inserted through the nose that is passed into the stomach. A Dobhoff Tube has the same basic principle except it is smaller in diameter and enters the first part of the small intestine called the Duodenum. The Dobhoff requires an X-ray to check for placement before the guide wire is removed. The Orogastric Tube may be ordered when a patient is unable to tolerate a tube placed in the nose or is on mechanical ventilation. The peg tube is usually reserved for long term enteral feedings when the patient is not expected to take anything by mouth.

The type of feedings ordered will depend upon the metabolic disorder. Specialized formulas will be provided according your nutritional needs. The amount of residuals left in the stomach should be checked on a routine basis to monitor if the patient is tolerating the feedings and reducing the risk of aspirating feedings into the lungs. Ask your healthcare provider how often the residuals will be checked. The head of the bed must be elevated at least thirty degrees to also reduce the risk of feedings entering the lungs.

PARENTERAL NUTRITION

Total Parenteral Nutrition is given intravenously. This type of nutrition is given when a patient is unable to tolerate feedings in the gastrointestinal tract. This type of feeding may be short or long term. The formulas will be ordered according to the patients needs. A PICC or central line which is an IV site in a main vein will be needed for administration. Lab tests including Lipids, Triglycerides, and Glucose will be monitored.

MY NUTRITION SCHEDULE

Date: ____________________ Enteral tube feedings: ___ yes, ___ no.

Current diet: ______________ Type of Enteral feedings: __________

Able to feed self: ___ yes, ___ no. Residuals: ____ yes, ____ no. If yes,

Breakfast % ________________ Amounts: _____, _____, _____, _____

Lunch % ____________________ Feedings Held: _____ yes, _____ no.

Dinner % ___________________ If Held, How Long: _________ Hours.

Snacks % ___________________ TPN: _____ yes, ____ no.

Fluid intake: __________ cc/ml TPN Rate: ______ cc/ml

Date: ____________________ Enteral tube feedings: ___ yes, ___ no.

Current diet: ______________ Type of Enteral feedings: __________

Able to feed self: ___ yes, ___ no. Residuals: ____ yes, ____ no. If yes,

Breakfast % ________________ Amounts: _____, _____, _____, _____

Lunch % ____________________ Feedings Held: _____ yes, _____ no.

Dinner % ___________________ If Held, How Long: _________ Hours.

Snacks % ___________________ TPN: _____ yes, ____ no.

Fluid intake: __________ cc/ml TPN Rate: ______ cc/ml

Date: ____________________ Enteral tube feedings: ___ yes, ___ no.

Current diet: ______________ Type of Enteral feedings: __________

Able to feed self: ___ yes, ___ no. Residuals: ____ yes, ____ no. If yes,

Breakfast % ________________ Amounts: _____, _____, _____, _____

Lunch % ____________________ Feedings Held: _____ yes, _____ no.

Dinner % ___________________ If Held, How Long: _________ Hours.

Snacks % ___________________ TPN: _____ yes, ____ no.

Fluid intake: __________ cc/ml TPN Rate: ______ cc/ml

MY NUTRITION SCHEDULE

Date: ______________________________

Current diet: ______________________

Able to feed self: ___ yes, ___ no.

Breakfast % _________________________

Lunch % _____________________________

Dinner % ____________________________

Snacks % ____________________________

Fluid intake: _______________ cc/ml

Enteral tube feedings: ____ yes, ___ no.

Type of Enteral feedings: ______________

Residuals: _____ yes, ____ no. If yes,

Amounts: ______, ______, ______, ______

Feedings Held: ______ yes, _____ no.

If Held, How Long: _________ Hours.

TPN: _____ yes, ____ no.

TPN Rate: _______ cc/ml

Date: ______________________________

Current diet: ______________________

Able to feed self: ___ yes, ___ no.

Breakfast % _________________________

Lunch % _____________________________

Dinner % ____________________________

Snacks % ____________________________

Fluid intake: _______________ cc/ml

Enteral tube feedings: ____ yes, ___ no.

Type of Enteral feedings: ______________

Residuals: _____ yes, ____ no. If yes,

Amounts: ______, ______, ______, ______

Feedings Held: ______ yes, _____ no.

If Held, How Long: _________ Hours.

TPN: _____ yes, ____ no.

TPN Rate: _______ cc/ml

Date: ______________________________

Current diet: ______________________

Able to feed self: ___ yes, ___ no.

Breakfast % _________________________

Lunch % _____________________________

Dinner % ____________________________

Snacks % ____________________________

Fluid intake: _______________ cc/ml

Enteral tube feedings: ____ yes, ___ no.

Type of Enteral feedings: ______________

Residuals: _____ yes, ____ no. If yes,

Amounts: ______, ______, ______, ______

Feedings Held: ______ yes, _____ no.

If Held, How Long: _________ Hours.

TPN: _____ yes, ____ no.

TPN Rate: _______ cc/ml

MY NUTRITION SCHEDULE

Date: ____________________

Current diet: ____________________

Able to feed self: ___ yes, ___ no.

Breakfast % ____________________

Lunch % ____________________

Dinner % ____________________

Snacks % ____________________

Fluid intake: __________ cc/ml

Enteral tube feedings: ___ yes, ___ no.

Type of Enteral feedings: __________

Residuals: _____ yes, ____ no. If yes,

Amounts: ______, ______, ______, ______

Feedings Held: ______ yes, _____ no.

If Held, How Long: _________ Hours.

TPN: _____ yes, ____ no.

TPN Rate: ______ cc/ml

Date: ____________________

Current diet: ____________________

Able to feed self: ___ yes, ___ no.

Breakfast % ____________________

Lunch % ____________________

Dinner % ____________________

Snacks % ____________________

Fluid intake: __________ cc/ml

Enteral tube feedings: ___ yes, ___ no.

Type of Enteral feedings: __________

Residuals: _____ yes, ____ no. If yes,

Amounts: ______, ______, ______, ______

Feedings Held: ______ yes, _____ no.

If Held, How Long: _________ Hours.

TPN: _____ yes, ____ no.

TPN Rate: ______ cc/ml

Date: ____________________

Current diet: ____________________

Able to feed self: ___ yes, ___ no.

Breakfast % ____________________

Lunch % ____________________

Dinner % ____________________

Snacks % ____________________

Fluid intake: __________ cc/ml

Enteral tube feedings: ___ yes, ___ no.

Type of Enteral feedings: __________

Residuals: _____ yes, ____ no. If yes,

Amounts: ______, ______, ______, ______

Feedings Held: ______ yes, _____ no.

If Held, How Long: _________ Hours.

TPN: _____ yes, ____ no.

TPN Rate: ______ cc/ml

MY NUTRITION SCHEDULE

Date: ______________________

Current diet: ______________________

Able to feed self: ___ yes, ___ no.

Breakfast % ______________________

Lunch % ______________________

Dinner % ______________________

Snacks % ______________________

Fluid intake: ____________ cc/ml

Enteral tube feedings: ___ yes, ___ no.

Type of Enteral feedings: __________

Residuals: _____ yes, ____ no. If yes,

Amounts: _____, _____, _____, _____

Feedings Held: _____ yes, _____ no.

If Held, How Long: _______ Hours.

TPN: _____ yes, ____ no.

TPN Rate: ______ cc/ml

Date: ______________________

Current diet: ______________________

Able to feed self: ___ yes, ___ no.

Breakfast % ______________________

Lunch % ______________________

Dinner % ______________________

Snacks % ______________________

Fluid intake: ____________ cc/ml

Enteral tube feedings: ___ yes, ___ no.

Type of Enteral feedings: __________

Residuals: _____ yes, ____ no. If yes,

Amounts: _____, _____, _____, _____

Feedings Held: _____ yes, _____ no.

If Held, How Long: _______ Hours.

TPN: _____ yes, ____ no.

TPN Rate: ______ cc/ml

Date: ______________________

Current diet: ______________________

Able to feed self: ___ yes, ___ no.

Breakfast % ______________________

Lunch % ______________________

Dinner % ______________________

Snacks % ______________________

Fluid intake: ____________ cc/ml

Enteral tube feedings: ___ yes, ___ no.

Type of Enteral feedings: __________

Residuals: _____ yes, ____ no. If yes,

Amounts: _____, _____, _____, _____

Feedings Held: _____ yes, _____ no.

If Held, How Long: _______ Hours.

TPN: _____ yes, ____ no.

TPN Rate: ______ cc/ml

MY NUTRITION SCHEDULE

Date: ______________________

Current diet: ______________

Able to feed self: ___ yes, ___ no.

Breakfast % ________________

Lunch % ____________________

Dinner % ___________________

Snacks % ___________________

Fluid intake: ____________ cc/ml

Enteral tube feedings: ___ yes, ___ no.

Type of Enteral feedings: __________

Residuals: ____ yes, ___ no. If yes,

Amounts: _____, _____, _____, _____

Feedings Held: _____ yes, _____ no.

If Held, How Long: ________ Hours.

TPN: ____ yes, ____ no.

TPN Rate: _____ cc/ml

Date: ______________________

Current diet: ______________

Able to feed self: ___ yes, ___ no.

Breakfast % ________________

Lunch % ____________________

Dinner % ___________________

Snacks % ___________________

Fluid intake: ____________ cc/ml

Enteral tube feedings: ___ yes, ___ no.

Type of Enteral feedings: __________

Residuals: ____ yes, ___ no. If yes,

Amounts: _____, _____, _____, _____

Feedings Held: _____ yes, _____ no.

If Held, How Long: ________ Hours.

TPN: ____ yes, ____ no.

TPN Rate: _____ cc/ml

Date: ______________________

Current diet: ______________

Able to feed self: ___ yes, ___ no.

Breakfast % ________________

Lunch % ____________________

Dinner % ___________________

Snacks % ___________________

Fluid intake: ____________ cc/ml

Enteral tube feedings: ___ yes, ___ no.

Type of Enteral feedings: __________

Residuals: ____ yes, ___ no. If yes,

Amounts: _____, _____, _____, _____

Feedings Held: _____ yes, _____ no.

If Held, How Long: ________ Hours.

TPN: ____ yes, ____ no.

TPN Rate: _____ cc/ml

MY NUTRITION SCHEDULE

Date: ______________________

Current diet: ______________________

Able to feed self: ___ yes, ___ no.

Breakfast % ______________________

Lunch % ______________________

Dinner % ______________________

Snacks % ______________________

Fluid intake: ____________ cc/ml

Enteral tube feedings: ___ yes, ___ no.

Type of Enteral feedings: __________

Residuals: ____ yes, ___ no. If yes,

Amounts: _____, _____, _____, _____

Feedings Held: _____ yes, _____ no.

If Held, How Long: _______ Hours.

TPN: ____ yes, ___ no.

TPN Rate: _____ cc/ml

Date: ______________________

Current diet: ______________________

Able to feed self: ___ yes, ___ no.

Breakfast % ______________________

Lunch % ______________________

Dinner % ______________________

Snacks % ______________________

Fluid intake: ____________ cc/ml

Enteral tube feedings: ___ yes, ___ no.

Type of Enteral feedings: __________

Residuals: ____ yes, ___ no. If yes,

Amounts: _____, _____, _____, _____

Feedings Held: _____ yes, _____ no.

If Held, How Long: _______ Hours.

TPN: ____ yes, ___ no.

TPN Rate: _____ cc/ml

Date: ______________________

Current diet: ______________________

Able to feed self: ___ yes, ___ no.

Breakfast % ______________________

Lunch % ______________________

Dinner % ______________________

Snacks % ______________________

Fluid intake: ____________ cc/ml

Enteral tube feedings: ___ yes, ___ no.

Type of Enteral feedings: __________

Residuals: ____ yes, ___ no. If yes,

Amounts: _____, _____, _____, _____

Feedings Held: _____ yes, _____ no.

If Held, How Long: _______ Hours.

TPN: ____ yes, ___ no.

TPN Rate: _____ cc/ml

MY NUTRITION SCHEDULE

Date: ______________________ Enteral tube feedings: ___ yes, ___ no.

Current diet: ________________ Type of Enteral feedings: __________

Able to feed self: ___ yes, ___ no. Residuals: ____ yes, ____ no. If yes,

Breakfast % __________________ Amounts: _____, _____, _____, _____

Lunch % _____________________ Feedings Held: _____ yes, _____ no.

Dinner % ____________________ If Held, How Long: ________ Hours.

Snacks % ____________________ TPN: ____ yes, ____ no.

Fluid intake: ____________ cc/ml TPN Rate: _____ cc/ml

Date: ______________________ Enteral tube feedings: ___ yes, ___ no.

Current diet: ________________ Type of Enteral feedings: __________

Able to feed self: ___ yes, ___ no. Residuals: ____ yes, ____ no. If yes,

Breakfast % __________________ Amounts: _____, _____, _____, _____

Lunch % _____________________ Feedings Held: _____ yes, _____ no.

Dinner % ____________________ If Held, How Long: ________ Hours.

Snacks % ____________________ TPN: ____ yes, ____ no.

Fluid intake: ____________ cc/ml TPN Rate: _____ cc/ml

Date: ______________________ Enteral tube feedings: ___ yes, ___ no.

Current diet: ________________ Type of Enteral feedings: __________

Able to feed self: ___ yes, ___ no. Residuals: ____ yes, ____ no. If yes,

Breakfast % __________________ Amounts: _____, _____, _____, _____

Lunch % _____________________ Feedings Held: _____ yes, _____ no.

Dinner % ____________________ If Held, How Long: ________ Hours.

Snacks % ____________________ TPN: ____ yes, ____ no.

Fluid intake: ____________ cc/ml TPN Rate: _____ cc/ml

MY NUTRITION SCHEDULE

Date: ______________________________

Current diet: ______________________

Able to feed self: ___ yes, ___ no.

Breakfast % ________________________

Lunch % ____________________________

Dinner % ___________________________

Snacks % ___________________________

Fluid intake: ________________ cc/ml

Enteral tube feedings: ____ yes, ___ no.

Type of Enteral feedings: ______________

Residuals: _____ yes, ____ no. If yes,

Amounts: ______, ______, ______, ______

Feedings Held: ______ yes, _____ no.

If Held, How Long: _________ Hours.

TPN: _____ yes, ____ no.

TPN Rate: _______ cc/ml

Date: ______________________________

Current diet: ______________________

Able to feed self: ___ yes, ___ no.

Breakfast % ________________________

Lunch % ____________________________

Dinner % ___________________________

Snacks % ___________________________

Fluid intake: ________________ cc/ml

Enteral tube feedings: ____ yes, ___ no.

Type of Enteral feedings: ______________

Residuals: _____ yes, ____ no. If yes,

Amounts: ______, ______, ______, ______

Feedings Held: ______ yes, _____ no.

If Held, How Long: _________ Hours.

TPN: _____ yes, ____ no.

TPN Rate: _______ cc/ml

Date: ______________________________

Current diet: ______________________

Able to feed self: ___ yes, ___ no.

Breakfast % ________________________

Lunch % ____________________________

Dinner % ___________________________

Snacks % ___________________________

Fluid intake: ________________ cc/ml

Enteral tube feedings: ____ yes, ___ no.

Type of Enteral feedings: ______________

Residuals: _____ yes, ____ no. If yes,

Amounts: ______, ______, ______, ______

Feedings Held: ______ yes, _____ no.

If Held, How Long: _________ Hours.

TPN: _____ yes, ____ no.

TPN Rate: _______ cc/ml

MY NUTRITION SCHEDULE

Date: ________________________ Enteral tube feedings: ___ yes, ___ no.
Current diet: ________________ Type of Enteral feedings: ___________
Able to feed self: ___ yes, ___ no. Residuals: ____ yes, ___ no. If yes,
Breakfast % __________________ Amounts: _____, _____, _____, _____
Lunch % ______________________ Feedings Held: _____ yes, _____ no.
Dinner % _____________________ If Held, How Long: _______ Hours.
Snacks % _____________________ TPN: ____ yes, ___ no.
Fluid intake: ___________ cc/ml TPN Rate: ______ cc/ml

Date: ________________________ Enteral tube feedings: ___ yes, ___ no.
Current diet: ________________ Type of Enteral feedings: ___________
Able to feed self: ___ yes, ___ no. Residuals: ____ yes, ___ no. If yes,
Breakfast % __________________ Amounts: _____, _____, _____, _____
Lunch % ______________________ Feedings Held: _____ yes, _____ no.
Dinner % _____________________ If Held, How Long: _______ Hours.
Snacks % _____________________ TPN: ____ yes, ___ no.
Fluid intake: ___________ cc/ml TPN Rate: ______ cc/ml

Date: ________________________ Enteral tube feedings: ___ yes, ___ no.
Current diet: ________________ Type of Enteral feedings: ___________
Able to feed self: ___ yes, ___ no. Residuals: ____ yes, ___ no. If yes,
Breakfast % __________________ Amounts: _____, _____, _____, _____
Lunch % ______________________ Feedings Held: _____ yes, _____ no.
Dinner % _____________________ If Held, How Long: _______ Hours.
Snacks % _____________________ TPN: ____ yes, ___ no.
Fluid intake: ___________ cc/ml TPN Rate: ______ cc/ml

MY NUTRITION SCHEDULE

Date: ____________________________

Current diet: ______________________

Able to feed self: ___ yes, ____ no.

Breakfast % _______________________

Lunch % __________________________

Dinner % _________________________

Snacks % _________________________

Fluid intake: ______________ cc/ml

Enteral tube feedings: ____ yes, ___ no.

Type of Enteral feedings: _____________

Residuals: _____ yes, ____ no. If yes,

Amounts: ______, ______, ______, _____

Feedings Held: ______ yes, _____ no.

If Held, How Long: _________ Hours.

TPN: _____ yes, ____ no.

TPN Rate: _______ cc/ml

Date: ____________________________

Current diet: ______________________

Able to feed self: ___ yes, ____ no.

Breakfast % _______________________

Lunch % __________________________

Dinner % _________________________

Snacks % _________________________

Fluid intake: ______________ cc/ml

Enteral tube feedings: ____ yes, ___ no.

Type of Enteral feedings: _____________

Residuals: _____ yes, ____ no. If yes,

Amounts: ______, ______, ______, _____

Feedings Held: ______ yes, _____ no.

If Held, How Long: _________ Hours.

TPN: _____ yes, ____ no.

TPN Rate: _______ cc/ml

Date: ____________________________

Current diet: ______________________

Able to feed self: ___ yes, ____ no.

Breakfast % _______________________

Lunch % __________________________

Dinner % _________________________

Snacks % _________________________

Fluid intake: ______________ cc/ml

Enteral tube feedings: ____ yes, ___ no.

Type of Enteral feedings: _____________

Residuals: _____ yes, ____ no. If yes,

Amounts: ______, ______, ______, _____

Feedings Held: ______ yes, _____ no.

If Held, How Long: _________ Hours.

TPN: _____ yes, ____ no.

TPN Rate: _______ cc/ml

BASIC UNDERSTANDING OF COMMON LAB TESTS

This is a list of the more commonly ordered lab tests. This is meant to give you a basic understanding. There are tests that are not commonly ordered and will not be listed. If a lab test is ordered for you that are not provided in this list, have your healthcare professional explain the purpose of the test. The first three are the most common. The rest will be listed in alphabetical order.

CBC or Complete Blood Count: This test is looking for the amount of White blood cells, Red blood cells, Hemoglobin, Hematocrit and Platelets. This test may be ordered with or without differential. The differential breaks down the amount of the five types of white blood cells and helps determine diagnosis. Hemoglobin carries oxygen to the tissues. Hematocrit is the percentage of red blood cells in whole blood. Platelets aid the body to help stop bleeding by sticking together to form a clot.

BMP or Basic Metabolic Panel: Includes Sodium, Potassium, Chloride, Carbon dioxide, Glucose, Bun or Blood Urea Nitrogen, and Creatinine. This test gives information about your kidney function, blood glucose, electrolytes and acid base balance.

CMP or Complete Metabolic Panel: It is a BMP with additional tests to look at proteins and liver function. This test also includes Calcium, Albumin, Total Protein, Alkaline Phosphatase or ALP, Alanine Aminotransferase or ALT, Aspartate Aminotransferase or AST, and Bilirubin.

ABG or Arterial Blood Gases: The blood is drawn from an artery or arterial line. This test measures the pH level or acidity, Partial Pressure of Oxygen, Partial Pressure of Carbon Dioxide, Bicarbonate, and oxygen saturation. Checks how well your lungs are able to move oxygen into the blood and remove carbon dioxide from the blood. This is a test that is frequently done if a patient is on mechanical ventilation.

Acute Hepatic Panel or LFT's: Includes ALT, AST, ALP, Total Bilirubin, Direct Bilirubin, Albumin and Total Protein. This test checks how well the liver is working and indicates if there is any liver damage.

Albumin: If low may indicate malnutrition, chronic inflammation or liver disease. Low levels may be seen in the elderly and people with Crohn's disease or Sprue. If the level is elevated it may indicate dehydration.

Ammonia: Indicated if a person is showing symptoms of confusion, excessive sleepiness, lethargic, coma or if the patient is having tremors. Elevated levels may indicate severe hepatitis or cirrhosis.

Amylase: Usually ordered with a lipase test. This is a blood test and also can be ordered as a urine test if also indicated. This test is for chronic or acute pancreatitis. Usually ordered if patient has severe abdominal pain, fever, loss of appetite, nausea and vomiting.

Bilirubin: Indicated if a person is jaundiced. If you have increased levels it may indicate Cirrhosis, Acute Hepatitis or gallstones. People in Sickle Cell Crisis and Hemolytic Disease will show an elevation.

Blood Cultures: Two sets of blood cultures usually ordered from different sites. This test is ordered to evaluate if a patient has bacteria in their blood. This blood test will inform the physician of the type of bacteria and to which antibiotics the organism is susceptible or resistant.

BNP or Brain Natriuretic Peptide: Indicates how well your heart is working. Increased levels indicated heart failure. This may be ordered if having difficulty breathing and swelling in the arm and/or legs is present.

Blood Urea Nitrogen or BUN: Indicates how well your kidneys are working. People with heart failure of dehydration will be elevated. A high protein diet will elevate the test. A low BUN indicates liver damage or disease.

BASIC UNDERSTANDING OF LAB TESTS CONTINUED

Calcium: High levels of blood calcium (Hypercalcemia) symptoms are weakness, poor appetite, nausea, vomiting, constipation, frequent urination, stomach and/or bone pain. Low levels of blood calcium (Hypocalcemia) symptoms are muscle cramps, spasms and/or twitches, tingling in hands or fingers and mouth, confusion and depression.

Cardiac Screen: Indicated if you are having a heart attack or a threatened heart attack, chest pain, shortness of breath and/or diaphoretic (sweating). And ECG or EKG will be done also. Elevated levels of CPK, CK, and Troponins indicate damage to the cardiac muscle. This test is often repeated over several hours for comparison. The first test may not show any damage to the heart muscle, this is normal. Damage will show in the second and third test.

Cholesterol: Checks the good cholesterol (High Density Lipoprotein or HDL) this helps keep cholesterol building up in you arteries. Checks the bad cholesterol (Low Density Lipoprotein) this builds up in your arteries and causes blockages. Triglycerides also play a part in causing blockages in your arteries. Cholesterol helps aid in the production of many hormones and helps produce bile acids that help your body break down fats that are in your diet.

Ck-mb: Ordered if patient has chest pain. This test will aid in determining heart attacks. Several tests will be drawn. It can usually be detected three to four hours after onset of chest pain if there is damage to cardiac muscle. The level will peak in about eighteen to twenty four hours. Usually returns to normal in about 72 hours. EKG, echocardiogram, and continuous monitoring will be ordered. Oxygen and medications to help prevent blood clots and improve blood flow will also be ordered.

Coagulation studies: Ordered if you have abnormal or prolonged bleeding. Patients on blood thinners will have blood drawn frequently (as per MD order) to monitor therapeutic levels. Test performed before any surgical procedure. It is very important to follow your physician's orders. Prothrombin Time (PT), Partial Thromboplastin Time (PTT), International Normalized Ratio (INR).

Creatinine Clearance: This is a twenty-four hour urine test that is kept on ice. A Serum Blood Creatinine may also be drawn. This is used to check kidney function. A low Creatinine may indicate dehydration, acute or chronic renal failure, Congestive Heart Failure, shock, End Stage Renal Disease, Glomerulonephritis, or Acute Nephrotic Syndrome.

D-dimer: Used to help detect if the body is clotting inappropriately. This test is ordered if a patient is having signs of Deep Vein Thrombosis (DVT). Signs are leg pain, tenderness, swelling, discoloration and swelling. This test is indicated if a patient has symptoms of a Pulmonary Embolism (PE). Symptoms include chest pain, difficulty breathing, lung pain when coughing and sometimes, pink or blood tinged sputum. This test is also used when a patient is thought to be in Disseminated Intravascular Coagulation (DIC).

Digoxin: This medication is used to treat Atrial Fibrillation, Atrial Flutter and sometimes heart failure. This must be closely monitored. ECG or EKG will be performed. A though level should be done. Levels are drawn to check therapeutic levels and for signs of toxicity.

Dilantin: This drug is used to treat seizures related to epilepsy. This test is used to check if possible drug interactions are present that may increase or decrease the effectiveness of the drug. Abrupt withdrawal may cause Status Epilepticus. Follow your physicians recommendations on dosages on do not miss a dose. Have your levels checked.

Disseminated Intravascular Coagulation Profile: This is when the body clots inappropriately and hemorrhages at the same time. This test includes PT, APTT, Fibrinogen, D-dimer, and ATIII activity.

Electrolyte Profile: Measures the Sodium, Potassium, Carbon Dioxide, And Chloride concentrations in the blood.

BASIC UNDERSTANDING OF LAB TESTS CONTINUED

Ferritin: This test is used to check for iron overload or deficiency. Used as an indicator for how much iron your body has stored for future use. Other test also ordered with this test may be Total Iron Binding Capacity, Serum Iron, Hemoglobin, and Hematocrit.

Fibrinogen: Used in testing your bloods ability to clot. This test is ordered if you have prolonged bleeding.

Folic Acid: This is one of your B vitamins. Folic acid aids in the production of red and white blood cells. This test may be used to check for malnutrition, anemia. This test is ordered in pregnancy. Birth defects can result if there is a deficiency of folic acid in pregnancy.

Gastric Occult Blood: Test if blood is present in the stool. A stool sample is required for this test. Blood in the stool may be from a rip or tear in the lining of the intestinal mucosa or rectum. This may be caused for constipation, polyps, or cancer. Overmedication from blood thinners, including aspirin may be the cause.

Gentamycin Level: Antibiotic used to treat Pseudomonas, Serratia, Proteus, and Gram Positive Staphylococcus. Have your healthcare provider discuss this medication and side effects with you. A peak and trough level should be ordered.

Hemoglobin/Hematocrit or H&H: Hemoglobin carries the oxygen to the tissues. Hematocrit is the percentage of red blood cells in whole blood. This test checks for anemia.

Ionized Calcium: Measures the free calcium in the blood. Usually a parathyroid hormone test will be performed at the same time. The parathyroid hormone and vitamin d maintain calcium levels in the blood. Test is used to check for kidney or thyroid disease. Symptoms of low blood calcium include: abdominal and muscle cramps, tingling in the hands and fingers, and numbness around the mouth, hands and feet. Symptoms of high blood calcium include: weakness, loss of appetite, fatigue, nausea, vomiting, abdominal pain, constipation, increased thirst, and frequent urination.

Lactic Acid: Tests for Lactic Acidosis. The lactic acid levels will increase in heart, kidney, and liver failure. Increased lactic acid is also associated with a severe infection known as sepsis. Symptoms for lactic acidosis include: increase in breathing rate, cool and clammy skin, excessive sweating, fruity or sweet breath, abdominal pain, nausea and/or vomiting, and even coma.

Lipid Profile or Lipid Panel: Ordered to assist in determining the risk of coronary heart disease. This test includes the following tests: Total Cholesterol, High Density Lipoprotein Cholesterol (HDL-C), known as your "good cholesterol", Low Density Lipoprotein Cholesterol (LDL-C), known as your "bad cholesterol", and triglycerides.

Liver Panel, Hepatic Panel, or LFT: Detects, evaluates, and monitors liver damage or disease. Includes the following tests: Alanine Aminotransferase (ALT): detects Hepatitis. Alkaline Phophatase (ALP): increases when bile ducts are blocked. Aspartate Aminotransferase (AST): enzyme found in liver, heart and muscles. Total Bilirubin: measures the Bilirubin in the blood. Direct Bilirubin: measures the conjugated form in the liver. Albumin: measures if the liver is producing enough of the main protein made by the liver. Total protein: measures proteins, Albumin, and antibodies in the blood. Other tests that may be ordered: Prothrombin Time (PT): detects bleeding disorders, Lactic Acid Dehydrogenase (LDH): screens for Hemolytic Anemia and liver disease, Gamma-Glutamyl Transferase (GGT): screens for liver disease and/or alcohol abuse. This test also screens for other abnormalities pertaining to other systems of the body including, but not limited to the following: heart, kidneys, brain, pulmonary, intestinal, and muscles.

BASIC UNDERSTANDING OF LAB TESTS CONTINUED

Magnesium: Ordered if a patient has low magnesium levels the patient will have muscle weakness, cramping, twitching, seizures, cardiac abnormalities, or confusion. This test is used to evaluate kidney problems, gastrointestinal disorders, or uncontrolled diabetes. It helps with diagnosing problems with Calcium, Potassium, Phosphorus, or Hypoparathyroidism. Causes of low magnesium: long term use of diuretics (water pills), diarrhea, Crohn's disease or Sprue, burns, post surgery, toxemia during pregnancy, diabetics, alcoholism. Causes of increased magnesium levels: dehydration, Hypothyroidism, kidney failure, Hyperparathyroidism, Addison's disease, onset of Diabetic Ketoacidosis, and Magnesium containing antacids or laxatives.

Myoglobin: Helps rule out heart attack. This test is drawn upon admission and approximately every two to three hours for twelve hours. Levels rise at two to three hours, peaks at approximately twelve hours and then returns to normal at twenty four hours. Not conclusive in determining a heart attack since Myoglobin is found in skeletal muscles. Heart attack will be confirmed with Troponin levels. Increased levels may be found in patients that have seizures, surgery, or muscular dystrophy.

Prealbumin: Renal Function Panel: Test the kidneys for proper function. Albumin, Blood Urea Nitrogen (BUN), Creatinine, Bun:Creatinine Ratio, Calcium, Chloride, Total Carbon Dioxide, Glucose, Phosphorus, Potassium, and Sodium.

Prothombin Time (PT), Partial Thromboplastin Time (PTT), International Normalized Ratio (INR): Ordered if a patient has abnormal or prolonged bleeding. Patients that are on blood thinners will have blood tests frequently (ordered per MD) to check therapeutic levels. Test performed before any surgical procedure. Always take medication as prescribed.

Renal Function Panel: Test the kidneys for proper function, Albumin, Blood Urea Nitrogen (BUN), Creatinine, Bun:Creatinine Ratio, Calcium, Chloride, Total Carbon Dioxide, Glucose, Phosphorus, Potassium, and Sodium.

Sedimentation Rate or ESR: Monitors inflammation in the body.

Serum Osmolality: Checks for dehydration or over hydration. This test evaluates amounts electrolytes and proteins in the blood. This test may be ordered if patient is having seizures or suspected ingestion of poisons.

Thyroid Panel: Evaluates thyroid disorders such as Hyperthyroidism or Hypothyroidism or thyroid replacement therapy.

Tobramycin Level: This is an antibiotic used to treat gram negative bacteria. Have your healthcare provider discuss side effects of this drug. A peak and trough level should be ordered.

Triglycerides: Used in assessing the risk of a heart attack.

Troponin Level: Ordered if patient is having chest pain. Levels are increased in heart failure Myocarditis, Pericarditis, and Rhabdomyolysis. This test is ordered with other cardiac tests. It is the preferred test for a suspected heart attack. This test is ordered upon admission and then six and twelve hours later.

Type and Screen or Type and Cross: This test is to determine blood type.

Uric Acid: Used to test for Gout and patients receiving chemotherapy or radiation treatments. Gout is a deposition of uric acid crystals in the fluids and tissues of joints.

Urinalysis: This is a urine test. This test will check for urinary tract infections and kidney disorders. It may be ordered in pregnancy and before surgery. Symptoms of a urinary tract infection include abdominal pain, back pain, frequent or painful urination, and blood in the urine.

Valproic Acid Level: Valproic acid is a medication used to help improve control seizures. A peak and trough level should be ordered.

BASIC UNDERSTANDING OF LAB TESTS CONTINUED

Vancomycin Level: Vancomycin is an antibiotic that treats serious bacterial infections such as Methacillin Resistant Staphylococcus Aureus or MRSA. It can be passed through breast milk. Must be monitored due to an overdose may cause acute renal failure. A peak and trough level should be done. Ask your healthcare provider for information regarding this medication.

Wound Culture: A test that is used to detect a specific bacterial or fungal infection in a wound. A viral culture can be ordered to detect if the wound is caused from a virus. Tell your healthcare provider if you are on antibiotics or have been taking antibiotics.

Note: A peak level is when the medication should be at its peak level of effectiveness. A trough level is when the medication is at the lowest concentration in the body and is usually drawn thirty minutes to one hour before a dose of medication is due.

Other lab tests ordered and results: ______________________________

IT'S ALL GREEK TO ME...UNDERSTANDING MEDICAL LANGUAGE

All too often medical professionals forget when speaking with patients and family members that we are not always speaking the same language. Medical professionals have their own terminology derived from the Latin language. This is a list of medical "lingo" that may be verbalized or written. I hope that this may assist you in decoding the confusion you may be experiencing. There are many other terms that are specialized according to the realm of practice. These may be covered in future publications. This is meant to give you a basic understanding.

AAA or triple A: Abdominal Aortic Aneurism.

A&O: Alert and Oriented.

ABD: Abdomen.

Abdomen: ABD.

Abdominal Aortic Aneurism: AAA or triple A.

ABG: Arterial Blood Gas.

Above the Knee Amputation: AKA.

Absolute Neutrophile Count: ANC.

A.C.: Before meals. This may be used in reference to medication administration or glucose monitoring.

Accucheck: Monitors your glucose levels. This requires blood from a finger stick.

ACE: Angiotensin-Converting Enzyme or Ace inhibitor. This is a cardiovascular medication used to treat Congestive Heart Failure, Hypertension, and other related diseases.

Ace Inhibitor: Ace or Angiotensin-Converting Enzyme. This is a cardiovascular medication used to treat Congestive Heart Failure, Hypertension, and other related diseases.

Acidosis: An increase in the level of acidity in the blood plasma. This happens when the pH level drops below 7.35. Acidosis can be respiratory or metabolic. An Arterial Blood Gas can determine Acidosis.

A.C.L.S.: Advanced Cardiac Life Support. Activities performed during cardiopulmonary arrest. This includes: chest compressions, medications, artificial ventilation, and electric shocks in an attempt to allow the heart to restart in a pattern that will sustain life.

Acquired Immune Deficiency Syndrome: AIDS.

Active Range of Motion: AROM.

Activities of Daily Living: ADL's.

Acute Lung Injury: ALI.

Acute Lymphoblastic Leukemia: A.L.L.

Acute Myelogenous Leukemia: AML.

Acute Respiratory Distress Syndrome: ARDS.

Ad Lib: As desired.

IT'S ALL GREEK TO ME...UNDERSTANDING MEDICAL LANGUAGE

ADL's: Activities of daily living.

ADR: Adverse reaction. This is an unexpected and/or dangerous reaction to a medication.

Advanced Cardiac Life Support: ACLS. Activities performed during cardiopulmonary arrest. This includes: chest compressions, medications, artificial ventilation, line insertions, and electric shocks in an attempt to allow the heart to restart in a pattern that will sustain life.

Adverse Event: AE.

Adverse Reaction: ADR. This is an unexpected and/or dangerous reaction to a medication.

AE: Adverse event.

Afebrile: Without fever.

A Fib: Atrial Fibrillation. This is the condition resulting from the upper portion of the heart or atria beating faster or quivering faster than the ventricles.

A Flutter: Atrial Flutter. This is a cardiac arrhythmia. The patient may feel a fluttering sensation in the chest.

Afterload: The pressure that the chambers of the heart have to create to force blood out of the chambers. If a chamber is not specified, it usually refers to the left ventricle.

After Meals: PC.

Against Medical Advice: AMA. You should understand that your insurance company may not pay your medical bill if you leave against medical advice.

AIDS: Acquired Immune Deficiency Syndrome.

AKA: Above the Knee Amputation.

Alcohol Intoxication: ETOH.

Alert and Oriented: A&O.

ALI: Acute Lung Injury.

A Line: Arterial Line. This gives an accurate real time blood pressure reading. This site allows blood samples to be taken for Arterial Blood Gases

Alkalosis: This occurs when the pH of the blood plasma is greater than 7.45. An Arterial Blood Gas can determine Alkalosis. Alkalosis can be respiratory or metabolic. Respiratory alkalosis is caused by hyperventilation. Metabolic Alkalosis is caused by vomiting, diuretics, alkali consumption, or endocrine disorders.

A.L.L.: Acute Lymphoblastic Leukemia or Acute Lymphocytic Leukemia.

AMA: Against Medical Advice. You should understand that your insurance company may not pay your medical bill if you leave against medical advice.

AMB: Ambulate. Meaning refers to the ability to walk or how a person walks.

Ambulate: AMB. Meaning refers to the ability to walk or how a person walks.

AML: Acute Myelogenous Leukemia.

AMP: Ampule.

IT'S ALL GREEK TO ME...UNDERSTANDING MEDICAL LANGUAGE

Ampule: AMP.

ANC: Absolute Neutrophil Count. This is the total percentage of Neutrophils in the body. Neutrophils are a type of White blood cells.

Anemia: A decreased level of Red blood cells.

Angiotensin-Converting Enzyme: ACE or Ace Inhibitor. This is a cardiovascular medication used to treat Congestive Heart Failure, Hypertension, and other related diseases.

Anoxic: When the patient is without the ability to get any oxygen to the lungs or circulatory system.

Anterior: The front side of the body.

Antiemetic: A type of medication used to decrease nausea.

Antithrombolytic Stockings: Ted hose. These are placed on the legs and are intended to decrease swelling in the legs and improve circulation.

AP & LAT: Anteroposterior and Lateral. This refers to a type of view from a radiological test.

Apnea: When you stop breathing for a period of greater than ten to thirty seconds. This usually occurs during sleep.

ARDS: Acute Respiratory Distress Syndrome. This condition is extremely serious and requires mechanical ventilation. This is often or fatal.

A.R.O.M. or AROM: Active Range of Motion.

Arterial Blood Gas: ABG.

Arterial Line: A Line. This gives an accurate real time blood pressure reading. This site allows blood samples to be taken for Arterial Blood Gases.

Art Line: Arterial line. This gives an accurate real time blood pressure reading. This site allows blood samples to be taken for Arterial Blood Gases.

ASA: Aspirin.

ASD: Atrial Septal Defect.

Aspirin: ASA.

As Desired: Ad lib.

Aspirate: This term has two meanings: the term can be interchangeably used with the term choking. The second meaning refers to the removal of an undesired substance through a suction device.

Asystole: No electrical activity or blood flow in the heart. This is commonly known as flat line.

Atelectasis: A condition where the lungs are fully inflating. Deep breathing and coughing exercises accompanied with a lung volume exerciser are recommended.

Atrial Fibrillation: The condition resulting from the upper portion of the heart or atria beating faster or quivering faster than the ventricles.

Atrial Flutter: A Flutter. This is a cardiac arrhythmia. The patient may feel a fluttering sensation in the chest.

IT'S ALL GREEK TO ME...UNDERSTANDING MEDICAL LANGUAGE

Atrial Septal Defect: ASD.

Axillary: Refers to the armpit.

Babinski: A neurological test to check for damage to the spinal cord.

Baker Act: Refers to a patient that is being held in the facility either voluntarily or involuntarily requiring emergency medical services and mental health evaluation and treatment.

Basal Metabolic Rate: BMR.

Baseline: This is a term that refers to what is normal for you regarding blood pressure, breathing patterns, or activity level.

Basic Life Support: BLS.

Basic Metabolic Panel: BMP. This blood test measures the levels of electrolytes present in the blood.

Bathroom Privileges: BRP.

Bedside Commode: BSC.

Before Meals: A.C.. This may be used in reference to medication administration or glucose monitoring.

Below the Knee Amputation: BKA.

Benign: A non-progressive or mild type of cancer or disease. This is typically harmless to your health.

Benzos: Benzodiazepines. This is a class of sedative psychoactive drugs.

Benzodiazepines: Benzos. This is a class of sedative psychoactive drugs.

Bicarb: Sodium Bicarbonate or NaHco3.

B.I.D.: Means two times or twice per day. This may be on you prescriptions or hear your healthcare professional speak this regarding your prescribed activities. This is also written as bid or b.i.d.

Bi-level Positive Airway Pressure: Bi-Pap. This machine assists with breathing.

Biopsy: BX.

Bi-pap: Bi-level Positive Airway Pressure. This machine assists with breathing.

Blood cultures: Blood CX. This blood test evaluates if any bacteria is present in the blood.

Blood CX: Blood Cultures. This blood test evaluates if any bacteria is present in the blood.

Blood Pressure: BP.

Blood Urea Nitrogen: BUN.

BLS: Basic Life Support.

BKA: Below the Knee Amputation.

BM: Bowel movement.

IT'S ALL GREEK TO ME...UNDERSTANDING MEDICAL LANGUAGE

BMP: Basic Metabolic Panel. This blood test measures the levels of electrolytes present in the blood.

BMR: Basal Metabolic Rate.

BMT: Bone Marrow Transplant.

BNP: Brain Natriuretic Peptide.

Body Surface Area: BSA.

Bolus: Refers to an amount of enteral feedings or medication given in larger amounts rather than a continual rate of flow.

Bone: Osteo.

Bone Marrow Transplant: BMT.

Both Eyes: OU.

Bowel Movement: BM.

B.P.: Blood pressure.

Brady: Refers to Bradycardia. Bradycardia is a heartbeat that is less than sixty beats per minute.

Bradycardia: Brady. Bradycardia is a heartbeat that is less than sixty beats per minute.

Brain Natriuretic Peptide: BNP.

Bronch: Refers to Bronchoscopy. This procedure uses a lighted scope to view the lungs, take biopsies, and remove fluid. This procedure also allows the Pulmonologist to view tumors, bleeding, or foreign bodies.

Bronchoscopy: Bronch. This procedure uses a lighted scope to view the lungs, take biopsies, and remove fluid. This procedure also allows the Pulmonologist to view tumors, bleeding, or foreign bodies.

BRP: Bathroom privileges.

BSA: Body surface area.

BSC: Bedside commode.

BX: Biopsy.

By Mouth: PO.

CA: Cancer.

CABG: Coronary Artery Bi-pass Graft Surgery.

CAD: Coronary Artery Disease.

Cancer: Ca.

Cap: Capsule.

Cap Refill: Capillary refill. This evaluates how quickly the capillaries are filling with blood.

IT'S ALL GREEK TO ME...UNDERSTANDING MEDICAL LANGUAGE

Capillary Refill: Cap refill. This evaluates how quickly the capillaries are filling with blood.

Capsule: Cap.

Carcinoembryonic Antigen: CEA. This is a tumor marker.

Carcinogen: This refers to anything that causes cancer.

Cardiac Cath: Cardiac Catheterization.

Cardiac Catheterization: Cardiac Cath.

Cardio: Refers to the heart.

Cardio-Pulmonary Resuscitation: CPR.

Cardiovert: Synchronized Electrical Cardioversion.

Cath: Usually refers to a Cardiac Catheterization or insertion of urinary catheter.

Cat Scan: Computerized Axial Tomography.

CBC: Complete Blood Count.

CC: A measurement of volume. It takes five cc's to equal one teaspoon or thirty cc's to make one ounce.

CCR: Complete Continuous Recovery.

CCU: Coronary or Critical Care Unit.

C Diff: Clostridium Difficile. This is a serious bacterium that causes serious intestinal complications, diarrhea, sepsis, and even death.

CEA: Carcinoembryonic Antigen. This is a tumor marker.

Central Line: Central Venous Catheter. This is a type of IV access that in inserted into a main vein in the body. Written consent must be obtained unless it is emergent and then two physicians must sign the consent.

Central Nervous System: CNS. This includes the brain, spinal column, and nervous system.

Central Venous Pressure: CVP. This is a direct measurement of the blood pressure in the Right Atrium and Vena Cava.

Cerebral Spinal Fluid: CSF.

Cerebrovascular Accident: CVA.

Certified Nursing Assistant: CNA.

Chest Tube: A flexible plastic tube that is inserted into the chest cavity to remove air, blood, or pus. It is connected to a collection chamber referred to as a Pleurovac. It is connected to wall suction or water seal.

Chest X-ray: CXR.

Cheyne Stokes: This is a type of abnormal breathing pattern.

CHF: Congestive Heart Failure.

Chronic Lymphocytic Leukemia: CLL.

Chronic Obstructive Pulmonary Disease: COPD.

CK-mb: A blood test ordered to determine if a patient has had a heart attack.

CLL: Chronic Lymphocytic Leukemia.

Clostridium Difficile: C diff. This is a serious bacterium that causes serious intestinal complications, diarrhea, sepsis, and even death.

Cm: 2.54 centimeters equals 1 inch.

CMO: Comfort measures only. Medications and life support is terminated.

CMP: Complete Metabolic Panel. This is a blood test that measures electrolytes, kidney, and liver function.

CMV: This abbreviation has two meanings. First: Conditional Mandatory Ventilation. The ventilator is completely breathing for the patient. Second: Cytomegalovirus.

CNA: Certified Nursing Assistant.

CNS: Central Nervous System. This includes the brain and nervous system. This refers to your brain, spinal column nerves.

C/O: Complains of.

Coags: Pronounced Co ags. This is a blood test for coagulation studies. It evaluates bleeding and clotting times.

Coagulation Studies: Coags. It evaluates bleeding and clotting times.

Coarse: A low pitched gurgling sound heard in the lungs upon inspiration and may be heard with the initiation of expiration. This is associated with Pulmonary Edema, Pneumonia, Pulmonary Fibrosis, Chronic Lung Disease, and patients with a depressed cough.

Code Blue: This is the code used when a patient is in need of immediate attention requiring resuscitation.

Code Pink: This is the code used when a pediatric patient is in need of immediate attention requiring resuscitation.

Comfort Measures Only: CMO. Medications and life support is terminated.

Complains Of: C/O.

Complete Blood Count: CBC.

Complete Continuous Recovery: CCR.

Complete Metabolic Panel: CMP. This is a blood test that measures electrolytes, kidney, and liver function.

Complete Remission: CR.

Computerized Axial Tomography: Cat scan.

Conditional Mandatory Ventilation: CMV.

Congestive Heart Failure: CHF.

Continue with: C/W.

Continuous Positive Airway Pressure: CPAP.

IT'S ALL GREEK TO ME...UNDERSTANDING MEDICAL LANGUAGE

Co-pay: The amount you will pay minus what your insurance does not cover.

COPD: Chronic Obstructive Pulmonary Disease.

Coronary Artery Bi-pass Graft Surgery: CABG.

Coronary Artery Disease: CAD.

Coronary Care: Critical Care Unit or CCU.

CPAP: Continuous Positive Airway Pressure.

CPR: Cardio-Pulmonary Resuscitation.

CR: Complete remission.

Crackles: A popping noise heard upon inspiration with a stethoscope.

Critical Care Unit or Coronary Care Unit: CCU.

CSF: Cerebral Spinal Fluid.

CT: Computerized Axial Tomography.

Cuff Pressure: The blood pressure taken by an inflatable cuff on the arm or leg.

CVA: Cerebrovascular Accident.

CVP: Central Venous Pressure. This is a direct measurement of the blood pressure in the Right Atrium and Vena Cava.

C/W: Continue with.

CX: Culture or chest depending on how the order is written.

CXR: Chest X-ray.

CX tube or Chest tube: A flexible plastic tube that is inserted into the chest cavity to remove air, blood, or pus. It is connected to a collection chamber referred to as a Pleurovac. It is connected to wall suction or water seal.

Cytomegalovirus: CMV.

D5, D10, D25, D50: The amount of dextrose in IV fluids. D25 treats pediatric patients with severely low blood glucose. D50 treats adult patients with severely low blood glucose.

DBP: Diastolic blood pressure.

D/C: Discontinue.

D&C: A procedure where the cervix is dilated and a curette is inserted into the uterus and tissue is removed.

Decub: Pronounced decube. This is a decubitis ulcer or another term for this is pressure ulcer.

Decubitis Ulcer: Decub or pressure ulcer.

Deep Vein Thrombosis: DVT or blood clot.

Defib: Defibrillation.

Defibrillation: Defib.

IT'S ALL GREEK TO ME...UNDERSTANDING MEDICAL LANGUAGE

Dehis: Dehisced. This refers to when a surgical wound opens or ruptures.

Dehisced: Dehis. This refers to when a surgical wound opens or ruptures.

Dehydrated: Dry. This refers to an excessive loss of fluid in the body.

Delirium Tremens: DT's. This is the process of withdrawal from alcohol, Benzodiazepines, or Barbiturates.

Diabetic Ketoacidosis: DKA. This condition happens when the body has high levels of Glucose, Acidosis, and Ketones.

Diagnosis: DX.

Diastolic Blood Pressure: DBP.

DIC: Disseminated Intravascular Coagulation.

Dig: Digoxin.

Digoxin: Dig.

Dilatation and Curettage: D&C.

Discontinue: D/C.

Disseminated Intravascular Coagulation: DIC.

Distal: The farthest point from one end to the other.

DKA: Diabetic Ketoacidosis. This condition happens when the body has high levels of Glucose, Acidosis, and Ketones.

DNR: Do not resuscitate.

Doll's Eyes: A neurological sign that tests functional integrity of the brainstem. A negative test indicates injury to the midbrain or pons.

Do Not Resuscitate: DNR.

Dressing: DSG.

Dry: Dehydrated.

DSG: Dressing.

DT's: Delirium Tremens is the process of withdrawal from alcohol, Benzodiazepines, or Barbiturates.

DVT: Deep Vein Thrombosis.

DX: Diagnosis.

Dysphagia: Difficulty or pain with swallowing.

Dyspneic: Difficulty in breathing or shortness of breath.

EBCT: Electron Beam Computed Tomography.

ECG: Electrocardiogram.

Echo: Echocardiogram.

Echocardiogram: Echo.

IT'S ALL GREEK TO ME...UNDERSTANDING MEDICAL LANGUAGE

E.D. or ED: Emergency Room Department.

Edema: Extra fluid that is in the tissues causing swelling.

EEG: Electroencephalogram.

EGD: Esophagogastroduodenoscopy. This is a lighted scope that is inserted through the mouth and passed into the upper portion of the small intestine.

E.J.: External Jugular.

Electrocardiogram: ECG.

Electroencephalogram: EEG.

Electron Beam Computed Tomography: EBCT.

Emergency Room Department: E.D. or ED.

End of Life: E.O.L.

Endotrachael Tube: ETT or ET Tube. The tube that is inserted into the trachea required for mechanical ventilation.

E.O.L.: End of life.

EPI: Epinephrine.

Epinephrine: EPI.

E.R.: Emergency Room.

Estimated Time of Arrival: ETA.

Esophagealgastroduodenoscopy: EGD.

ESR: Sedimentation Rate.

E.T.A.: Estimated Time of Arrival.

ETOH: Alcohol intoxication.

ET Tube: Endotrachael Tube. The tube that is inserted into the trachea required for mechanical ventilation.

Eval: Evaluate.

Evaluate: Eval.

Every: q.

Exam: Examination.

Examination: Exam.

Febrile: Fever.

Femoral: Refers to the femoral artery. When a patient has a femoral central line, it is usually referred to as a femoral.

Femoral Artery: Femoral. When a patient has a femoral central line, it is usually referred to as a femoral.

Fever: Febrile.

IT'S ALL GREEK TO ME...UNDERSTANDING MEDICAL LANGUAGE

FFP: Fresh Frozen Plasma. This is a blood product.

Flexiseal: This is type of rectal tube used to collect stool. This is also used to help prevent skin and tissue breakdown on the buttocks and perineal area.

Flush: This is typically normal saline in a syringe that either flushes medication into the IV or keeps the IV site patent.

Foley: A type of urinary catheter.

Fowlers: This is a semi-upright sitting position with the head of the bed at forty-five to sixty degrees. The knees may or may not be slightly bent for comfort.

Fresh Frozen Plasma: FFP. This is a blood product.

Full Code: All attempts to resuscitate will be administered.

Gait: The manner in which a person walks.

Gastroesophageal Reflux Disease: GERD.

Gastrointestinal: GI. This is the digestive system.

Gastrostomy Tube: G Tube. This is a tube used for feedings and medication administration. This may also be connected to suction to empty stomach contents.

Genitourinary: GU. This is the reproductive and urinary system.

GERD: Gastroesophageal Reflux Disease.

GFR: Glomerular Filtration Rate. This is a blood test used to determine the kidneys ability to filter out waste products from the body.

GI: Gastrointestinal. This is the digestive system.

Glomerular Filtration Rate: GFR. This is a blood test used to determine the kidneys ability to filter out waste products from the body.

Grade: This gives information regarding growth rate of cancer and gives information about the tendency of the tumor spreading. Grade 1 has the most differentiated cells and is the least abnormal. Grade 2 has moderately differentiated cells. Grade 3 has the poorest differentiated cells and the greatest abnormality. Grade IV is fast growing and looks different from normal cells.

Graft Versus Host Disease or GVHD: A disease that is caused when the cells from a donated stem cell graft attack the transplant patient.

Gram Stain: A test used to determine if the bacteria is gram positive or gram negative. This helps determine which antibiotics are needed to treat the infection.

GTT: Means drops. This refers to the measurement amount of oral, ear, eye drop administration.

G Tube: Refers to a gastrostomy tube used for feedings and medication administration. This may also be connected to suction to empty stomach contents.

GU: Genitourinary. This is the reproductive and urinary system.

GVHD or Graft Versus Host Disease: A disease that is caused when the cells from a donated stem cell graft attack the transplant patient.

H: Hour or hours. Example: Your prescribed activity or medication is q8h or q8h, meaning every eight hours.

H&H: Hemoglobin and Hematocrit.

H30, h45, h60, h90: This refers to the degree of the head of the bed should be elevated. These are examples. The head of the bed can be set from zero to ninety degrees.

Halo: This has three meanings: Meaning one: The diffuse ring seen around lights. Meaning two: The depigmented area of the skin around a mole. Meaning three: A circular metal brace fixed to the skull with pins.

Hco3: Bicarbonate.

Head of bed: HOB.

Health Insurance Portability and Accountability Act: HIPAA. This protects a patient's privacy and information. Contact information if you feel you rights have violated are as follows: on your computer type in HIPAA violations, you will have to download forms and email them to ocrcomplaint@hhs.gov or call 1-866-627-7748.

Hemothorax: A collection of blood in the pleural space around the lung.

Heplock: Refers to an IV site that may or may not be accessed.

Hickman: This is an intravenous catheter that is used for long term use. It is used for the administration of chemotherapy or dialysis.

High Blood Pressure: Hypertension or HTN.

HIPAA: Health Insurance Portability and Accountability Act. This protects a patient's privacy and information. Contact information if you feel you rights have violated are as follows: on your computer type in HIPAA violations, you will have to download forms and email them to ocrcomplaint@hhs.gov or call 1-866-627-7748.

History: HX.

HIV: Human Immunodeficiency Virus.

H.O.B.: Head of bed.

Homans: This is a simple test used to evaluate the possibility of a blood clot in the legs.

Hour: H.

Hours of Sleep: HS. This is usually ordered for glucose monitoring and administration of medications.

HS: Hours of sleep. This is usually ordered for glucose monitoring and administration of medications.

HTN: Hypertension or high blood pressure.

Human Immunodeficiency Virus: HIV.

HX: History. This refers to a patient's medical history.

HYO: Hypotension or low blood pressure.

Hypertension: HTN or high blood pressure.

Hypotension: HYO or low blood pressure.

Hypoxic: A condition that occurs when the body is deprived of adequate oxygen supply.

IBS: Irritable Bowel Syndrome.

ICP: The measurement of intracranial pressure.

ICU: Intensive Care Unit.

I.D.: Infectious Disease. This usually refers to the physician monitoring infections.

IJ: Internal Jugular. This is one of the main veins in the neck.

IM: Intramuscular injection.

Immediate: Stat.

IMV: Intermittent Mechanical Ventilation. This is a mechanical ventilation setting. It is used for weaning.

Incentive Spirometer: I.S. This is a simple appliance that helps improve lung volumes. It is sometimes referred to as a lung exerciser.

Infant Respiratory Distress Syndrome: IRDS. This is a deficiency of surfactant in premature infants.

Infectious Disease: I.D. This usually refers to the physician monitoring infections.

INH: Inhaler.

Inhaler: INH.

Intensive Care Unit: ICU.

Intermittent Mechanical Ventilation: IMV. This is a mechanical ventilation setting. It is used for weaning.

Internal Jugular: IJ. This is one of the main veins in the neck.

Intracranial Pressure: ICP.

Intravenous: IV.

Intravenous Fluids: IVF.

Intravenous Piggyback: IVPB.

I&O: Input and output.

IRDS: Infant Respiratory Distress Syndrome. This is a deficiency of surfactant in premature infants.

Irritable bowel syndrome: IBS.

I.S.: Incentive Spirometer. This is a simple appliance that helps improve lung volumes. It is sometimes referred to as a lung exerciser.

Isolation Precautions: Precautions. This assists in decreasing the transmissions of infectious agents in the healthcare setting. This can be contact, respiratory, and/or reverse isolation for patients with very low immune systems. The equipment includes gown, gloves, and mask.

I.V. or IV: Intravenous.

IVF: Intravenous fluids.

IT'S ALL GREEK TO ME...UNDERSTANDING MEDICAL LANGUAGE

IVPB: Intravenous piggyback. These are IV medications that are in addition to the main IV fluids.

Jackson-Pratt Drain: JP. This is a bulb drain that is compressed to create constant suction to remove excess fluid. The appearance resembles a hand grenade.

Jaundice: This is a condition when the skin turns yellow caused from an abnormal liver function.

JCAHO: Joint Commission on Accreditation of Healthcare Organizations. This is who you report to if you have a complaint about the facility. Email address is www.jointcommision.org or call at 800-994-6610.

Jejunostomy Tube: J Tube. A tube inserted into the Jejunum which is located in the small intestine. This is used for administration of feedings and medications. A feeding pump must be used.

Joint Commission on Accreditation of Healthcare Organizations: JCAHO. This is who you report to if you have a complaint about the facility. Email address is www.jointcommision.org or call at 800-994-6610.

JP: Jackson-Pratt Drain. This is a bulb drain that is compressed to create constant suction to remove excess fluid. The appearance resembles a hand grenade.

J Tube: Jejunostomy Tube. A tube inserted into the Jejunum which is located in the small intestine. This is used for administration of feedings and medications. A feeding pump must be used.

Jugular Venous Distension: JVD. With jugular venous distension you will visualize the pronounced internal jugular vein in the neck fill with blood with every beat of the heart. The neck should be positioned at a forty-five degree angle for viewing. This is an indicator of increased jugular venous pressure, right sided heart failure, and many other cardiac abnormalities. This should be interpreted by healthcare professionals only.

JVD: Jugular venous distension. With JVD, you will visualize the pronounced internal jugular vein in the neck fill with blood with every beat of the heart. The neck should be positioned at a forty-five degree angle for viewing. This is an indicator of increased jugular venous pressure, right sided heart failure, and many other cardiac abnormalities. This should be interpreted by healthcare professionals only.

K: Potassium.

KCL: Potassium.

Ketones: A bi-product of your body when it burns stored fat for energy. This can be seen in many conditions such as diabetics, pregnancy, starvation, illness, stress, and exercise. The signs of Ketoacidosis are fatigue, increased thirst, fruity but unpleasant breath, dry mouth, decreased appetite, nausea/vomiting, increased urination, and dry flushed skin.

Kg: Kilogram. 2.2 pounds equal 1 Kilogram of weight.

Kilogram: Kg. 2.2 pounds equal 1 Kilogram of weight.

Kussmaul: A deep and labored breathing pattern in which the patient is hyperventilating. This is seen in patients with severe Metabolic Acidosis, especially Diabetic Ketoacidosis. This may be seen in renal failure. This is the body attempting to blow off excess Carbon Dioxide.

Laboratory Tests: Labs.

Labs: Laboratory tests.

IT'S ALL GREEK TO ME...UNDERSTANDING MEDICAL LANGUAGE

LAC or L.A.C.: Left Antecubital area. This is the area of the inside or front of the elbow. This may refer to an IV site.

Lactated Ringers: LR. This is a type of intravenous fluid.

Lateral: Side lying position or a side view on a test.

Lavage: This means to wash out something. This could refer to respiratory, stomach, or wound.

LCS: Low Continuous Suction.

Left Antecubital: LAC or L.A.C. This is the area of the inside or front of the elbow. This may refer to an IV site.

Left Eye: OS.

Left Lower Extremity: LLE. This refers to the left leg.

Left Lower Lobe of the Lung: LLL.

Left Lower Quadrant: LLQ. This refers to the abdomen.

Left Upper Lobe of the Lung: LUL.

Left Upper Quadrant: LUQ. This refers to the abdomen.

Left Ventricular Assist Device: LVAD.

Level of Consciousness: LOC.

Levo: Levophed. This medication is used to increase blood pressure.

Levophed: Levo. This medication is used to increase blood pressure.

LFT's: Liver Function Test.

Lip Line: A term used to measure where an endotracheal tube is placed and secured for ventilation.

LIS: Low Intermittent Suction.

Liver Function Test: LFT's.

LLE: Left Lower Extremity. This refers to the left leg.

LLL: Left Lower Lobe of the lung.

LLQ: Left Lower Quadrant. This refers to the abdomen.

L.O.C.: Level of consciousness.

Low Blood Pressure: Hypotension or HYO.

Low Continuous Suction: LCS.

Low Intermittent Suction: LIS.

LP or Lumbar Puncture: The removal of cerebral spinal fluid through a small needle inserted into the lower area of the spinal column. This test is examined for abnormal cells.

LR: Lactated Ringers. This is a type of intravenous fluid.

IT'S ALL GREEK TO ME...UNDERSTANDING MEDICAL LANGUAGE

LUE: Left Upper Extremity. This refers to the left arm.

LUL: Left Upper Lobe of the lung.

Lumbar Puncture or LP: The removal of Cerebral Spinal Fluid through a small needle inserted into the lower area of the spinal column. This test is examined for abnormal cells.

L.U.Q. or LUQ: Left Upper Quadrant. This refers to the abdomen.

LVAD: Left Ventricular Assist Device.

Mag: Magnesium.

Magnesium: Mag.

Magnetic Resonance Angiography: MRA.

Magnetic Resonance Imaging: MRI.

Malignant: This refers to cancer cells present in the tissues.

M.A.P. or MAP: Mean Arterial Pressure. This is the perfusion pressure seen in the organs of the body. A map greater than sixty is preferred for blood flow to the organs.

MAR: Medication Administration Record. This is the record used determine what medications will be and have been administered.

Mastectomy: MX.

Mcg: Microgram. A measurement used in administering medications at very specific dosages.

MDR: Multiple Drug Resistant.

Mean Arterial Pressure: MAP. This is the perfusion pressure seen in the organs of the body. A map greater than sixty is preferred for blood flow to the organs.

Medial: This pertains to the middle or center of the body. This is used as a reference point.

Medical Surgical Unit or floor: Med Surg.

Med Surg: Medical Surgical Unit or floor.

Medication Administration Record: MAR. This is the record used determine what medications will be and have been administered.

Melanoma: A serious form of cancer that spreads easily throughout the body. This type of cancer begins in the skin.

mEq: Molar Equivalent. This is a unit amount of a medication or substance.

Metastatic Cancer: METS. This means the cancer has spread from one part of the body to another part of the body. Survival rates greatly decrease.

Methicillin-Resistant Staphylococcus Aureus: MRSA. This can be hospital acquired. You should be swabbed upon admission to determine if you had this before entering the hospital. There are very few antibiotics that can treat the infection. Vancomycin and Zyvox can still treat the infection at the current time, although once acquired there are no guarantees of successful recovery. MRSA can be fatal. Good hand washing and wearing gloves will help reduce the chances of infection.

IT'S ALL GREEK TO ME...UNDERSTANDING MEDICAL LANGUAGE

Mets: Metastatic Cancer. This means the cancer has spread from one part of the body to another part of the body. Survival rates greatly decrease.

M.I.: Myocardial Infarction. This is a term used for heart attack.

Microgram: mcg. A measurement used in administering medications at very specific dosages.

Milliliter: ml. This is a unit of measurement.

Millimole: mm. This is a unit of measurement.

Ml: Milliliter. This is a unit of measurement.

mM: Millimole. This is a unit of measurement.

Molar Equivalent: mEq. This is a unit amount of a medication or substance.

MRA: Magnetic Resonance Angiography.

MRI.: Magnetic Resonance Imaging.

MRSA: This is sometimes pronounced Mersa. MRSA is the acronym for Methicillin-Resistant Staphylococcus Aureus. This can be hospital acquired. You should be swabbed upon admission to determine if you had this before entering the hospital. There are very few antibiotics that can treat the infection. Vancomycin and Zyvox can still treat the infection at the present time, although once acquired there are no guarantees of successful recovery. MRSA can be fatal. Good hand washing and wearing gloves will help reduce the chances of infection.

Multiple Drug Resistant: MDR.

Multi-vitamin: MVI.

MVI: Multi-vitamin.

MX: Mastectomy.

Na: Sodium.

Nadir: The lowest point that the white blood cell counts drop after chemotherapy. This usually occurs seven to ten days after chemotherapy.

NaHco3: Sodium Bicarbonate or Bicarb.

Nasal Cannula: A low flow oxygenation administration device. This is a tube with two prongs that fit into the opening of the nose and is secured around the ears to deliver oxygen to the patient. The prongs always are turned downward. Oxygen can humidified for comfort if requested and is prescribed by the physician. Never use petroleum products or have anything flammable around oxygen.

Nasogastric tube: NG or NGT.

NC: Nasal cannula.

Neo: Neosynephrine.

Neonatal Intensive Care Unit: NICU.

Neosynephrine: Neo.

Neuro: Neurologic.

IT'S ALL GREEK TO ME...UNDERSTANDING MEDICAL LANGUAGE

Neurologic: Neuro.

Neurological Intensive Care Unit: NICU.

Neuropathy: This refers to damage to the nerves resulting in pain, numbness, and tingling.

Neutropenia: This is an abnormally low amount of Neutrophils. This is a type of white blood cell.

Ng: NGT or Nasogastric Tube. A tube inserted through the nose into the stomach for administration of feedings and medications. It can also be used to empty the stomach contents when connected to suction.

NGT: Nasogasrtic Tube.

NICU: Neurological Intensive Care Unit or Neonatal Intensive Care Unit.

Night: NOC.

Nitro: Nitroglycerine. Medication used for angina or chest pain.

Nitroglycerine: Nitro. Medication used for angina or chest pain.

NKA: No Known Allergies.

NKDA: No Known Drug Allergies.

NOC: Night.

No Known Allergies: NKA.

No Known Drug Allergies: NKDA.

Non-Rebreather: A type of mask used to deliver oxygen.

Normal Saline: NS.

Nosocomial Infections: Infections acquired during your hospital or inpatient stay. This is an infection that you did not have prior to your admission.

Nothing By Mouth: NPO.

NPO: Nothing by mouth.

NS: Normal Saline.

Nuclear Medicine: Nuc Med.

Nuc Med: Nuclear Medicine.

O2 sats: The amount of oxygen circulating in your blood.

O.B. or OB: Obstetrics.

Ob & Gyn: Obstetrics and Gynaecology.

Obstetrics and Gynaecology: Ob & Gyn.

Occupational Therapy: OT.

O.D: Right eye.

OG: Oralgastric Tube. A tube inserted through the mouth into the stomach for administration of feedings and medications. It can also used to empty the stomach when connected to suction.

Ointment: Oint.

O.O.B. or OOB: Out of bed.

O/P: Outpatient.

OP: Ova and Parasite. This test requires a stool sample. It is used to test for parasites or parasite eggs in the gastrointestinal tract.

Operating Room: O.R. / OR.

O.R. / OR: Operating Room.

Oralgastric Tube: OG. A tube inserted through the mouth into the stomach for administration of feedings and medications. It can also used to empty the stomach when connected to suction.

Orthostatic Hypotension: This condition happens when your blood pressure suddenly falls upon standing or coming to a raised position. Lightheadedness, dizziness, blurred vision, headache, and even fainting or momentary blindness may occur.

O.S.: Left eye.

Osteo: Bone.

Ostomy: A surgically created opening used for the purpose of discharging waste from the body. There are many different types of ostomies. Some examples are: Colostomy, Ileostomy, Nephrostomy, and Urostomy.

O.T.: Occupational Therapy.

O.U.: Both eyes.

Out of bed: OOB.

Outpatient: O/P.

Ova and Parasite: OP. This test requires a stool sample. It is used to test for parasites or parasite eggs in the gastrointestinal tract.

P.A.C. Or PAC: Premature atrial contraction.

Pacer: Pacemaker.

Pacemaker: Pacer.

Packed Red Blood Cells: PRBC's.

P.A.C.U. or PACU: Post Anesthesia Care Unit. This is usually referred to as the recovery room.

Paradoxical effect: This is essentially the opposite desired effect from a medication.

Partial Pressure of Carbon Dioxide: PCO2. This is a part of the Arterial Blood Gas.

Partial Pressure of Oxygen: PO2.

Partial Thromboplastin Time: PTT.

Passive Range of Motion: PROM.

P.A.T. or PAT: Premature Atrial Tachycardia. This happens when the heart beats 160-200 beats per minute. It usually begins and ends abruptly.

Patient: PT.

Patient Care Technician: PCT. They assist the nursing staff in providing care for the patient.

Patient Controlled Analgesia: PCA. This is the medication pump controlled by the patient that is used to deliver pain medications.

PAWP: Pulmonary Artery Wedge Pressure. Measure the mean left atrial pressure in the heart. A central intravenous line is required.

PC: After meals. Usually refers to medication administration.

PCA: Patient Controlled Analgesia. This is the medication pump controlled by the patient that is used to deliver pain medications.

PCO2: Partial Pressure of Carbon Dioxide. This is a part of the arterial blood gas.

PCT: Patient Care Technician. They assist the nursing staff in providing care for the patient.

P.C.U. or PCU: Progressive Care Unit. This is a step down from the intensive care unit.

P.E.: Pulmonary Embolism. This is a blockage caused by a blood clot, fat embolism, or air embolism. This is a blockage in the pulmonary artery or its branches. This is a very serious condition requiring immediate attention. Symptoms include rapid and labored breathing, chest pain with inspiration, low oxygen saturations, rapid heart rate, and a feeling of heart "skipping or fluttering."

Pediatric Intensive Care Unit: PICU.

PEEP: Positive End Expiratory Pressure. This is one of the settings used in mechanical ventilation. It helps keep the alveoli, which is the small sacs needed for oxygenation from collapsing.

PEG: Percutaneous Endoscopic Gastrostomy Tube. A tube inserted into the stomach through the abdominal wall. This is used for administration of medications and feedings.

Peptic Ulcer Disease: PUD.

Percutaneous Endoscopic Gastrostomy Tube: PEG. A tube inserted into the stomach through the abdominal wall. This is used for administration of medications and feedings.

Percutaneous Transluminal Coronary Angioplasty: PTCA.

Peri Area: Perineal area. The area between the scrotum or vagina to the anus.

Perineal Area: Peri area. The area between the scrotum or vagina to the anus.

Peripherally Inserted Central Catheter: PICC. This is an IV access that may be used for prolonged periods of time. It is used for medication administration and blood can also be removed from the port for tests. This reduces the amount of times the patient needs to be stuck. Consent must be obtained. Confirmation of placement is made by x-ray. New IV tubing should be hung and labeled with date to be changed before connecting it to the patient.

Perm A Cath: A large bore catheter used to administer chemotherapy.

IT'S ALL GREEK TO ME...UNDERSTANDING MEDICAL LANGUAGE

PERRL: Pupils, equal, round, reactive to light. This is a neurological test.

Pet Scan: Positron Emission Tomography. This is a nuclear medicine imaging test that uses small amount of radiation to detect cancers, heart disease, certain diseases, and abnormalities in the body.

PH or pH: Measures the acidity or alkaline base balance in the body.

PHOS: Phosphorus.

Phosphorus: PHOS.

Physical Therapy: P.T.

PICC: Peripherally Inserted Central Catheter. This is an IV access that may be used for prolonged periods of time. It is used for medication administration and blood can also be removed from the port for tests. This reduces the amount of times the patient needs to be stuck. Consent must be obtained. Confirmation of placement is made by X-ray. New IV tubing should be hung and labeled with date to be changed before connecting it to the patient.

P.I.C.U. or PICU: Pediatric Intensive Care Unit.

Piggyback: This is an IV medication that is connected to the patient in addition to the maintenance fluids.

Pleural Effusions: This refers to an excess of fluid in the pleural space in the chest.

PN or PNE: Pneumonia.

Pneumonia: PN or PNE.

Pneumo: This usually refers to a Pneumothorax. This is commonly called a collapsed lung. It is when air enters the pleural cavity in the chest outside the lung.

Pneumothorax: Pneumo. This is commonly called a collapsed lung. It is when air enters the pleural cavity in the chest outside the lung.

PO: By mouth.

P.O.A. or POA: Power of Attorney.

PO2: Partial Pressure of Oxygen. This is a part of an Arterial Blood Gas.

Port or Port A Cath: A port surgically implanted underneath the skin on the chest and inserted into a main vein. This is used mainly for chemotherapy administration.

Positive End Expiratory Pressure: PEEP. This is one of the settings used in mechanical ventilation. It helps keep the alveoli, which is the small sacs needed for oxygenation from collapsing.

Positron Emission Tomography: Pet Scan. This is a nuclear medicine imaging test that uses small amount of radiation to detect cancers, heart disease, certain diseases, and abnormalities in the body.

Post Anesthesia Care Unit: PACU. This is usually referred to as the recovery room.

Posterior: The backside of the body.

Post Op: Post operative or the period after surgery.

Post Operative: Post Op.

IT'S ALL GREEK TO ME...UNDERSTANDING MEDICAL LANGUAGE

Potassium: K or KCL.

Power of Attorney: P.O.A or POA.

Precautions: Isolation Precautions. This assists in decreasing the transmissions of infectious agents in the healthcare setting. This can be contact, respiratory, and/or reverse isolation for patients with very low immune systems. The equipment includes gown, gloves, and mask.

Premature Atrial Contraction: P.A.C. or PAC.

Premature Atrial Tachycardia: P.A.T. or PAT. This happens when the heart beats 160-200 beats per minute. It usually begins and ends abruptly.

Premature Ventricular Contraction: PVC.

Pre Op: The period of time before surgery.

Prescription: RX.

Pressors: The medications used to increase blood pressure.

Pressure Support: This refers to a setting during mechanical ventilation that decreases the workload of breathing.

Pressure Support Ventilation: PSV. It assists in the inspiratory phase when a patient is on mechanical ventilation.

Privacy Code: This is the number or code that is assigned to you. In accordance with HIPAA no one can receive information regarding your condition or if you are even in the facility without having authorization. This is the code or number you give to people if you want to have access to your condition.

Progressive care unit: PCU. This is a step down from the intensive care unit.

P.R.O.M. or PROM: Passive Range of Motion.

Prone: Face down position.

Prothrombin Time: PT.

Protocol: A detailed plan of a medical treatment, experiment, or procedure related to the clinical trials of cancer patients.

Proximal: A reference point such as a point of attachment that is closest to the midline of the body.

PRN: As needed. This refers to activities and medications. Example: Give Ativan 1mg IV q4h prn for anxiety, translated meaning give Ativan 1 milligram intravenously every four hours as needed for anxiety.

Psych: Psychiatric Therapy. This refers to the treatment of various conditions of the mind.

Psychiatric Therapy: Psych. This refers to the treatment of various conditions of the mind.

PSV: Pressure Support Ventilation. It assists in the inspiratory phase when a patient is on mechanical ventilation.

PT: Patient.

P.T.: Physical Therapy.

PTCA: Percutaneous Transluminal Coronary Angioplasty.

PTT: Partial Thromboplastin Time.

P.U.D. or PUD: Peptic Ulcer Disease.

Pulmonary Artery Wedge Pressure: PAWP. Measure the mean left atrial pressure in the heart. A central intravenous line is required.

Pulmonary Embolism: PE. This is a blockage caused by a blood clot, fat embolism, or air embolism. This is a blockage in the Pulmonary Artery or its branches. This is a very serious condition requiring immediate attention. Symptoms include rapid and labored breathing, chest pain with inspiration, low oxygen saturations, rapid heart rate, and a feeling of heart "skipping or fluttering."

PVC: Premature Ventricular Contraction.

"Q or q": "Every." Examples: This medication is ordered, "q day or qd," meaning every day. Another example is "q6 or q6," meaning every six hours. When your medical professional speaks with you, they may not always add hours at the end of the sentence.

QID: Four times per day. This may be on your prescriptions or hear your healthcare professional speak of this regarding your prescribed activities. This is also written as qid or q.i.d..

Quinton: A large bore catheter used for Hemodialysis.

Rales: A clicking or rattling sound heard with a stethoscope with inspiration.

Range Of Motion: ROM.

RBC: Red blood cell.

Rectal Tube: A tube inserted into the rectum to collect stool and prevent skin breakdown.

Red Blood Cell: RBC.

Regression: This refers to the shrinkage of cancer and the reduction of signs and symptoms related to a response to treatment.

Rehab: Rehabilitation Services. This includes speech, physical, occupational, massage, and respiratory services.

Rehabilitation Services: Rehab. This includes speech, physical, occupational, massage, and respiratory services.

Relapse: This refers to a recurrence of a disease after an apparent recovery.

Remission: This can be partial or complete disappearance of cancer.

Residuals: This refers to the amount of contents in the stomach that is aspirated or removed when monitoring a patient's feedings. Healthcare professionals monitor this to evaluate if a patient is tolerating tube feedings. Depending on the rate and the amount aspirated, the residuals may or may not be re-fed to the patient.

Respiratory Therapy: RT.

Reverse Trendelenburg: The position of lying on your back with your head higher than your feet.

Rhonchi: The coarse rattling sound heard during auscultation. This can be heard during inspiration or expiration.

IT'S ALL GREEK TO ME...UNDERSTANDING MEDICAL LANGUAGE

Right eye: O.D.

Right Lower Extremity: R.L.E. or RLE. This refers to the right leg.

Right Lower Lobe: R.L.L or RLL.

Right Lower Quadrant: R.L.Q. or RLQ. This refers to the right leg.

Right Upper Extremity: R.U.E. or RUE. This refers to the right arm.

Right Upper Lobe of the Lung: R.U.L. or RUL. This refers to the right upper lobe of the lung.

Right Upper Quadrant: R.U.Q. or RUQ. This refers to the abdomen.

R.L.E. or RLE: Right Lower Extremity. This refers to the right leg.

R.L.L. or RLL: Right Lower Lobe of the Lung.

R.L.Q. or RLQ: Right Lower Quadrant. This refers to the right leg.

R.O.M. or ROM: Range Of Motion.

RT: Respiratory Therapy.

R.U.E. or RUE: Right Upper Extremity. This refers to the right arm.

R.U.L. or RUL: Right Upper Lobe of the Lung.

R.U.Q. or RUQ: Right Upper Quadrant. This refers to the abdomen.

RX: Prescription.

SB: Sinus Brady. This is when the heart rate is below sixty beats per minute and is a normal rhythm pattern.

SCD: Sequential Compression Devices. This device is worn on the legs. It is designed to improve blood flow and decrease edema and blood clots.

Scrub The Hub: A term used as a reminder to clean the ports before accessing the IV site. This should be done for ten seconds.

Sedimentation rate: ESR.

Semi-Fowlers: The position of lying on the back with the head of the bed slightly elevated.

Semi-Private Room: This is a room that is shared by two patients. Make sure that if you are placed in this type of room that your roommate is not isolation precautions for an infection that you do not already have.

Sepsis: An acute inflammation of the whole body. This condition is very serious. It can be characterized by either a decreased or increased white blood cell count and lower than average or high body temperatures. An increase in respiratory and heart rates will also be noted. This type of patient needs to be closely observed in the critical care unit.

Sequential Compression Devices: SCD. This device is worn on the legs. It is designed to improve blood flow and decrease edema and blood clots.

Shock: This is a major medical emergency. This condition is a sudden drop in blood flow throughout the body. Types of shock: Cardiogenic, Hypovolemic, and Septic.

Short of breath: SOB.

Side effect: A change in condition of a person health resulting from medication.

SIDS: Sudden Infant Death Syndrome.

Signs and Symptoms: SS.

Sims: This position requires the patient to be lying on their left side and chest, the right knee and thigh is drawn up toward the chest and the left arm is behind the back. Used for vaginal, colorectal examinations, and enemas.

SIMV: Synchronized Intermittent Mechanical Ventilation. This is a mechanical ventilator setting. This is a setting that is used for weaning. A patient can take breaths on their own while receiving a specific number of mechanical breaths.

Sinus Bradycardia: Sinus Brady, Brady, or SB. This is when the heart rate is below sixty beats per minute.

Sinus Rhythm: This is the normal rhythm of the heart. The normal heart rate is between 60-100 per minute.

Sinus Tachycardia: Sinus Tach or Tachy. This is a normal heart rhythm that is beating greater than 100 beats per minute.

SIRS: Systemic Inflammatory Response Syndrome. This condition is when the body is in an acute inflammatory state.

S.O.B.: Short of breath.

Sodium: NA.

Sodium Bicarbonate: Sodium bicarb or NaHco3.

Speech: Speech-Language Therapy.

Speech-Language Therapy: Speech.

SR: Sinus rhythm. This is the normal heart rhythm seen on an ECG, EKG, or monitor. It means the electrical system in your heart is functioning in a normal pathway.

SS: Signs and symptoms.

STAT: Immediate.

Stoma: This is the actual end of the opening made for removal of waste from the body. The site should be a pink healthy color. A bluish purple color may suggest blood flow is not getting to site. This should be seen by your medical professional as soon as possible.

Subclavian: The two large veins located just under the Clavicle. This term usually refers to a central line that is inserted into the Subclavian for medication administration.

Subcutaneous: Sub Q. This refers to the tissue under the skin. It is also a term used for a type of injection.

Sub Q: Subcutaneous. This refers to the tissue under the skin. It is also a term used for a type of injection.

Supine: This position is lying on your back, face up.

Supraventricular Tachycardia: SVT. This is a rapid heart rate originating above the ventricles.

SVR: Systemic Vascular Resistance.

SVT: Supraventricular Tachycardia. This is a rapid heart rate originating above the ventricles.

Swan Ganz: An intravenous catheter used for hemodynamic monitoring.

SX: Suction.

Synchronized Electrical Cardioversion: Cardiovert.

Synchronized Intermittent Mechanical Ventilation: SIMV. This is a mechanical ventilator setting. This is a setting that is used for weaning. A patient can take breaths on their own while receiving a specific number of mechanical breaths.

Systemic Inflammatory Response Syndrome: SIRS. This condition is when the body is in an acute inflammatory state.

Systemic Vascular Resistance: SVR.

Tab: Tablet.

Tablet: Tab.

Tachy: Increased respirations or heart rate.

Tachycardia: A heart rate greater than one hundred beats per minute.

Tachypnea: Rapid respirations.

TB: Tuberculosis.

T&C: Type and Cross. This is the blood test to determine blood type.

Tech: Technician.

Technician: Tech.

Ted hose: Antithrombolytic Stockings. These are placed on the legs and are intended to decrease swelling in the legs and improve circulation.

T.E.E. or TEE: Transesophageal Echocariogram. This procedure requires the patient to pass an echo transducer through the mouth and into the esophagus. This offers a better image over a standard echocardiogram of the heart.

Temp: Temperature.

Temperature: Temp.

Temporal Mandibular Joint: TMJ.

Terminally Cleaned: The process in which your room has had all the surfaced cleaned with a germicidal disinfectant and a new privacy curtain has been hung.

Thrombocytopenia: This is a condition resulting from an abnormal low platelet level, typically under 100,000. Bleeding and bruising can occur.

T.I.A.: Transient Ischemic Attack. This is a mini stroke and a warning sign of an impending stroke.

TID: Three times per day. This may be on your prescriptions or hear your healthcare professional speak this regarding your prescribed activities. This is also written as tid or t.i.d..

IT'S ALL GREEK TO ME...UNDERSTANDING MEDICAL LANGUAGE

TLC: Triple Lumen Catheter. This is a type of central intravenous catheter for medication administration, blood withdrawals for labs, and hemodynamic monitoring.

Tmax: Temperature.

TMJ: Temporomandibular Joint.

Total Parenteral Nutrition: TPN. This is nutrition that is fed intravenously.

TPN: Total Parenteral Nutrition. This is nutrition that is fed intravenously.

Trach: The term used for Tracheostomy.

Tracheostomy: Trach.

Trach mask: A mask designed to assist in the delivery of oxygen for a person that has a Trachoestomy.

Transesophageal Echocariogram: T.E.E or TEE. This procedure requires the patient to pass an echo transducer through the mouth and into the esophagus. This offers a better image over a standard echocardiogram of the heart.

Transient Ischemic Attack: T.I.A. This is a mini stroke and a warning sign of an impending stroke.

Treatment: TX.

Trendelenburg: This is a position that requires the patient to lay on their back with the head of the bed lower than the lower extremities. This position is often used when a patient's blood pressure is low.

Triple A: Abdominal aortic aneurism.

Triple Lumen Catheter: TLC. This is a type of central intravenous catheter for medication administration, blood withdrawals for labs, and hemodynamic monitoring.

Tunneling: This is open wounds that have separated into the soft tissues. This is a potential site for infection.

TX: Treatment.

Type and Cross: T&C. This is the blood test to determine blood type.

Type and Screen: T&S. This is the blood test to determine blood type.

UA: Urinalysis. This is a urine test.

Ultrasound: US.

Unit dose: A single dose of medication.

Urinalysis: UA. This is a urine test.

Urinary tract infection: UTI.

Urine CX or Urine Culture: A urine test that is used to test for bacteria.

UTI: Urinary Tract Infection.

VAD or Vascular Access Device: This is a type of catheter or port surgically placed under the skin on the chest for administration of chemotherapy.

Vanco: Vancomycin.

Vancomycin: Vanco.

Vancomycin Resistance Enterococcus: VRE. This can be a life threatening infection. Good hand washing and wearing gloves can help reduce the risk of transmission.

VAP: Ventilator Acquired Pneumonia.

Vascular Access Device: VAD. This is a type of catheter or port surgically placed under the skin on the chest for administration of chemotherapy.

Vent: Ventilator.

Venti: Venturi mask.

Ventilator: Vent.

Ventilator Acquired Pneumonia: VAP.

Ventricular Fibrillation: V Fib. This is a cardiac arrhythmia needing immediate attention.

Ventricular Septal Defect: VSD.

Ventricular Tachycardia: V Tach. This is a cardiac arrhythmia needing immediate attention.

Venturi Mask: Venti.

V Fib: Ventricular Fibrillation. This is a cardiac arrhythmia needing immediate attention.

Vitals: Vital signs.

Vital Signs: Vitals.

Vital Signs Stable: VSS.

VRE: Vancomycin Resistance Enterococcus. This can be a life threatening infection. Good hand washing and wearing gloves can help reduce the risk of transmission.

VSD: Ventricular Septal Defect.

VSS: Vital Signs Stable.

V Tach: Ventricular Tachycardia. This is a cardiac arrhythmia needing immediate attention.

WBC: White blood cell.

Well approximated: Refers to the edges of a wound or incision that is pink, healthy, healing, and not open.

White blood cell: WBC.

Within normal limits: WNL.

Without distress: W.O.D. or WOD.

WNL: Within Normal Limits.

W.O.D. or WOD: Without distress.

Wound CX or Wound Culture: A test that evaluates if a wound is infected with bacteria or fungus.

IT'S ALL GREEK TO ME...UNDERSTANDING MEDICAL LANGUAGE

Wound Vac: Wound vacuum. This is a type of suction device that creates a negative pressure directly over a wound to promote drainage and promote healing.

Symbols: the medical professional community uses several symbols in communication. Here are a few of the most common. The symbol for the word "with" is a line drawn over the letter c. This is usually done in lower case. The symbol for the word "change" is a triangle. The symbol for "left" is the letter "L" encompassed in a circle. The symbol for "right" is the letter "R" encompassed in a circle.

ABBREVIATIONS USED DURING MY HOSPITAL STAY AND THEIR MEANINGS:

ENTERING THE EMERGENCY ROOM

I need a translator: _____ yes, _____ no. Language: ______________________________.

I am hearing impaired: _____ yes, _____ no. Interpreter needed: _____ yes, _____ no.

Date and time I entered emergency room: ______________________________.

Reason I came into the emergency room: ______________________________

______________________________.

My signs and symptoms: ______________________________

______________________________.

Date, time, and duration of signs and symptoms: ______________________________.

Pain: _____ yes, _____ no. Describe pain and location: ______________________________

______________________________.

Any activity that increases pain: _____ yes, _____ no.

Chest pain: _____ yes, _____ no. Describe: ______________________________.

Pain exacerbated by: ______________________________

______________________________.

Physician names: __________, __________, __________, __________.

Nurse's names: __________, __________, __________, __________.

Time nurse entered the room: _______ am/pm, _______ am/pm, _______ am/pm,

_______ am/pm, _______ am/pm, _______ am/pm, _______ am/pm, _______ am/pm.

Activities performed by nurse: ______________________________

____

______________________________.

Times physicians entered the room: _____ am/pm, _____ am/pm, _____ am/pm, _____ am/pm.

Activities performed by physician(s): ______________________________

____

______________________________.

Physical examination: _____ yes, _____ no.

By whom: ______________________ when: ______________________.

Re-examined: _____ yes, _____ no.

By whom: ______________________ when: ______________________.

ENTERING THE EMERGENCY ROOM

Lab tests ordered: ______________, ______________, ______________, ______________,
______________, ______________, ______________, ______________, ______________.

Electrocardiogram: _____ yes, _____ no. Results: ______________________________.

X-Ray: _____ yes, _____ no. Location: ______________________________________.

Cat scan: _____ yes, _____ no. Contrast: _____ yes, _____ no. Oral: _____, IV _____.

Area scanned: ____.

MRI: _____ yes, _____ no. Contrast: _____ yes, _____ no. Type: ______________.

Area scanned: ____.

List other scans and results: ____
____
____.

Oxygen: _____ yes, _____ no. Route of delivery: ____________ amount: ____________

Vital signs: Temperature-Temp, Pulse-P, Respirations-R, Blood Pressure-B/P, Oxygen-O2

Time: _______ am/pm Temp ______, P ______, R ______, B/P ________, O2 ______%

Time: _______ am/pm Temp ______, P ______, R ______, B/P ________, O2 ______%.

Time: _______ am/pm Temp ______, P ______, R ______, B/P ________, O2 ______%

Time: _______ am/pm Temp ______, P ______, R ______, B/P ________, O2 ______%

Time: _______ am/pm Temp ______, P ______, R ______, B/P ________, O2 ______%

Time: _______ am/pm Temp ______, P ______, R ______, B/P ________, O2 ______%

Time: _______ am/pm Temp ______, P ______, R ______, B/P ________, O2 ______%

Time: _______ am/pm Temp ______, P ______, R ______, B/P ________, O2 ______%

Time: _______ am/pm Temp ______, P ______, R ______, B/P ________, O2 ______%

Time: _______ am/pm Temp ______, P ______, R ______, B/P ________, O2 ______%

Admitted to room: _____ yes, _____ no. Time of transfer: _____ am/pm. Room # ______

My diagnosis: ____

Code blue: _______ yes, _______ no. Resuscitated: _______ yes, _______ no.

Patient expired: _____ yes, _____ no. Length of Code Pink / Blue : _______ minutes.

MD name(s): ____

MEDICAL JOURNAL FOR ______________________________

DATE ____________________, DAY NUMBER ______________

VISITS FROM MY DOCTORS TODAY

Goals for today: ______________________________
____
____.

Things to discuss with my doctor(s): ______________
____
____

Dr.__________ came in at ____ am/pm. Left at _____ am/pm.
We discussed __________________________________.
Did doctor examine patient: _____ yes, _____ no.
Wash hands before touching patient: _____ yes, _____ no.
Wear gloves: ____ yes, ___ no. Clean stethoscope: ____ yes, ____ no.
Wear gown and mask (precautions only):____ yes, _____ no.
Wash hands before leaving the room: _____ yes, _____ no.

Dr.__________ came in at ____ am/pm. Left at _____ am/pm.
We discussed __________________________________.
Did doctor examine patient: _____ yes, _____ no.
Wash hands before touching patient: _____ yes, _____ no.
Wear gloves: ____ yes, ___ no. Clean stethoscope: ____ yes, ____ no.
Wear gown and mask (precautions only):____ yes, _____ no.
Wash hands before leaving the room: _____ yes, _____ no.

Dr.__________ came in at ____ am/pm. Left at _____ am/pm.
We discussed __________________________________.
Did doctor examine patient: _____ yes, _____ no.
Wash hands before touching patient: _____ yes, _____ no.
Wear gloves: ____ yes, ___ no. Clean stethoscope: ____ yes, ____ no.
Wear gown and mask (precautions only):____ yes, _____ no.
Wash hands before leaving the room: _____ yes, _____ no.

Dr.__________ came in at ____ am/pm. Left at _____ am/pm.
We discussed __________________________________.
Did doctor examine patient: _____ yes, _____ no.
Wash hands before touching patient: _____ yes, _____ no.
Wear gloves: ____ yes, ___ no. Clean stethoscope: ____ yes, ____ no.
Wear gown and mask (precautions only):____ yes, _____ no.
Wash hands before leaving the room: _____ yes, _____ no.

Dr.__________ came in at ____ am/pm. Left at _____ am/pm.
We discussed __________________________________.
Did doctor examine patient: _____ yes, _____ no.
Wash hands before touching patient: _____ yes, _____ no.
Wear gloves: ____ yes, ___ no. Clean stethoscope: ____ yes, ____ no.
Wear gown and mask (precautions only):____ yes, _____ no.
Wash hands before leaving the room: _____ yes, _____ no.

NURSING CARE FOR ________________________________

DATE __________________, DAY NUMBER __________________

INITIAL DAY SHIFT EXAM:

My nurse has _____ # of patients. CNA ___yes, ___no. Charge nurse ____________
Nurse ______________ RN/LPN came in at _________ am/pm. Left at _________ am/pm.
Did nurse wash hands and wear gloves before touching patient: ______ yes, ______ no.
Wash hands after touching patient and before leaving the room: ______ yes, ______ no.
Don't hesitate to request staff to wash their hands. This will help decrease the risk of spreading potentially lethal germs.
Did nurse wear protective gear (isolation precautions only): ______ yes, ______ no.
Did nurse provide oral care (to be done every two hours if unable to provide for self, also decreases risk of pneumonia, infections, and aspiration): ______ yes, _____ no.
If able to provide own oral care, then supplies at bedside: _______ yes, ________ no.
Was patient repositioned (every two hours if unable to turn self): _____ yes _____ no.
Head of bed at ________ degrees. This is important for patients on ventilators or on tube feedings. Anything less than thirty degrees places patients at risk for aspiration of stomach contents into the lungs causing aspiration pneumonia.
Checked for incontinence and skin breakdown: _____ yes, _____ no.
Patient's linens wet or soiled: _____ yes, ____ no. Linens changed: ____ yes, ____ no.
Time linens changed: _______ am/pm. Any skin redness or breakdown: ____ yes, ____ no.
If yes, what stage is pressure ulcer: ________. Acquired when: _______________.
List wounds not associated with pressure ulcers and how acquired: ______________
____.
Mattress type: ____.
Specialty mattresses are important to help prevent pressure ulcers)
If patient on ventilator or has tracheostomy, suction performed: _____ yes, ______ no.
Did nurse listen to lung sounds: _____ yes, _____ no.
Does patient have chest tubes: ____ yes, ____ no. Functioning _____ yes, _____ no.
Bowel sounds: _______ yes, _______ no. Bowel sounds active: ______ yes, ______ no.
Neurological exam: _____ yes, _____ no. Follow commands: _______ yes, _______ no.
Is patient alert and oriented to person, place, time, and events: _____ yes, _____ no.
If confused, patient is not oriented to: ____ person, ____ place, ____ time, ____ event.
Confusion began (time and date): ____.
Glasgow coma scale (checks conscious scale of patient): __________________________.
Intracranial pressure monitoring: ______ yes, ______ no.
If yes, pressure is at ________ mm mercury. (Normal is one to fifteen).
Moves extremities: ___ yes, ___ no.
Paralysis: (inability to move extremities) ______ yes, ______ no.
If yes, extremities affected and when paralysis began: __________________________.
Is patient in pain: ____ yes, ____ no. Describe pain and location _______________.
Patient able to eat: ____ yes, ____ no. What type of diet? _____________________.
If patient on tube feedings list type: ______________ at ____________ cc/ml per hour.
Nausea ____, vomiting _____. If so, describe: ___________________________________.
Patient has: Nasal gastric tube ______, Dobhoff tube _____, Peg or gastric tube _____.
When was feeding tube placed and what site: _____________________________________.
Catheter for draining urine: ____ yes, ____ no. If so, when placed: _____________.
Find out policy for allowed time to remain in bladder. Too long may cause infections.)
IV site(s) where: _____________________________ when placed: ____________________.
IV fluids (types and rates): ________________________, __________________________,
__________________, __________________________, __________________________,
Is patient on oxygen: _____ yes, _____ no. If so, how much and route delivered (see oxygen routes): ____.
If patient on ventilator, list settings (see list on ventilator settings): _______
____
Vital signs: temp _____, pulse _____, resp _____, b/p _____, o2 _____%,
current weight _____ pounds, _____ kg. Glucose level: ____________________
Insulin coverage: ____ yes, ____ no. Insulin type: __________, # of units: _____.

NURSING CARE CONTINUED FOR ____________________
DATE ____________________, DAY NUMBER ____________________

FOLLOWING EXAMINATIONS FOR DAY SHIFT:

Nurse ____________, CNA ____________, in at _____ am/pm. Left at ______ am/pm.
Wash hands and wear gloves before touching patient: _______ yes, _______ no.
Wash hands before leaving room: ___ yes, ___ no. Wear protective gear: __ yes, __ no.
Clean stethoscope: __ yes, __ no. Oral care: __ yes, __ no. Suctioned: __ yes, __ no.
Repositioned: ___ yes, ___ no. Turned to: ___ left, ___ right, ___ backside ___.
Head of bed at: ________ degrees. Incontinence/skin breakdown: ____ yes, ____ no.
Linens wet or soiled: ______ yes, ______ no. Linens changed: ______ yes, ______ no.
Dressing changed: _____ yes, _____ no. Location: ________________________.
IV site checked: _____ yes, _______ no. IV tubing labeled: _____ yes, _____ no.
IV fluids at: ____.
Pain level (0-10 scale.0-no pain, 10 intolerable): ____________________.
Location of pain: ____________. Medicated for pain: ____ yes, ___ no.
Patient is alert/oriented: ____ yes, ____ no. New confusion: ___ yes, ___ no.
Vital signs: temp ____, pulse ____, resp _____, b/p _____, 02 ____ %, ___ liters.
Glucose level: _____. Insulin: ___ yes, ___ no. Type: ___________ # of units ____.

Nurse ____________, CNA ____________, in at _____ am/pm. Left at ______ am/pm.
Wash hands and wear gloves before touching patient: _______ yes, _______ no.
Wash hands before leaving room: ___ yes, ___ no. Wear protective gear: __ yes, __ no.
Clean stethoscope: __ yes, __ no. Oral care: __ yes, __ no. Suctioned: __ yes, __ no.
Repositioned: ___ yes, ___ no. Turned to: ___ left, ___ right, ___ backside ___.
Head of bed at: ________ degrees. Incontinence/skin breakdown: ____ yes, ____ no.
Linens wet or soiled: ______ yes, ______ no. Linens changed: ______ yes, ______ no.
Dressing changed: _____ yes, _____ no. Location: ________________________.
IV site checked: _____ yes, _______ no. IV tubing labeled: _____ yes, _____ no.
IV fluids at: ____.
Pain level (0-10 scale.0-no pain, 10 intolerable): ____________________.
Location of pain: ____________. Medicated for pain: ____ yes, ___ no.
Patient is alert/oriented: ____ yes, ____ no. New confusion: ___ yes, ___ no.
Vital signs: temp ____, pulse ____, resp _____, b/p _____, 02 ____ %, ___ liters.
Glucose level: _____. Insulin: ___ yes, ___ no. Type: ___________ # of units ____.

Nurse ____________, CNA ____________, in at _____ am/pm. Left at ______ am/pm.
Wash hands and wear gloves before touching patient: _______ yes, _______ no.
Wash hands before leaving room: ___ yes, ___ no. Wear protective gear: __ yes, __ no.
Clean stethoscope: __ yes, __ no. Oral care: __ yes, __ no. Suctioned: __ yes, __ no.
Repositioned: ___ yes, ___ no. Turned to: ___ left, ___ right, ___ backside ___.
Head of bed at: ________ degrees. Incontinence/skin breakdown: ____ yes, ____ no.
Linens wet or soiled: ______ yes, ______ no. Linens changed: ______ yes, ______ no.
Dressing changed: _____ yes, _____ no. Location: ________________________.
IV site checked: _____ yes, _______ no. IV tubing labeled: _____ yes, _____ no.
IV fluids at: ____.
Pain level (0-10 scale.0-no pain, 10 intolerable): ____________________.
Location of pain: ____________. Medicated for pain: ____ yes, ___ no.
Patient is alert/oriented: ____ yes, ____ no. New confusion: ___ yes, ___ no.
Vital signs: temp ____, pulse ____, resp _____, b/p _____, 02 ____ %, ___ liters.
Glucose level: _____. Insulin: ___ yes, ___ no. Type: ___________ # of units ____.

NURSING CARE CONTINUED FOR ______________________
DATE ____________________, DAY NUMBER ____________________

FOLLOWING EXAMINATIONS FOR DAY SHIFT:

Nurse ____________, CNA ____________, in at _____ am/pm. Left at ______ am/pm.
Wash hands and wear gloves before touching patient: ______ yes, ______ no.
Wash hands before leaving room: ___ yes, ___ no. Wear protective gear: __ yes, __ no.
Clean stethoscope: __ yes, __ no. Oral care: __ yes, __ no. Suctioned: __ yes, __ no.
Repositioned: ___ yes, ___ no. Turned to: ___ left, ___ right, ___ backside ___.
Head of bed at: _______ degrees. Incontinence/skin breakdown: ____ yes, ____ no.
Linens wet or soiled: ____ yes, ____ no. Linens changed: _____ yes, _____ no.
Dressing changed: ____ yes, ____ no. Location: ______________________.
IV site checked: _____ yes, _____ no. IV tubing labeled: _____ yes, _____no.
IV fluids at: ____.
Pain level (0-10 scale.0-no pain, 10 intolerable): ____________________.
Location of pain: ____________. Medicated for pain: _____ yes, ___ no.
Patient is alert/oriented: ___ yes, ___ no. New confusion: ____ yes, ___ no.
Vital signs: temp ___, pulse ____, resp ____, b/p _____, 02 _____ %, ____ liters.
Glucose level: _____. Insulin: ___ yes, ___ no. Type: ____________ # of units ____.

Nurse ____________, CNA ____________, in at _____ am/pm. Left at ______ am/pm.
Wash hands and wear gloves before touching patient: ______ yes, ______ no.
Wash hands before leaving room: ___ yes, ___ no. Wear protective gear: __ yes, __ no.
Clean stethoscope: __ yes, __ no. Oral care: __ yes, __ no. Suctioned: __ yes, __ no.
Repositioned: ___ yes, ___ no. Turned to: ___ left, ___ right, ___ backside ___.
Head of bed at: _______ degrees. Incontinence/skin breakdown: ____ yes, ____ no.
Linens wet or soiled: ____ yes, ____ no. Linens changed: _____ yes, _____ no.
Dressing changed: ____ yes, ____ no. Location: ______________________.
IV site checked: _____ yes, _____ no. IV tubing labeled: _____ yes, _____no.
IV fluids at: ____.
Pain level (0-10 scale.0-no pain, 10 intolerable): ____________________.
Location of pain: ____________. Medicated for pain: _____ yes, ___ no.
Patient is alert/oriented: ___ yes, ___ no. New confusion: ____ yes, ___ no.
Vital signs: temp ___, pulse ____, resp ____, b/p _____, 02 _____ %, ____ liters.
Glucose level: _____. Insulin: ___ yes, ___ no. Type: ____________ # of units ____.

Nurse ____________, CNA ____________, in at _____ am/pm. Left at ______ am/pm.
Wash hands and wear gloves before touching patient: ______ yes, ______ no.
Wash hands before leaving room: ___ yes, ___ no. Wear protective gear: __ yes, __ no.
Clean stethoscope: __ yes, __ no. Oral care: __ yes, __ no. Suctioned: __ yes, __ no.
Repositioned: ___ yes, ___ no. Turned to: ___ left, ___ right, ___ backside ___.
Head of bed at: _______ degrees. Incontinence/skin breakdown: ____ yes, ____ no.
Linens wet or soiled: ____ yes, ____ no. Linens changed: _____ yes, _____ no.
Dressing changed: ____ yes, ____ no. Location: ______________________.
IV site checked: _____ yes, _____ no. IV tubing labeled: _____ yes, _____no.
IV fluids at: ____.
Pain level (0-10 scale.0-no pain, 10 intolerable): ____________________.
Location of pain: ____________. Medicated for pain: _____ yes, ___ no.
Patient is alert/oriented: ___ yes, ___ no. New confusion: ____ yes, ___ no.
Vital signs: temp ___, pulse ____, resp ____, b/p _____, 02 _____ %, ____ liters.
Glucose level: _____. Insulin: ___ yes, ___ no. Type: ____________ # of units ____.

NURSING CARE FOR ______________________________________

DATE ____________________, DAY NUMBER ____________________

INITIAL NIGHT SHIFT EXAM:

My nurse has _____ # of patients. CNA ___yes, ___no. Charge nurse _____________
Nurse __________ RN/LPN came in at __________ am/pm. Left at _________ am/pm.
Did nurse wash hands and wear gloves before touching patient: _____ yes, _____ no.
Wash hands after touching patient and before leaving the room: _____ yes, _____ no.
Don't hesitate to request staff to wash their hands. This will help decrease the risk of spreading potentially lethal germs.
Did nurse wear protective gear (isolation precautions only): _______ yes, _____ no.
Did nurse provide oral care (to be done every two hours if unable to provide for self, also decreases risk of pneumonia, infections, and aspiration): ______ yes, _____ no.
If able to provide own oral care, then supplies at bedside: _______ yes, _______ no.
Was patient repositioned (every two hours if unable to turn self): _____ yes _____ no.
Head of bed at ________ degrees. This is important for patients on ventilators or on tube feedings. Anything less than thirty degrees places patients at risk for aspiration of stomach contents into the lungs causing aspiration pneumonia.
Checked for incontinence and skin breakdown: _____ yes, _____ no.
Patient's linens wet or soiled: ____ yes, ____ no. Linens changed: ____ yes, ____ no.
Time linens changed: _______ am/pm. Any skin redness or breakdown: ____ yes, ____ no.
If yes, what stage is pressure ulcer: ______. Acquired when: _________________.
List wounds not associated with pressure ulcers and how acquired: _______________
____.
Mattress type: ____.
Specialty mattresses are important to help prevent pressure ulcers)
If patient on ventilator or has tracheostomy, suction performed: _____ yes, _____ no.
Did nurse listen to lung sounds: _____ yes, _____ no.
Does patient have chest tubes: ____ yes, ____ no. Functioning _____ yes, _____ no.
Bowel sounds: ______ yes, ______ no. Bowel sounds active: ______ yes, ______ no.
Neurological exam: _____ yes, _____ no. Follow commands: ______ yes, ______ no.
Is patient alert and oriented to person, place, time, and events: ____yes, _____ no.
If confused, patient is not oriented to: ___ person, ___ place, ___ time, ___ event.
Confusion began (time and date): _______________________________________.
Glasgow coma scale (checks conscious scale of patient): ______________________.
Intracranial pressure monitoring: ____ yes, ____ no.
If yes, pressure is at _________ mm mercury. (Normal is one to fifteen).
Moves extremities: ___ yes, ___ no.
Paralysis: (inability to move extremities) ______ yes, ______ no.
If yes, extremities affected and when paralysis began: ________________________
Is patient in pain: ____ yes, ____ no. Describe pain and location ______________
Patient able to eat: ___ yes, ____ no. What type of diet? ____________________
If patient on tube feedings list type: __________ at _________ cc/ml per hour.
Nausea ____, vomiting ____. If so, describe: _________________________________
Patient has: Nasal gastric tube ____, Dobhoff tube _____, Peg or gastric tube ______
When was feeding tube placed and what site: _____________________________.
Catheter for draining urine: ____ yes, ____ no. If so, when placed: ___________.
Find out policy for allowed time to remain in bladder. Too long may cause infections.)
IV site(s) where: ____________________ when placed: __________________.
IV fluids (types and rates): ______________, ______________, ______________,
______________, ______________, ______________, ______________,
Is patient on oxygen: ____ yes, ____ no. If so, how much and route delivered (see oxygen routes): ____.
If patient on ventilator, list settings (see list on ventilator settings): _________
____.
Vital signs: temp _____, pulse _____, resp _____, b/p _____, o2 _____%,
current weight _____ pounds, _____ kg. Glucose level: _____
Insulin coverage: ____ yes, ____ no. Insulin type: ___________, # of units: _____.

NURSING CARE CONTINUED FOR ______________________________
DATE ____________________, DAY NUMBER ____________________

FOLLOWING EXAMINATIONS FOR NIGHT SHIFT:

Nurse ______________, CNA ______________, in at _____ am/pm. Left at _______ am/pm.
Wash hands and wear gloves before touching patient: _______ yes, _______ no.
Wash hands before leaving room: ___ yes, ___ no. Wear protective gear: __ yes, __ no.
Clean stethoscope: __ yes, __ no. Oral care: __ yes, __ no. Suctioned: __ yes, __ no.
Repositioned: ___ yes, ___ no. Turned to: ___ left, ___ right, ___ backside ___.
Head of bed at: ________ degrees. Incontinence/skin breakdown: ____ yes, ____ no.
Linens wet or soiled: _____ yes, _____ no. Linens changed: _____ yes, _____ no.
Dressing changed: ____ yes, ____ no. Location: ______________________________.
IV site checked: _____ yes, _____ no. IV tubing labeled: _____ yes, _____no.
IV fluids at: ____.
Pain level (0-10 scale.0-no pain, 10 intolerable): _____________________________.
Location of pain: ____________________. Medicated for pain: ____ yes, ____ no.
Patient is alert/oriented: ___ yes, ____ no. New confusion: ____ yes, ____ no.
Vital signs: temp ____, pulse _____, resp _____, b/p ______, 02 _____ %,____ liters.
Glucose level: _____. Insulin: ___ yes, ___ no. Type: ______________ # of units ____.

Nurse ______________, CNA ______________, in at _____ am/pm. Left at _______ am/pm.
Wash hands and wear gloves before touching patient: _______ yes, _______ no.
Wash hands before leaving room: ___ yes, ___ no. Wear protective gear: __ yes, __ no.
Clean stethoscope: __ yes, __ no. Oral care: __ yes, __ no. Suctioned: __ yes, __ no.
Repositioned: ___ yes, ___ no. Turned to: ___ left, ___ right, ___ backside ___.
Head of bed at: ________ degrees. Incontinence/skin breakdown: ____ yes, ____ no.
Linens wet or soiled: _____ yes, _____ no. Linens changed: _____ yes, _____ no.
Dressing changed: ____ yes, ____ no. Location: ______________________________.
IV site checked: _____ yes, _____ no. IV tubing labeled: _____ yes, _____no.
IV fluids at: ____.
Pain level (0-10 scale.0-no pain, 10 intolerable): _____________________________.
Location of pain: ____________________. Medicated for pain: ____ yes, ____ no.
Patient is alert/oriented: ___ yes, ____ no. New confusion: ____ yes, ____ no.
Vital signs: temp ____, pulse _____, resp _____, b/p ______, 02 _____ %,____ liters.
Glucose level: _____. Insulin: ___ yes, ___ no. Type: ______________ # of units ____.

Nurse ______________, CNA ______________, in at _____ am/pm. Left at _______ am/pm.
Wash hands and wear gloves before touching patient: _______ yes, _______ no.
Wash hands before leaving room: ___ yes, ___ no. Wear protective gear: __ yes, __ no.
Clean stethoscope: __ yes, __ no. Oral care: __ yes, __ no. Suctioned: __ yes, __ no.
Repositioned: ___ yes, ___ no. Turned to: ___ left, ___ right, ___ backside ___.
Head of bed at: ________ degrees. Incontinence/skin breakdown: ____ yes, ____ no.
Linens wet or soiled: _____ yes, _____ no. Linens changed: _____ yes, _____ no.
Dressing changed: ____ yes, ____ no. Location: ______________________________.
IV site checked: _____ yes, _____ no. IV tubing labeled: _____ yes, _____no.
IV fluids at: ____.
Pain level (0-10 scale.0-no pain, 10 intolerable): _____________________________.
Location of pain: ____________________. Medicated for pain: ____ yes, ____ no.
Patient is alert/oriented: ___ yes, ____ no. New confusion: ____ yes, ____ no.
Vital signs: temp ____, pulse _____, resp _____, b/p ______, 02 _____ %,____ liters.
Glucose level: _____. Insulin: ___ yes, ___ no. Type: ______________ # of units ____.

NURSING CARE CONTINUED FOR ____________________
DATE ____________________, DAY NUMBER ____________________

FOLLOWING EXAMINATIONS FOR NIGHT SHIFT:

Nurse ______________, CNA ______________, in at _____ am/pm. Left at _____ am/pm.
Wash hands and wear gloves before touching patient: ________ yes, ________ no.
Wash hands before leaving room: ___ yes, ___ no. Wear protective gear: __ yes, __ no.
Clean stethoscope: __ yes, __ no. Oral care: __ yes, __ no. Suctioned: __ yes, __ no.
Repositioned: ___ yes, ___ no. Turned to: ___ left, ___ right, ___ backside ___.
Head of bed at: _______ degrees. Incontinence/skin breakdown: ____ yes, ____ no.
Linens wet or soiled: _____ yes, _____ no. Linens changed: _____ yes, _____ no.
Dressing changed: ____ yes, ____ no. Location: ______________________________.
IV site checked: _____ yes, _____ no. IV tubing labeled: _____ yes, _____no.
IV fluids at: ____.
Pain level (0-10 scale.0-no pain, 10 intolerable): ______________.
Location of pain: ______________. Medicated for pain: _____ yes, _____ no.
Patient is alert/oriented: ____ yes, ____ no. New confusion: ____ yes, ____ no.
Vital signs: temp ____, pulse _____, resp _____, b/p ______, 02 _____ %, _____ liters.
Glucose level: _____. Insulin: ___ yes, ___ no. Type: ______________ # of units ____.

Nurse ______________, CNA ______________, in at _____ am/pm. Left at _____ am/pm.
Wash hands and wear gloves before touching patient: ________ yes, ________ no.
Wash hands before leaving room: ___ yes, ___ no. Wear protective gear: __ yes, __ no.
Clean stethoscope: __ yes, __ no. Oral care: __ yes, __ no. Suctioned: __ yes, __ no.
Repositioned: ___ yes, ___ no. Turned to: ___ left, ___ right, ___ backside ___.
Head of bed at: _______ degrees. Incontinence/skin breakdown: ____ yes, ____ no.
Linens wet or soiled: _____ yes, _____ no. Linens changed: _____ yes, _____ no.
Dressing changed: ____ yes, ____ no. Location: ______________________________.
IV site checked: _____ yes, _____ no. IV tubing labeled: _____ yes, _____no.
IV fluids at: ____.
Pain level (0-10 scale.0-no pain, 10 intolerable): ______________.
Location of pain: ______________. Medicated for pain: _____ yes, _____ no.
Patient is alert/oriented: ____ yes, ____ no. New confusion: ____ yes, ____ no.
Vital signs: temp ____, pulse _____, resp _____, b/p ______, 02 _____ %, _____ liters.
Glucose level: _____. Insulin: ___ yes, ___ no. Type: ______________ # of units ____.

Nurse ______________, CNA ______________, in at _____ am/pm. Left at _____ am/pm.
Wash hands and wear gloves before touching patient: ________ yes, ________ no.
Wash hands before leaving room: ___ yes, ___ no. Wear protective gear: __ yes, __ no.
Clean stethoscope: __ yes, __ no. Oral care: __ yes, __ no. Suctioned: __ yes, __ no.
Repositioned: ___ yes, ___ no. Turned to: ___ left, ___ right, ___ backside ___.
Head of bed at: _______ degrees. Incontinence/skin breakdown: ____ yes, ____ no.
Linens wet or soiled: _____ yes, _____ no. Linens changed: _____ yes, _____ no.
Dressing changed: ____ yes, ____ no. Location: ______________________________.
IV site checked: _____ yes, _____ no. IV tubing labeled: _____ yes, _____no.
IV fluids at: ____.
Pain level (0-10 scale.0-no pain, 10 intolerable): ______________.
Location of pain: ______________. Medicated for pain: _____ yes, _____ no.
Patient is alert/oriented: ____ yes, ____ no. New confusion: ____ yes, ____ no.
Vital signs: temp ____, pulse _____, resp _____, b/p ______, 02 _____ %, _____ liters.
Glucose level: _____. Insulin: ___ yes, ___ no. Type: ______________ # of units ____.

MEDICATION ADMINISTRATION LIST FOR ____________________
DATE ______________ DAY NUMBER ______________________

List the medication for each day. Routes of administration: oral, thru feeding tube, intravenous (IV), intramuscular (IM), subcutaneous (SQ), epidural or a catheter in your spinal column, rectal, topical, eye drops, and ear drops.

Medication: ______________ Route: ______________ Time: __________
Medication: ______________ Route: ______________ Time: __________
Medication: ______________ Route: ______________ Time: __________
Medication: ______________ Route: ______________ Time: __________
Medication: ______________ Route: ______________ Time: __________
Medication: ______________ Route: ______________ Time: __________
Medication: ______________ Route: ______________ Time: __________
Medication: ______________ Route: ______________ Time: __________
Medication: ______________ Route: ______________ Time: __________
Medication: ______________ Route: ______________ Time: __________
Medication: ______________ Route: ______________ Time: __________
Medication: ______________ Route: ______________ Time: __________
Medication: ______________ Route: ______________ Time: __________
Medication: ______________ Route: ______________ Time: __________
Medication: ______________ Route: ______________ Time: __________
Medication: ______________ Route: ______________ Time: __________
Medication: ______________ Route: ______________ Time: __________
Medication: ______________ Route: ______________ Time: __________
Medication: ______________ Route: ______________ Time: __________
Medication: ______________ Route: ______________ Time: __________
Medication: ______________ Route: ______________ Time: __________
Medication: ______________ Route: ______________ Time: __________
Medication: ______________ Route: ______________ Time: __________
Medication: ______________ Route: ______________ Time: __________
Medication: ______________ Route: ______________ Time: __________
Medication: ______________ Route: ______________ Time: __________
Medication: ______________ Route: ______________ Time: __________
Medication: ______________ Route: ______________ Time: __________
Medication: ______________ Route: ______________ Time: __________
Medication: ______________ Route: ______________ Time: __________
Medication: ______________ Route: ______________ Time: __________
Medication: ______________ Route: ______________ Time: __________
Medication: ______________ Route: ______________ Time: __________
Medication: ______________ Route: ______________ Time: __________
Medication: ______________ Route: ______________ Time: __________
Medication: ______________ Route: ______________ Time: __________
Medication: ______________ Route: ______________ Time: __________
Medication: ______________ Route: ______________ Time: __________
Medication: ______________ Route: ______________ Time: __________
Medication: ______________ Route: ______________ Time: __________
Medication: ______________ Route: ______________ Time: __________
Medication: ______________ Route: ______________ Time: __________
Medication: ______________ Route: ______________ Time: __________
Medication: ______________ Route: ______________ Time: __________
Medication: ______________ Route: ______________ Time: __________
Medication: ______________ Route: ______________ Time: __________
Medication: ______________ Route: ______________ Time: __________
Medication: ______________ Route: ______________ Time: __________
Medication: ______________ Route: ______________ Time: __________
Medication: ______________ Route: ______________ Time: __________
Medication: ______________ Route: ______________ Time: __________
Medication: ______________ Route: ______________ Time: __________
Medication: ______________ Route: ______________ Time: __________
Medication: ______________ Route: ______________ Time: __________

NOTES FOR DAY NUMBER ________________________

DATE ________________________

MEDICAL JOURNAL FOR ______________________________

DATE __________________, DAY NUMBER _______________

VISITS FROM MY DOCTORS TODAY

Goals for today: ____

____

____.

Things to discuss with my doctor(s): ____________________________________

____

____

Dr.____________ came in at _____ am/pm. Left at _____ am/pm.
We discussed ____.
Did doctor examine patient: _____ yes, _____ no.
Wash hands before touching patient: _____ yes, _____ no.
Wear gloves: ____ yes, ___ no. Clean stethoscope: ____ yes, ____ no.
Wear gown and mask (precautions only):____ yes, _____ no.
Wash hands before leaving the room: _____ yes, _____ no.

Dr.____________ came in at _____ am/pm. Left at _____ am/pm.
We discussed ____.
Did doctor examine patient: _____ yes, _____ no.
Wash hands before touching patient: _____ yes, _____ no.
Wear gloves: ____ yes, ___ no. Clean stethoscope: ____ yes, ____ no.
Wear gown and mask (precautions only):____ yes, _____ no.
Wash hands before leaving the room: _____ yes, _____ no.

Dr.____________ came in at _____ am/pm. Left at _____ am/pm.
We discussed ____.
Did doctor examine patient: _____ yes, _____ no.
Wash hands before touching patient: _____ yes, _____ no.
Wear gloves: ____ yes, ___ no. Clean stethoscope: ____ yes, ____ no.
Wear gown and mask (precautions only):____ yes, _____ no.
Wash hands before leaving the room: _____ yes, _____ no.

Dr.____________ came in at _____ am/pm. Left at _____ am/pm.
We discussed ____.
Did doctor examine patient: _____ yes, _____ no.
Wash hands before touching patient: _____ yes, _____ no.
Wear gloves: ____ yes, ___ no. Clean stethoscope: ____ yes, ____ no.
Wear gown and mask (precautions only):____ yes, _____ no.
Wash hands before leaving the room: _____ yes, _____ no.

Dr.____________ came in at _____ am/pm. Left at _____ am/pm.
We discussed ____.
Did doctor examine patient: _____ yes, _____ no.
Wash hands before touching patient: _____ yes, _____ no.
Wear gloves: ____ yes, ___ no. Clean stethoscope: ____ yes, ____ no.
Wear gown and mask (precautions only):____ yes, _____ no.
Wash hands before leaving the room: _____ yes, _____ no.

NURSING CARE FOR ________________________________

DATE ____________________, DAY NUMBER ____________________

INITIAL DAY SHIFT EXAM:

My nurse has ______ # of patients. CNA ___yes, ___no. Charge nurse ________________
Nurse _______________ RN/LPN came in at _________ am/pm. Left at __________ am/pm.
Did nurse wash hands and wear gloves before touching patient: ______ yes, ______ no.
Wash hands after touching patient and before leaving the room: ______ yes, ______ no.
Don't hesitate to request staff to wash their hands. This will help decrease the risk of spreading potentially lethal germs.
Did nurse wear protective gear (isolation precautions only): ______ yes, ______ no.
Did nurse provide oral care (to be done every two hours if unable to provide for self, also decreases risk of pneumonia, infections, and aspiration): ______ yes, ______ no.
If able to provide own oral care, then supplies at bedside: _______ yes, _______ no.
Was patient repositioned (every two hours if unable to turn self): _____ yes _____ no.
Head of bed at __________ degrees. This is important for patients on ventilators or on tube feedings. Anything less than thirty degrees places patients at risk for aspiration of stomach contents into the lungs causing aspiration pneumonia.
Checked for incontinence and skin breakdown: _____ yes, _____ no.
Patient's linens wet or soiled: _____ yes, ____ no. Linens changed: ____ yes, ____ no.
Time linens changed: ________ am/pm. Any skin redness or breakdown: ____ yes, ____ no.
If yes, what stage is pressure ulcer: ________. Acquired when: ________________.
List wounds not associated with pressure ulcers and how acquired: ________________
____
Mattress type: ____
Specialty mattresses are important to help prevent pressure ulcers)
If patient on ventilator or has tracheostomy, suction performed: _____ yes, _____ no.
Did nurse listen to lung sounds: _____ yes, _____ no.
Does patient have chest tubes: ____ yes, ____ no. Functioning _____ yes, _____ no.
Bowel sounds: _______ yes, _______ no. Bowel sounds active: ______ yes, ______ no.
Neurological exam: ______ yes, ______ no. Follow commands: ______ yes, ______ no.
Is patient alert and oriented to person, place, time, and events: ____ yes, ____ no.
If confused, patient is not oriented to: ___ person, ___ place, ___ time, ___ event.
Confusion began (time and date): ____.
Glasgow coma scale (checks conscious scale of patient): _________________________.
Intracranial pressure monitoring: _____ yes, _____ no.
If yes, pressure is at ________ mm mercury. (Normal is one to fifteen).
Moves extremities: ___ yes, ___ no.
Paralysis: (inability to move extremities) ______ yes, ______ no.
If yes, extremities affected and when paralysis began: _________________________.
Is patient in pain: ____ yes, ____ no. Describe pain and location ______________.
Patient able to eat: _____ yes, _____ no. What type of diet? ____________________.
If patient on tube feedings list type: ________________ at ______ cc/ml per hour.
Nausea ____, vomiting ____. If so, describe: ____________________________________.
Patient has: Nasal gastric tube ______, Dobhoff tube _____, Peg or gastric tube ____.
When was feeding tube placed and what site: _____________________________________.
Catheter for draining urine: ____ yes, ____ no. If so, when placed: _____________.
Find out policy for allowed time to remain in bladder. Too long may cause infections.)
IV site(s) where: _________________ when placed: _______________________________.
IV fluids (types and rates): _________________, _________________, ______________,
________________, ________________, ________________, ________________, _________,
Is patient on oxygen: _____ yes, _____ no. If so, how much and route delivered (see oxygen routes): ____.
If patient on ventilator, list settings (see list on ventilator settings): _________
____.
Vital signs: temp ______, pulse ______, resp ______, b/p ______, o2 ______%,
current weight ______ pounds, ______ kg. Glucose level: ______
Insulin coverage: ____ yes, ____ no. Insulin type: ____________, # of units: ______.

NURSING CARE CONTINUED FOR ______________________
DATE ____________________, DAY NUMBER ______________________

FOLLOWING EXAMINATIONS FOR DAY SHIFT:

Nurse ____________, CNA ____________, in at _____ am/pm. Left at ______ am/pm.
Wash hands and wear gloves before touching patient: ______ yes, ______ no.
Wash hands before leaving room: ___ yes, ___ no. Wear protective gear: __ yes, __ no.
Clean stethoscope: __ yes, __ no. Oral care: __ yes, __ no. Suctioned: __ yes, __ no.
Repositioned: ___ yes, ___ no. Turned to: ___ left, ___ right, ___ backside ___.
Head of bed at: _______ degrees. Incontinence/skin breakdown: ____ yes, ___ no.
Linens wet or soiled: _____ yes, _____ no. Linens changed: _____ yes, ______ no.
Dressing changed: ____ yes, ____ no. Location: ______________________.
IV site checked: _____ yes, _____ no. IV tubing labeled: _____ yes, _____no.
IV fluids at: ____.
Pain level (0-10 scale.0-no pain, 10 intolerable): ____________________.
Location of pain: ________________. Medicated for pain: _____ yes, ____ no.
Patient is alert/oriented: ____ yes, ____ no. New confusion: ____ yes, ____ no.
Vital signs: temp ____, pulse _____, resp _____, b/p _____, 02 _____ %, ___ liters.
Glucose level: _____. Insulin: ___ yes, ___ no. Type: ____________ # of units ____.

Nurse ____________, CNA ____________, in at _____ am/pm. Left at ______ am/pm.
Wash hands and wear gloves before touching patient: ______ yes, ______ no.
Wash hands before leaving room: ___ yes, ___ no. Wear protective gear: __ yes, __ no.
Clean stethoscope: __ yes, __ no. Oral care: __ yes, __ no. Suctioned: __ yes, __ no.
Repositioned: ___ yes, ___ no. Turned to: ___ left, ___ right, ___ backside ___.
Head of bed at: _______ degrees. Incontinence/skin breakdown: ____ yes, ____ no.
Linens wet or soiled: _____ yes, _____ no. Linens changed: _____ yes, ______ no.
Dressing changed: ____ yes, ____ no. Location: ______________________.
IV site checked: _____ yes, _____ no. IV tubing labeled: _____ yes, _____no.
IV fluids at: ____.
Pain level (0-10 scale.0-no pain, 10 intolerable): ____________________.
Location of pain: ________________. Medicated for pain: _____ yes, ____ no.
Patient is alert/oriented: ____ yes, ____ no. New confusion: ____ yes, ____ no.
Vital signs: temp ____, pulse _____, resp _____, b/p _____, 02 _____ %, ___ liters.
Glucose level: _____. Insulin: ___ yes, ___ no. Type: ____________ # of units ____.

Nurse ____________, CNA ____________, in at _____ am/pm. Left at ______ am/pm.
Wash hands and wear gloves before touching patient: ______ yes, ______ no.
Wash hands before leaving room: ___ yes, ___ no. Wear protective gear: __ yes, __ no.
Clean stethoscope: __ yes, __ no. Oral care: __ yes, __ no. Suctioned: __ yes, __ no.
Repositioned: ___ yes, ___ no. Turned to: ___ left, ___ right, ___ backside ___.
Head of bed at: _______ degrees. Incontinence/skin breakdown: ____ yes, ____ no.
Linens wet or soiled: _____ yes, _____ no. Linens changed: _____ yes, ______ no.
Dressing changed: ____ yes, ____ no. Location: ______________________.
IV site checked: _____ yes, _____ no. IV tubing labeled: _____ yes, _____no.
IV fluids at: ____.
Pain level (0-10 scale.0-no pain, 10 intolerable): ____________________.
Location of pain: ________________. Medicated for pain: _____ yes, ____ no.
Patient is alert/oriented: ____ yes, ____ no. New confusion: ____ yes, ____ no.
Vital signs: temp ____, pulse _____, resp _____, b/p _____, 02 _____ %, ____ liters.
Glucose level: _____. Insulin: ___ yes, ___ no. Type: ____________ # of units ____.

NURSING CARE CONTINUED FOR ______________________
DATE ____________________, DAY NUMBER ________________

FOLLOWING EXAMINATIONS FOR DAY SHIFT:

Nurse ______________, CNA ______________, in at _____ am/pm. Left at ______ am/pm.
Wash hands and wear gloves before touching patient: ______ yes, ______ no.
Wash hands before leaving room: ___ yes, ___ no. Wear protective gear: __ yes, __ no.
Clean stethoscope: __ yes, __ no. Oral care: __ yes, __ no. Suctioned: __ yes, __ no.
Repositioned: ___ yes, ___ no. Turned to: ___ left, ___ right, ___ backside ___.
Head of bed at: _______ degrees. Incontinence/skin breakdown: ___ yes, ___ no.
Linens wet or soiled: _____ yes, _____ no. Linens changed: _____ yes, _____ no.
Dressing changed: ____ yes, ____ no. Location: ______________________________.
IV site checked: _____ yes, _____ no. IV tubing labeled: _____ yes, _____no.
IV fluids at: ____.
Pain level (0-10 scale.0-no pain, 10 intolerable): ____________________________.
Location of pain: ______________. Medicated for pain: ____ yes, ____ no.
Patient is alert/oriented: ____ yes, ____ no. New confusion: ____ yes, ____ no.
Vital signs: temp ____, pulse ____, resp ____, b/p ____, 02 ____%, ____ liters.
Glucose level: _____. Insulin: ___ yes, ___ no. Type: __________ # of units ___.

Nurse ______________, CNA ______________, in at _____ am/pm. Left at ______ am/pm.
Wash hands and wear gloves before touching patient: ______ yes, ______ no.
Wash hands before leaving room: ___ yes, ___ no. Wear protective gear: __ yes, __ no.
Clean stethoscope: __ yes, __ no. Oral care: __ yes, __ no. Suctioned: __ yes, __ no.
Repositioned: ___ yes, ___ no. Turned to: ___ left, ___ right, ___ backside ___.
Head of bed at: _______ degrees. Incontinence/skin breakdown: ___ yes, ___ no.
Linens wet or soiled: _____ yes, _____ no. Linens changed: _____ yes, _____ no.
Dressing changed: ____ yes, ____ no. Location: ______________________________.
IV site checked: _____ yes, _____ no. IV tubing labeled: _____ yes, _____no.
IV fluids at: ____.
Pain level (0-10 scale.0-no pain, 10 intolerable): ____________________________.
Location of pain: ______________. Medicated for pain: ____ yes, ____ no.
Patient is alert/oriented: ____ yes, ____ no. New confusion: ____ yes, ____ no.
Vital signs: temp ____, pulse ____, resp ____, b/p ____, 02 ____%, ____ liters.
Glucose level: _____. Insulin: ___ yes, ___ no. Type: __________ # of units ___.

Nurse ______________, CNA ______________, in at _____ am/pm. Left at ______ am/pm.
Wash hands and wear gloves before touching patient: ______ yes, ______ no.
Wash hands before leaving room: ___ yes, ___ no. Wear protective gear: __ yes, __ no.
Clean stethoscope: __ yes, __ no. Oral care: __ yes, __ no. Suctioned: __ yes, __ no.
Repositioned: ___ yes, ___ no. Turned to: ___ left, ___ right, ___ backside ___.
Head of bed at: _______ degrees. Incontinence/skin breakdown: ___ yes, ___ no.
Linens wet or soiled: _____ yes, _____ no. Linens changed: _____ yes, _____ no.
Dressing changed: ____ yes, ____ no. Location: ______________________________.
IV site checked: _____ yes, _____ no. IV tubing labeled: _____ yes, _____no.
IV fluids at: ____.
Pain level (0-10 scale.0-no pain, 10 intolerable): ____________________________.
Location of pain: ______________. Medicated for pain: ____ yes, ____ no.
Patient is alert/oriented: ____ yes, ____ no. New confusion: ____ yes, ____ no.
Vital signs: temp ____, pulse ____, resp ____, b/p ____, 02 ____%, ____ liters.
Glucose level: _____. Insulin: ___ yes, ___ no. Type: __________ # of units ___.

NURSING CARE FOR ______________________________

DATE ____________________, DAY NUMBER ________________________

INITIAL NIGHT SHIFT EXAM:

My nurse has _____ # of patients. CNA ___yes, ___no. Charge nurse ______________
Nurse ______________ RN/LPN came in at _________ am/pm. Left at _________ am/pm.
Did nurse wash hands and wear gloves before touching patient: ______ yes, ______ no.
Wash hands after touching patient and before leaving the room: ______ yes, ______ no.
Don't hesitate to request staff to wash their hands. This will help decrease the risk of spreading potentially lethal germs.
Did nurse wear protective gear (isolation precautions only): ______ yes, ______ no.
Did nurse provide oral care (to be done every two hours if unable to provide for self, also decreases risk of pneumonia, infections, and aspiration): ______ yes, ______ no.
If able to provide own oral care, then supplies at bedside: ______ yes, ______ no.
Was patient repositioned (every two hours if unable to turn self): _____ yes _____ no.
Head of bed at _______ degrees. This is important for patients on ventilators or on tube feedings. Anything less than thirty degrees places patients at risk for aspiration of stomach contents into the lungs causing aspiration pneumonia.
Checked for incontinence and skin breakdown: ____ yes, _____ no.
Patient's linens wet or soiled: _____ yes, ____ no. Linens changed: ____ yes, ____ no.
Time linens changed: _______ am/pm. Any skin redness or breakdown: ____ yes, ____ no.
If yes, what stage is pressure ulcer: _______. Acquired when: _______________.
List wounds not associated with pressure ulcers and how acquired: _______________
____.
Mattress type: ____.
Specialty mattresses are important to help prevent pressure ulcers)
If patient on ventilator or has tracheostomy, suction performed: _____ yes, _____ no.
Did nurse listen to lung sounds: _____ yes, _____ no.
Does patient have chest tubes: ____ yes, ____ no. Functioning _____ yes, _____ no.
Bowel sounds: ______ yes, ______ no. Bowel sounds active: ______ yes, ______ no.
Neurological exam: _____ yes, ______ no. Follow commands: ______ yes, ______ no.
Is patient alert and oriented to person, place, time, and events: _____ yes, _____ no.
If confused, patient is not oriented to: ____ person, ___ place, ___ time, ___ event.
Confusion began (time and date): ____.
Glasgow coma scale (checks conscious scale of patient): ______________________.
Intracranial pressure monitoring: ______ yes, ______ no.
If yes, pressure is at ________ mm mercury. (Normal is one to fifteen).
Moves extremities: ___ yes, ___ no.
Paralysis: (inability to move extremities) ______ yes, ______ no.
If yes, extremities affected and when paralysis began: _______________________.
Is patient in pain: _____ yes, _____ no. Describe pain and location ______________.
Patient able to eat: ____ yes, ____ no. What type of diet? ______________________.
If patient on tube feedings list type: ____________ at ___________ cc/ml per hour.
Nausea ____, vomiting ____. If so, describe: _________________________________.
Patient has: Nasal gastric tube ______, Dobhoff tube _____, Peg or gastric tube _____.
When was feeding tube placed and what site: ___________________________________.
Catheter for draining urine: ____ yes, ____ no. If so, when placed: ___________.
Find out policy for allowed time to remain in bladder. Too long may cause infections.)
IV site(s) where: ______________________ when placed: ________________________.
IV fluids (types and rates): _______________________, __________________________,
_____________________, ____________________________, _____________________________.
Is patient on oxygen: _____ yes, _____ no. If so, how much and route delivered (see oxygen routes): ____.
If patient on ventilator, list settings (see list on ventilator settings): _________
____.
Vital signs: temp _____, pulse _____, resp _____, b/p _____, o2 _____%,
current weight _____ pounds, _____ kg. Glucose level: ______
Insulin coverage: ____ yes, ____ no. Insulin type: ____________, # of units: _____.

NURSING CARE CONTINUED FOR ________________________
DATE ____________________, DAY NUMBER ____________________

FOLLOWING EXAMINATIONS FOR NIGHT SHIFT:

Nurse ______________, CNA ______________, in at _____ am/pm. Left at ______ am/pm.
Wash hands and wear gloves before touching patient: ______ yes, ______ no.
Wash hands before leaving room: ___ yes, ___ no. Wear protective gear: __ yes, __ no.
Clean stethoscope: __ yes, __ no. Oral care: __ yes, __ no. Suctioned: __ yes, __ no.
Repositioned: ___ yes, ___ no. Turned to: ___ left, ___ right, ___ backside ___.
Head of bed at: ___ degrees. Incontinence/skin breakdown: ___ yes, ___ no.
Linens wet or soiled: ___ yes, ___ no. Linens changed: ____ yes, ___ no.
Dressing changed: ____ yes, ____ no. Location: ____________________.
IV site checked: _____ yes, _____ no. IV tubing labeled: _____ yes, ____ no.
IV fluids at: ______________________________________.
Pain level (0-10 scale.0-no pain, 10 intolerable): ________________.
Location of pain: _______________. Medicated for pain: ____ yes, ____ no.
Patient is alert/oriented: ____ yes, ____ no. New confusion: ___ yes, ___ no.
Vital signs: temp ____, pulse ____, resp _____, b/p _____, O2 ____ %, ___ liters.
Glucose level: _____. Insulin: ___ yes, ___ no. Type: ____________ # of units ____.

Nurse ______________, CNA ______________, in at _____ am/pm. Left at ______ am/pm.
Wash hands and wear gloves before touching patient: ______ yes, ______ no.
Wash hands before leaving room: ___ yes, ___ no. Wear protective gear: __ yes, __ no.
Clean stethoscope: __ yes, __ no. Oral care: __ yes, __ no. Suctioned: __ yes, __ no.
Repositioned: ___ yes, ___ no. Turned to: ___ left, ___ right, ___ backside ___.
Head of bed at: ___ degrees. Incontinence/skin breakdown: ___ yes, ___ no.
Linens wet or soiled: ___ yes, ___ no. Linens changed: ____ yes, ___ no.
Dressing changed: ____ yes, ____ no. Location: ____________________.
IV site checked: _____ yes, _____ no. IV tubing labeled: _____ yes, ____ no.
IV fluids at: ______________________________________.
Pain level (0-10 scale.0-no pain, 10 intolerable): ________________.
Location of pain: _______________. Medicated for pain: ____ yes, ____ no.
Patient is alert/oriented: ____ yes, ____ no. New confusion: ___ yes, ___ no.
Vital signs: temp ____, pulse ____, resp _____, b/p _____, O2 ____ %, ___ liters.
Glucose level: _____. Insulin: ___ yes, ___ no. Type: ____________ # of units ____.

Nurse ______________, CNA ______________, in at _____ am/pm. Left at ______ am/pm.
Wash hands and wear gloves before touching patient: ______ yes, ______ no.
Wash hands before leaving room: ___ yes, ___ no. Wear protective gear: __ yes, __ no.
Clean stethoscope: __ yes, __ no. Oral care: __ yes, __ no. Suctioned: __ yes, __ no.
Repositioned: ___ yes, ___ no. Turned to: ___ left, ___ right, ___ backside ___.
Head of bed at: ___ degrees. Incontinence/skin breakdown: ___ yes, ___ no.
Linens wet or soiled: ___ yes, ___ no. Linens changed: ____ yes, ___ no.
Dressing changed: ____ yes, ____ no. Location: ____________________.
IV site checked: _____ yes, _____ no. IV tubing labeled: _____ yes, ____ no.
IV fluids at: ______________________________________.
Pain level (0-10 scale.0-no pain, 10 intolerable): ________________.
Location of pain: _______________. Medicated for pain: ____ yes, ____ no.
Patient is alert/oriented: ____ yes, ____ no. New confusion: ___ yes, ___ no.
Vital signs: temp ____, pulse ____, resp _____, b/p _____, O2 ____ %, ___ liters.
Glucose level: _____. Insulin: ___ yes, ___ no. Type: ____________ # of units ____.

NURSING CARE CONTINUED FOR ______________________

DATE ____________________, DAY NUMBER ______________________

FOLLOWING EXAMINATIONS FOR NIGHT SHIFT:

Nurse _____________, CNA _____________, in at _____ am/pm. Left at ______ am/pm.
Wash hands and wear gloves before touching patient: _______ yes, _______ no.
Wash hands before leaving room: ___ yes, ___ no. Wear protective gear: __ yes, __ no.
Clean stethoscope: __ yes, __ no. Oral care: __ yes, __ no. Suctioned: __ yes, __ no.
Repositioned: ___ yes, ___ no. Turned to: ___ left, ___ right, ___ backside ___.
Head of bed at: ______ degrees. Incontinence/skin breakdown: ____ yes, ____ no.
Linens wet or soiled: _____ yes, _____ no. Linens changed: _____ yes, _____ no.
Dressing changed: ____ yes, ____ no. Location: _______________________.
IV site checked: _____ yes, _____ no. IV tubing labeled: _____ yes, _____no.
IV fluids at: ____.
Pain level (0-10 scale.0-no pain, 10 intolerable): _______________.
Location of pain: ______________. Medicated for pain: _____ yes, ____ no.
Patient is alert/oriented: ____ yes, ____ no. New confusion: ____ yes, ____ no.
Vital signs: temp ____, pulse _____, resp ______, b/p ______, 02 _____ %, ____ liters.
Glucose level: _____. Insulin: ___ yes, ___ no. Type: ______________ # of units ____.

Nurse _____________, CNA _____________, in at _____ am/pm. Left at ______ am/pm.
Wash hands and wear gloves before touching patient: _______ yes, _______ no.
Wash hands before leaving room: ___ yes, ___ no. Wear protective gear: __ yes, __ no.
Clean stethoscope: __ yes, __ no. Oral care: __ yes, __ no. Suctioned: __ yes, __ no.
Repositioned: ___ yes, ___ no. Turned to: ___ left, ___ right, ___ backside ___.
Head of bed at: ______ degrees. Incontinence/skin breakdown: ____ yes, ____ no.
Linens wet or soiled: _____ yes, _____ no. Linens changed: _____ yes, _____ no.
Dressing changed: ____ yes, ____ no. Location: _______________________.
IV site checked: _____ yes, _____ no. IV tubing labeled: _____ yes, _____no.
IV fluids at: ____.
Pain level (0-10 scale.0-no pain, 10 intolerable): _______________.
Location of pain: ______________. Medicated for pain: _____ yes, ____ no.
Patient is alert/oriented: ____ yes, ____ no. New confusion: ____ yes, ____ no.
Vital signs: temp ____, pulse _____, resp ______, b/p ______, 02 _____ %, ____ liters.
Glucose level: _____. Insulin: ___ yes, ___ no. Type: ______________ # of units ____.

Nurse _____________, CNA _____________, in at _____ am/pm. Left at ______ am/pm.
Wash hands and wear gloves before touching patient: _______ yes, _______ no.
Wash hands before leaving room: ___ yes, ___ no. Wear protective gear: __ yes, __ no.
Clean stethoscope: __ yes, __ no. Oral care: __ yes, __ no. Suctioned: __ yes, __ no.
Repositioned: ___ yes, ___ no. Turned to: ___ left, ___ right, ___ backside ___.
Head of bed at: ______ degrees. Incontinence/skin breakdown: ____ yes, ____ no.
Linens wet or soiled: _____ yes, _____ no. Linens changed: _____ yes, _____ no.
Dressing changed: ____ yes, ____ no. Location: _______________________.
IV site checked: _____ yes, _____ no. IV tubing labeled: _____ yes, _____no.
IV fluids at: ____.
Pain level (0-10 scale.0-no pain, 10 intolerable): _______________.
Location of pain: ______________. Medicated for pain: _____ yes, ____ no.
Patient is alert/oriented: ____ yes, ____ no. New confusion: ____ yes, ____ no.
Vital signs: temp ____, pulse _____, resp ______, b/p ______, 02 _____ %, ____ liters.
Glucose level: _____. Insulin: ___ yes, ___ no. Type: ______________ # of units ____.

MEDICATION ADMINISTRATION LIST FOR ____________________
DATE ________________ DAY NUMBER ____________________

List the medication for each day. Routes of administration: oral, thru feeding tube, intravenous (IV), intramuscular (IM), subcutaneous (SQ), epidural or a catheter in your spinal column, rectal, topical, eye drops, and ear drops.

Medication: ________________ Route: ________________ Time: ____________
Medication: ________________ Route: ________________ Time: ____________
Medication: ________________ Route: ________________ Time: ____________
Medication: ________________ Route: ________________ Time: ____________
Medication: ________________ Route: ________________ Time: ____________
Medication: ________________ Route: ________________ Time: ____________
Medication: ________________ Route: ________________ Time: ____________
Medication: ________________ Route: ________________ Time: ____________
Medication: ________________ Route: ________________ Time: ____________
Medication: ________________ Route: ________________ Time: ____________
Medication: ________________ Route: ________________ Time: ____________
Medication: ________________ Route: ________________ Time: ____________
Medication: ________________ Route: ________________ Time: ____________
Medication: ________________ Route: ________________ Time: ____________
Medication: ________________ Route: ________________ Time: ____________
Medication: ________________ Route: ________________ Time: ____________
Medication: ________________ Route: ________________ Time: ____________
Medication: ________________ Route: ________________ Time: ____________
Medication: ________________ Route: ________________ Time: ____________
Medication: ________________ Route: ________________ Time: ____________
Medication: ________________ Route: ________________ Time: ____________
Medication: ________________ Route: ________________ Time: ____________
Medication: ________________ Route: ________________ Time: ____________
Medication: ________________ Route: ________________ Time: ____________
Medication: ________________ Route: ________________ Time: ____________
Medication: ________________ Route: ________________ Time: ____________
Medication: ________________ Route: ________________ Time: ____________
Medication: ________________ Route: ________________ Time: ____________
Medication: ________________ Route: ________________ Time: ____________
Medication: ________________ Route: ________________ Time: ____________
Medication: ________________ Route: ________________ Time: ____________
Medication: ________________ Route: ________________ Time: ____________
Medication: ________________ Route: ________________ Time: ____________
Medication: ________________ Route: ________________ Time: ____________
Medication: ________________ Route: ________________ Time: ____________
Medication: ________________ Route: ________________ Time: ____________
Medication: ________________ Route: ________________ Time: ____________
Medication: ________________ Route: ________________ Time: ____________
Medication: ________________ Route: ________________ Time: ____________
Medication: ________________ Route: ________________ Time: ____________
Medication: ________________ Route: ________________ Time: ____________
Medication: ________________ Route: ________________ Time: ____________
Medication: ________________ Route: ________________ Time: ____________
Medication: ________________ Route: ________________ Time: ____________
Medication: ________________ Route: ________________ Time: ____________
Medication: ________________ Route: ________________ Time: ____________
Medication: ________________ Route: ________________ Time: ____________
Medication: ________________ Route: ________________ Time: ____________
Medication: ________________ Route: ________________ Time: ____________
Medication: ________________ Route: ________________ Time: ____________
Medication: ________________ Route: ________________ Time: ____________
Medication: ________________ Route: ________________ Time: ____________
Medication: ________________ Route: ________________ Time: ____________
Medication: ________________ Route: ________________ Time: ____________

NOTES FOR DAY NUMBER ______________________

DATE ______________________

MEDICAL JOURNAL FOR ______________________________

DATE ________________, DAY NUMBER ______________

VISITS FROM MY DOCTORS TODAY

Goals for today: ____

____

____.

Things to discuss with my doctor(s): ___________________________

____

____.

Dr.____________ came in at ____ am/pm. Left at ____ am/pm.
We discussed ____.
Did doctor examine patient: ____ yes, ____ no.
Wash hands before touching patient: ____ yes, ____ no.
Wear gloves: ____ yes, ___ no. Clean stethoscope: ____ yes, ____ no.
Wear gown and mask (precautions only):____ yes, ____ no.
Wash hands before leaving the room: ____ yes, ____ no.

Dr.____________ came in at ____ am/pm. Left at ____ am/pm.
We discussed ____.
Did doctor examine patient: ____ yes, ____ no.
Wash hands before touching patient: ____ yes, ____ no.
Wear gloves: ____ yes, ___ no. Clean stethoscope: ____ yes, ____ no.
Wear gown and mask (precautions only):____ yes, ____ no.
Wash hands before leaving the room: ____ yes, ____ no.

Dr.____________ came in at ____ am/pm. Left at ____ am/pm.
We discussed ____.
Did doctor examine patient: ____ yes, ____ no.
Wash hands before touching patient: ____ yes, ____ no.
Wear gloves: ____ yes, ___ no. Clean stethoscope: ____ yes, ____ no.
Wear gown and mask (precautions only):____ yes, ____ no.
Wash hands before leaving the room: ____ yes, ____ no.

Dr.____________ came in at ____ am/pm. Left at ____ am/pm.
We discussed ____.
Did doctor examine patient: ____ yes, ____ no.
Wash hands before touching patient: ____ yes, ____ no.
Wear gloves: ____ yes, ___ no. Clean stethoscope: ____ yes, ____ no.
Wear gown and mask (precautions only):____ yes, ____ no.
Wash hands before leaving the room: ____ yes, ____ no.

Dr.____________ came in at ____ am/pm. Left at ____ am/pm.
We discussed ____.
Did doctor examine patient: ____ yes, ____ no.
Wash hands before touching patient: ____ yes, ____ no.
Wear gloves: ____ yes, ___ no. Clean stethoscope: ____ yes, ____ no.
Wear gown and mask (precautions only):____ yes, ____ no.
Wash hands before leaving the room: ____ yes, ____ no.

NURSING CARE FOR ______________________________

DATE ________________, DAY NUMBER ________________

INITIAL DAY SHIFT EXAM:

My nurse has _____ # of patients. CNA ___yes, ___no. Charge nurse ____________
Nurse ______________ RN/LPN came in at ________ am/pm. Left at _________ am/pm.
Did nurse wash hands and wear gloves before touching patient: ______ yes, ______ no.
Wash hands after touching patient and before leaving the room: ______ yes, ______ no.
Don't hesitate to request staff to wash their hands. This will help decrease the risk of spreading potentially lethal germs.
Did nurse wear protective gear (isolation precautions only): ______ yes, ______ no.
Did nurse provide oral care (to be done every two hours if unable to provide for self, also decreases risk of pneumonia, infections, and aspiration): ______ yes, ______ no.
If able to provide own oral care, then supplies at bedside: _______ yes, _______ no.
Was patient repositioned (every two hours if unable to turn self): _____ yes _____ no.
Head of bed at ________ degrees. This is important for patients on ventilators or on tube feedings. Anything less than thirty degrees places patients at risk for aspiration of stomach contents into the lungs causing aspiration pneumonia.
Checked for incontinence and skin breakdown: _____ yes, _____ no.
Patient's linens wet or soiled: _____ yes, ___ no. Linens changed: ____ yes, ____ no.
Time linens changed: _______ am/pm. Any skin redness or breakdown: ____ yes, ____ no.
If yes, what stage is pressure ulcer: ________. Acquired when: _______________.
List wounds not associated with pressure ulcers and how acquired: _______________
____.
Mattress type: ____.
Specialty mattresses are important to help prevent pressure ulcers)
If patient on ventilator or has tracheostomy, suction performed: _____ yes, ______ no.
Did nurse listen to lung sounds: ____ yes, _____ no.
Does patient have chest tubes: ____ yes, ____ no. Functioning _____ yes, ______ no.
Bowel sounds: _______ yes, _______ no. Bowel sounds active: ______ yes, _______ no.
Neurological exam: ______ yes, ______ no. Follow commands: _______ yes, _______ no.
Is patient alert and oriented to person, place, time, and events: _____ yes, _____ no.
If confused, patient is not oriented to: ____ person, ___ place, ___ time, ___ event.
Confusion began (time and date): ______________________________________.
Glasgow coma scale (checks conscious scale of patient): _____________________.
Intracranial pressure monitoring: _____ yes, _____ no.
If yes, pressure is at ________ mm mercury. (Normal is one to fifteen).
Moves extremities: ___ yes, ___ no.
Paralysis: (inability to move extremities) _______ yes, _______ no.
If yes, extremities affected and when paralysis began: ______________________.
Is patient in pain: ____ yes, ____ no. Describe pain and location ______________.
Patient able to eat: ____ yes, ____ no. What type of diet? ______________________.
If patient on tube feedings list type: _____________ at ___________ cc/ml per hour.
Nausea ____, vomiting _____. If so, describe: _____________________________.
Patient has: Nasal gastric tube ______, Dobhoff tube _____, Peg or gastric tube _____.
When was feeding tube placed and what site: ____________________________________.
Catheter for draining urine: ___ yes, ____ no. If so, when placed: ____________.
Find out policy for allowed time to remain in bladder. Too long may cause infections.)
IV site(s) where: ___________________________ when placed: ________________.
IV fluids (types and rates): _____________________, ___________________________,
_________________________, ________________________, __________________________,
Is patient on oxygen: _____ yes, _____ no. If so, how much and route delivered
(see oxygen routes): ____.
If patient on ventilator, list settings (see list on ventilator settings): _____________
____.
Vital signs: temp _____, pulse _____, resp _____, b/p _____, o2 _____%,
current weight ______ pounds, ______ kg. Glucose level: _______________.
Insulin coverage: ____ yes, ____ no. Insulin type: ___________, # of units: ______.

NURSING CARE CONTINUED FOR ______________________
DATE ______________________, DAY NUMBER ______________________

FOLLOWING EXAMINATIONS FOR DAY SHIFT:

Nurse ___________, CNA ___________, in at _____ am/pm. Left at _______ am/pm.
Wash hands and wear gloves before touching patient: _______ yes, _______ no.
Wash hands before leaving room: __ yes, __ no. Wear protective gear: __ yes, __ no.
Clean stethoscope: yes, no. Oral care: __ yes, __ no. Suctioned: __ yes, __ no.
Repositioned: ___ yes, ___ no. Turned to: __ left, __ right, ___ backside ___.
Head of bed at: _______ degrees. Incontinence/skin breakdown: _____ yes, ___ no.
Linens wet or soiled: _____ yes, _____ no. Linens changed: _____ yes, _____ no.
Dressing changed: ____ yes, ____ no. Location: ______________________.
IV site checked: _____ yes, _____ no. IV tubing labeled: _____ yes, _____ no.
IV fluids at: ____.
Pain level (0-10 scale.0-no pain, 10 intolerable): ______________________.
Location of pain: ______________. Medicated for pain: _____ yes, _____ no.
Patient is alert/oriented: ___ yes, ___ no. New confusion: _____ yes, _____ no
Vital signs: temp ____, pulse ____, resp ____, b/p ____, 02 ____ %, ____ liters.
Glucose level: _____. Insulin: ___ yes, ___ no. Type: __________ # of units ____.

Nurse ___________, CNA ___________, in at _____ am/pm. Left at _______ am/pm.
Wash hands and wear gloves before touching patient: _______ yes, _______ no.
Wash hands before leaving room: __ yes, __ no. Wear protective gear: __ yes, __ no.
Clean stethoscope: yes, no. Oral care: __ yes, __ no. Suctioned: __ yes, __ no.
Repositioned: ___ yes, ___ no. Turned to: __ left, __ right, ___ backside ___.
Head of bed at: _______ degrees. Incontinence/skin breakdown: _____ yes, ___ no.
Linens wet or soiled: _____ yes, _____ no. Linens changed: _____ yes, _____ no.
Dressing changed: ____ yes, ____ no. Location: ______________________.
IV site checked: _____ yes, _____ no. IV tubing labeled: _____ yes, _____ no.
IV fluids at: ____.
Pain level (0-10 scale.0-no pain, 10 intolerable): ______________________.
Location of pain: ______________. Medicated for pain: _____ yes, _____ no.
Patient is alert/oriented: ___ yes, ___ no. New confusion: _____ yes, _____ no.
Vital signs: temp ____, pulse ____, resp ____, b/p ____, 02 ____ %, ____ liters.
Glucose level: _____. Insulin: ___ yes, ___ no. Type: __________ # of units ____.

Nurse ___________, CNA ___________, in at _____ am/pm. Left at _______ am/pm.
Wash hands and wear gloves before touching patient: _______ yes, _______ no.
Wash hands before leaving room: __ yes, __ no. Wear protective gear: __ yes, __ no.
Clean stethoscope: yes, no. Oral care: __ yes, __ no. Suctioned: __ yes, __ no.
Repositioned: ___ yes, ___ no. Turned to: __ left, __ right, ___ backside ___.
Head of bed at: _______ degrees. Incontinence/skin breakdown: _____ yes, ___ no.
Linens wet or soiled: _____ yes, _____ no. Linens changed: _____ yes, _____ no.
Dressing changed: ____ yes, ____ no. Location: ______________________.
IV site checked: _____ yes, _____ no. IV tubing labeled: _____ yes, _____ no.
IV fluids at: ____.
Pain level (0-10 scale.0-no pain, 10 intolerable): ______________________.
Location of pain: ______________. Medicated for pain: _____ yes, _____ no.
Patient is alert/oriented: ___ yes, ___ no. New confusion: _____ yes, _____ no.
Vital signs: temp ____, pulse ____, resp ____, b/p ____, 02 ____ %, ____ liters.
Glucose level: _____. Insulin: ___ yes, ___ no. Type: __________ # of units ____.

NURSING CARE CONTINUED FOR ____________________
DATE ____________________, DAY NUMBER ____________________

FOLLOWING EXAMINATIONS FOR DAY SHIFT:

Nurse ______________, CNA ______________, in at _____ am/pm. Left at ______ am/pm.
Wash hands and wear gloves before touching patient: ______ yes, ______ no.
Wash hands before leaving room: ___ yes, ___ no. Wear protective gear: __ yes, __ no.
Clean stethoscope: __ yes, __ no. Oral care: __ yes, __ no. Suctioned: __ yes, __ no.
Repositioned: ___ yes, ___ no. Turned to: ___ left, ___ right, ___ backside ___.
Head of bed at: _______ degrees. Incontinence/skin breakdown: ____ yes, ____ no.
Linens wet or soiled: _____ yes, _____ no. Linens changed: _____ yes, ______ no.
Dressing changed: ____ yes, ____ no. Location: ____________________.
IV site checked: _____ yes, _____ no. IV tubing labeled: _____ yes, _____no.
IV fluids at: ____________________.
Pain level (0-10 scale.0-no pain, 10 intolerable): ____________________.
Location of pain: __________. Medicated for pain: _____ yes, ____ no.
Patient is alert/oriented: ____ yes, ____ no. New confusion: ____ yes, ____ no.
Vital signs: temp ____, pulse _____, resp ______, b/p _____, 02 _____ %, ____ liters.
Glucose level: _____. Insulin: ___ yes, ___ no. Type: ______________ # of units ____.

Nurse ______________, CNA ______________, in at _____ am/pm. Left at ______ am/pm.
Wash hands and wear gloves before touching patient: ______ yes, ______ no.
Wash hands before leaving room: ___ yes, ___ no. Wear protective gear: __ yes, __ no.
Clean stethoscope: __ yes, __ no. Oral care: __ yes, __ no. Suctioned: __ yes, __ no.
Repositioned: ___ yes, ___ no. Turned to: ___ left, ___ right, ___ backside ___.
Head of bed at: _______ degrees. Incontinence/skin breakdown: ____ yes, ____ no.
Linens wet or soiled: _____ yes, _____ no. Linens changed: _____ yes, ______ no.
Dressing changed: ____ yes, ____ no. Location: ____________________.
IV site checked: _____ yes, _____ no. IV tubing labeled: _____ yes, _____no.
IV fluids at: ____________________.
Pain level (0-10 scale.0-no pain, 10 intolerable): ____________________.
Location of pain: __________. Medicated for pain: _____ yes, ____ no.
Patient is alert/oriented: ____ yes, ____ no. New confusion: ____ yes, ____ no.
Vital signs: temp ____, pulse _____, resp ______, b/p _____, 02 _____ %, ____ liters.
Glucose level: _____. Insulin: ___ yes, ___ no. Type: ______________ # of units ____.

Nurse ______________, CNA ______________, in at _____ am/pm. Left at ______ am/pm.
Wash hands and wear gloves before touching patient: ______ yes, ______ no.
Wash hands before leaving room: ___ yes, ___ no. Wear protective gear: __ yes, __ no.
Clean stethoscope: __ yes, __ no. Oral care: __ yes, __ no. Suctioned: __ yes, __ no.
Repositioned: ___ yes, ___ no. Turned to: ___ left, ___ right, ___ backside ___.
Head of bed at: _______ degrees. Incontinence/skin breakdown: ____ yes, ____ no.
Linens wet or soiled: _____ yes, _____ no. Linens changed: _____ yes, ______ no.
Dressing changed: ____ yes, ____ no. Location: ____________________.
IV site checked: _____ yes, _____ no. IV tubing labeled: _____ yes, _____no.
IV fluids at: ____________________.
Pain level (0-10 scale.0-no pain, 10 intolerable): ____________________.
Location of pain: __________. Medicated for pain: _____ yes, ____ no.
Patient is alert/oriented: ____ yes, ____ no. New confusion: ____ yes, ____ no.
Vital signs: temp ____, pulse _____, resp ______, b/p _____, 02 _____ %, ____ liters.
Glucose level: _____. Insulin: ___ yes, ___ no. Type: ______________ # of units ____.

NURSING CARE FOR ______________________________

DATE ____________________, DAY NUMBER ____________________

INITIAL NIGHT SHIFT EXAM:

My nurse has _____ # of patients. CNA ___yes, ___no. Charge nurse ______________
Nurse ____________ RN/LPN came in at _________ am/pm. Left at _________ am/pm.
Did nurse wash hands and wear gloves before touching patient: _____ yes, _____ no.
Wash hands after touching patient and before leaving the room: _____ yes, _____ no.
Don't hesitate to request staff to wash their hands. This will help decrease the risk of spreading potentially lethal germs.
Did nurse wear protective gear (isolation precautions only): _____ yes, _____ no.
Did nurse provide oral care (to be done every two hours if unable to provide for self, also decreases risk of pneumonia, infections, and aspiration): _____ yes, _____ no.
If able to provide own oral care, then supplies at bedside: _____ yes, _____ no.
Was patient repositioned (every two hours if unable to turn self): ____yes ____ no.
Head of bed at ________ degrees. This is important for patients on ventilators or on tube feedings. Anything less than thirty degrees places patients at risk for aspiration of stomach contents into the lungs causing aspiration pneumonia.
Checked for incontinence and skin breakdown: ____ yes, ____ no.
Patient's linens wet or soiled: ___ yes,___ no. Linens changed: ____ yes, ____ no.
Time linens changed: _______ am/pm. Any skin redness or breakdown: ____ yes, ____ no.
If yes, what stage is pressure ulcer: ______. Acquired when: ______________.
List wounds not associated with pressure ulcers and how acquired: ______________
____
Mattress type: ____
Specialty mattresses are important to help prevent pressure ulcers)
If patient on ventilator or has tracheostomy, suction performed: ____ yes, ____ no.
Did nurse listen to lung sounds: ____ yes, ____ no.
Does patient have chest tubes: ____ yes, ____ no. Functioning _____ yes, _____ no.
Bowel sounds: ______ yes, ______ no. Bowel sounds active: _____ yes, _____ no.
Neurological exam: _____ yes, _____ no. Follow commands: _____ yes, _____ no.
Is patient alert and oriented to person, place, time, and events: _____ yes, _____ no.
If confused, patient is not oriented to: ___ person, ___ place, ___ time, ___ event.
Confusion began (time and date): ____.
Glasgow coma scale (checks conscious scale of patient): _________________________.
Intracranial pressure monitoring: ____ yes, ____ no.
If yes, pressure is at ________ mm mercury. (Normal is one to fifteen).
Moves extremities: ____ yes, ____ no.
Paralysis: (inability to move extremities) ____ yes, ____ no.
If yes, extremities affected and when paralysis began: _____________________.
Is patient in pain: ___ yes, ___ no. Describe pain and location ________________.
Patient able to eat: ___ yes, ___ no. What type of diet? ______________________.
If patient on tube feedings list type: __________ at __________ cc/ml per hour.
Nausea ____, vomiting ____. If so, describe: ______________________________.
Patient has: Nasal gastric tube _____, Dobhoff tube _____, Peg or gastric tube _____
When was feeding tube placed and what site: ______________________________.
Catheter for draining urine: ____ yes, ____ no. If so, when placed: ____________.
Find out policy for allowed time to remain in bladder. Too long may cause infections.)
IV site(s) where: ________________________ when placed: ____________________.
IV fluids (types and rates): ____________, ____________, ____________, ____________, ____________, ____________,
Is patient on oxygen: ____ yes, ____ no. If so, how much and route delivered (see oxygen routes): ____.
If patient on ventilator, list settings (see list on ventilator settings): _________
____.
Vital signs: temp _____, pulse _____, resp _____, b/p _____, o2 _____%, current weight _____ pounds, _____ kg. Glucose level: _____
Insulin coverage: ____ yes, ____ no. Insulin type: ___________, # of units: _____.

NURSING CARE CONTINUED FOR ______________________________
DATE ______________________, DAY NUMBER _________________________

FOLLOWING EXAMINATIONS FOR NIGHT SHIFT:

Nurse _____________, CNA _____________, in at _____ am/pm. Left at _______ am/pm.
Wash hands and wear gloves before touching patient: _______ yes, _______ no.
Wash hands before leaving room: ___ yes, ___ no. Wear protective gear: __ yes, __ no.
Clean stethoscope: __ yes, __ no. Oral care: __ yes, __ no. Suctioned: __ yes, __ no.
Repositioned: ___ yes, ___ no. Turned to: ___ left, ___ right, ___ backside ___.
Head of bed at: _______ degrees. Incontinence/skin breakdown: ____ yes, ____ no.
Linens wet or soiled: _____ yes, _____ no. Linens changed: _____ yes, _____ no.
Dressing changed: ____ yes, ____ no. Location: _______________________________.
IV site checked: _____ yes, _____ no. IV tubing labeled: _____ yes, _____no.
IV fluids at: ____.
Pain level (0-10 scale.0-no pain, 10 intolerable): __________________________.
Location of pain: ____________________. Medicated for pain: ____ yes, ____ no.
Patient is alert/oriented: ____ yes, ____ no. New confusion: ____ yes, ____ no.
Vital signs: temp ____, pulse ____, resp _____, b/p ______, 02 _____ %, ____ liters.
Glucose level: _____. Insulin: ___ yes, ___ no. Type: ____________ # of units ____.

Nurse _____________, CNA _____________, in at _____ am/pm. Left at _______ am/pm.
Wash hands and wear gloves before touching patient: _______ yes, _______ no.
Wash hands before leaving room: ___ yes, ___ no. Wear protective gear: __ yes, __ no.
Clean stethoscope: __ yes, __ no. Oral care: __ yes, __ no. Suctioned: __ yes, __ no.
Repositioned: ___ yes, ___ no. Turned to: ___ left, ___ right, ___ backside ___.
Head of bed at: _______ degrees. Incontinence/skin breakdown: ____ yes, ____ no.
Linens wet or soiled: _____ yes, _____ no. Linens changed: _____ yes, _____ no.
Dressing changed: ____ yes, ____ no. Location: _______________________________.
IV site checked: _____ yes, _____ no. IV tubing labeled: _____ yes, _____no.
IV fluids at: ____.
Pain level (0-10 scale.0-no pain, 10 intolerable): __________________________.
Location of pain: ____________________. Medicated for pain: ____ yes, ____ no.
Patient is alert/oriented: ____ yes, ____ no. New confusion: ____ yes, ____ no.
Vital signs: temp ____, pulse ____, resp _____, b/p ______, 02 _____ %, ____ liters.
Glucose level: _____. Insulin: ___ yes, ___ no. Type: ____________ # of units ____.

Nurse _____________, CNA _____________, in at _____ am/pm. Left at _______ am/pm.
Wash hands and wear gloves before touching patient: _______ yes, _______ no.
Wash hands before leaving room: ___ yes, ___ no. Wear protective gear: __ yes, __ no.
Clean stethoscope: __ yes, __ no. Oral care: __ yes, __ no. Suctioned: __ yes, __ no.
Repositioned: ___ yes, ___ no. Turned to: ___ left, ___ right, ___ backside ___.
Head of bed at: _______ degrees. Incontinence/skin breakdown: ____ yes, ____ no.
Linens wet or soiled: _____ yes, _____ no. Linens changed: _____ yes, _____ no.
Dressing changed: ____ yes, ____ no. Location: _______________________________.
IV site checked: _____ yes, _____ no. IV tubing labeled: _____ yes, _____no.
IV fluids at: ____.
Pain level (0-10 scale.0-no pain, 10 intolerable): __________________________.
Location of pain: ____________________. Medicated for pain: ____ yes, ____ no.
Patient is alert/oriented: ____ yes, ____ no. New confusion: ____ yes, ____ no.
Vital signs: temp ____, pulse ____, resp _____, b/p ______, 02 _____ %, ____ liters.
Glucose level: _____. Insulin: ___ yes, ___ no. Type: ____________ # of units ____.

NURSING CARE CONTINUED FOR ______________________
DATE ____________________, DAY NUMBER ____________________

FOLLOWING EXAMINATIONS FOR NIGHT SHIFT:

Nurse ______________, CNA ______________, in at _____ am/pm. Left at _______ am/pm.
Wash hands and wear gloves before touching patient: _________ yes, _______ no.
Wash hands before leaving room: ___ yes, ___ no. Wear protective gear: __ yes, __ no.
Clean stethoscope: __ yes, __ no. Oral care: __ yes, __ no. Suctioned: __ yes, __ no.
Repositioned: ___ yes, ___ no. Turned to: ___ left, ___ right, ___ backside ___.
Head of bed at: _______ degrees. Incontinence/skin breakdown: ____ yes, ____ no.
Linens wet or soiled: _____ yes, _____ no. Linens changed: _____ yes, _____ no.
Dressing changed: ____ yes, ____ no. Location: ____________________________.
IV site checked: _____ yes, _____ no. IV tubing labeled: _____ yes, _____no.
IV fluids at: ____.
Pain level (0-10 scale.0-no pain, 10 intolerable): ________________________.
Location of pain: ______________. Medicated for pain: ____ yes, ____ no.
Patient is alert/oriented: ____ yes, ____ no. New confusion: ____ yes, ____ no.
Vital signs: temp ____, pulse _____, resp _____, b/p _____, 02 ____ %, ____ liters.
Glucose level: _____. Insulin: ___ yes, ___ no. Type: ______________ # of units ___.

Nurse ______________, CNA ______________, in at _____ am/pm. Left at _______ am/pm.
Wash hands and wear gloves before touching patient: _________ yes, _______ no.
Wash hands before leaving room: ___ yes, ___ no. Wear protective gear: __ yes, __ no.
Clean stethoscope: __ yes, __ no. Oral care: __ yes, __ no. Suctioned: __ yes, __ no.
Repositioned: ___ yes, ___ no. Turned to: ___ left, ___ right, ___ backside ___.
Head of bed at: _______ degrees. Incontinence/skin breakdown: ____ yes, ____ no.
Linens wet or soiled: _____ yes, _____ no. Linens changed: _____ yes, _____ no.
Dressing changed: ____ yes, ____ no. Location: ____________________________.
IV site checked: _____ yes, _____ no. IV tubing labeled: _____ yes, _____no.
IV fluids at: ____.
Pain level (0-10 scale.0-no pain, 10 intolerable): ________________________.
Location of pain: ______________. Medicated for pain: ____ yes, ____ no.
Patient is alert/oriented: ____ yes, ____ no. New confusion: ____ yes, ____ no.
Vital signs: temp ____, pulse _____, resp _____, b/p _____, 02 ____ %, ____ liters.
Glucose level: _____. Insulin: ___ yes, ___ no. Type: ______________ # of units ___.

Nurse ______________, CNA ______________, in at _____ am/pm. Left at _______ am/pm.
Wash hands and wear gloves before touching patient: _________ yes, _______ no.
Wash hands before leaving room: ___ yes, ___ no. Wear protective gear: __ yes, __ no.
Clean stethoscope: __ yes, __ no. Oral care: __ yes, __ no. Suctioned: __ yes, __ no.
Repositioned: ___ yes, ___ no. Turned to: ___ left, ___ right, ___ backside ___.
Head of bed at: _______ degrees. Incontinence/skin breakdown: ____ yes, ____ no.
Linens wet or soiled: _____ yes, _____ no. Linens changed: _____ yes, _____ no.
Dressing changed: ____ yes, ____ no. Location: ____________________________.
IV site checked: _____ yes, _____ no. IV tubing labeled: _____ yes, _____no.
IV fluids at: ____.
Pain level (0-10 scale.0-no pain, 10 intolerable): ________________________.
Location of pain: ______________. Medicated for pain: ____ yes, ____ no.
Patient is alert/oriented: ____ yes, ____ no. New confusion: ____ yes, ____ no.
Vital signs: temp ____, pulse _____, resp _____, b/p _____, 02 ____ %, ____ liters.
Glucose level: _____. Insulin: ___ yes, ___ no. Type: ______________ # of units ___.

MEDICATION ADMINISTRATION LIST FOR ____________________
DATE ______________ DAY NUMBER ____________________

List the medication for each day. Routes of administration: oral, thru feeding tube, intravenous (IV), intramuscular (IM), subcutaneous (SQ), epidural or a catheter in your spinal column, rectal, topical, eye drops, and ear drops.

Medication:	Route:	Time:

NOTES FOR DAY NUMBER ____________________

DATE ____________________

MEDICAL JOURNAL FOR ______________________________

DATE ____________________, DAY NUMBER _______________

VISITS FROM MY DOCTORS TODAY

Goals for today: ____

____

____.

Things to discuss with my doctor(s): ____________________________

____

____

Dr.____________ came in at _____ am/pm. Left at _____ am/pm.
We discussed ____.
Did doctor examine patient: _____ yes, _____ no.
Wash hands before touching patient: _____ yes, _____ no.
Wear gloves: ____ yes, ___ no. Clean stethoscope: ____ yes, ____ no.
Wear gown and mask (precautions only):____ yes, _____ no.
Wash hands before leaving the room: _____ yes, _____ no.

Dr.____________ came in at _____ am/pm. Left at _____ am/pm.
We discussed ____.
Did doctor examine patient: _____ yes, _____ no.
Wash hands before touching patient: _____ yes, _____ no.
Wear gloves: ____ yes, ___ no. Clean stethoscope: ____ yes, ____ no.
Wear gown and mask (precautions only):____ yes, _____ no.
Wash hands before leaving the room: _____ yes, _____ no.

Dr.____________ came in at _____ am/pm. Left at _____ am/pm.
We discussed ____.
Did doctor examine patient: _____ yes, _____ no.
Wash hands before touching patient: _____ yes, _____ no.
Wear gloves: ____ yes, ___ no. Clean stethoscope: ____ yes, ____ no.
Wear gown and mask (precautions only):____ yes, _____ no.
Wash hands before leaving the room: _____ yes, _____ no.

Dr.____________ came in at _____ am/pm. Left at _____ am/pm.
We discussed ____.
Did doctor examine patient: _____ yes, _____ no.
Wash hands before touching patient: _____ yes, _____ no.
Wear gloves: ____ yes, ___ no. Clean stethoscope: ____ yes, ____ no.
Wear gown and mask (precautions only):____ yes, _____ no.
Wash hands before leaving the room: _____ yes, _____ no.

Dr.____________ came in at _____ am/pm. Left at _____ am/pm.
We discussed ____.
Did doctor examine patient: _____ yes, _____ no.
Wash hands before touching patient: _____ yes, _____ no.
Wear gloves: ____ yes, ___ no. Clean stethoscope: ____ yes, ____ no.
Wear gown and mask (precautions only):____ yes, _____ no.
Wash hands before leaving the room: _____ yes, _____ no.

NURSING CARE FOR ________________________________

DATE ____________________, DAY NUMBER ______________________

INITIAL DAY SHIFT EXAM:

My nurse has ______ # of patients. CNA ___yes, ___no. Charge nurse ____________
Nurse ______________ RN/LPN came in at __________ am/pm. Left at __________ am/pm.
Did nurse wash hands and wear gloves before touching patient: ______ yes, ______ no.
Wash hands after touching patient and before leaving the room: ______ yes, ______no.
Don't hesitate to request staff to wash their hands. This will help decrease the risk of spreading potentially lethal germs.
Did nurse wear protective gear (isolation precautions only): _______ yes, ______ no.
Did nurse provide oral care (to be done every two hours if unable to provide for self, also decreases risk of pneumonia, infections, and aspiration): ______ yes, ______ no.
If able to provide own oral care, then supplies at bedside: _______ yes, ______ no.
Was patient repositioned (every two hours if unable to turn self): _____yes _____ no.
Head of bed at _________ degrees. This is important for patients on ventilators or on tube feedings. Anything less than thirty degrees places patients at risk for aspiration of stomach contents into the lungs causing aspiration pneumonia.
Checked for incontinence and skin breakdown: ____ yes, ____ no.
Patient's linens wet or soiled: ____ yes, ____ no. Linens changed: ____ yes, ____ no.
Time linens changed: ________ am/pm. Any skin redness or breakdown: ____ yes, ____ no.
If yes, what stage is pressure ulcer: _______. Acquired when: _____________________.
List wounds not associated with pressure ulcers and how acquired: ________________
____.
Mattress type: ____.
Specialty mattresses are important to help prevent pressure ulcers)
If patient on ventilator or has tracheostomy, suction performed: _____ yes, _____ no.
Did nurse listen to lung sounds: ______ yes, ______ no.
Does patient have chest tubes: ____ yes, ____ no. Functioning _____ yes, _____ no.
Bowel sounds: _______ yes, _______ no. Bowel sounds active: ______ yes, ______ no.
Neurological exam: ______ yes, ______ no. Follow commands: ______ yes, ______ no.
Is patient alert and oriented to person, place, time, and events: ____ yes, ____ no.
If confused, patient is not oriented to: ___ person, ___ place, ___ time, ___ event.
Confusion began (time and date): ____.
Glasgow coma scale (checks conscious scale of patient): ________________________.
Intracranial pressure monitoring: _____ yes, _____ no.
If yes, pressure is at ________ mm mercury. (Normal is one to fifteen).
Moves extremities: ___ yes, ___ no.
Paralysis: (inability to move extremities) ______ yes, ______ no.
If yes, extremities affected and when paralysis began: __________________________
Is patient in pain: ____ yes, ____ no. Describe pain and location _______________
Patient able to eat: ____ yes, ____ no. What type of diet? ______________________
If patient on tube feedings list type: __________ at ________ cc/ml per hour.
Nausea ____, vomiting ____. If so, describe: ____________________________________.
Patient has: Nasal gastric tube ______, Dobhoff tube _____, Peg or gastric tube ____.
When was feeding tube placed and what site: _____________________________________.
Catheter for draining urine: ____ yes, ____ no. If so, when placed: __________.
Find out policy for allowed time to remain in bladder. Too long may cause infections.)
IV site(s) where: _______________ when placed: _____________________.
IV fluids (types and rates): ____,
____,
Is patient on oxygen: _____ yes, _____ no. If so, how much and route delivered (see oxygen routes): ____.
If patient on ventilator, list settings (see list on ventilator settings): _________
____.
Vital signs: temp ______, pulse ______, resp ______, b/p ______, o2 ______%,
current weight ______ pounds, ______ kg. Glucose level: ______
Insulin coverage: ____ yes, ____ no. Insulin type: ____________, # of units: ______.

NURSING CARE CONTINUED FOR ______________________
DATE ______________, DAY NUMBER ______________

FOLLOWING EXAMINATIONS FOR DAY SHIFT:

Nurse ____________, CNA ____________, in at _____ am/pm. Left at ______ am/pm.
Wash hands and wear gloves before touching patient: ______ yes, ______ no.
Wash hands before leaving room: ___ yes, ___ no. Wear protective gear: __ yes, __ no.
Clean stethoscope: __ yes, __ no. Oral care: __ yes, __ no. Suctioned: __ yes, __ no.
Repositioned: ___ yes, ___ no. Turned to: ___ left, ___ right, ___ backside ___.
Head of bed at: _______ degrees. Incontinence/skin breakdown: ____ yes, ____ no.
Linens wet or soiled: _____ yes, _____ no. Linens changed: _____ yes, ______ no.
Dressing changed: ____ yes, ____ no. Location: ______________________.
IV site checked: _____ yes, _____ no. IV tubing labeled: _____ yes, _____no.
IV fluids at: ______________________________________.
Pain level (0-10 scale.0-no pain, 10 intolerable): ______________________.
Location of pain: ______________. Medicated for pain: _____ yes, ____ no.
Patient is alert/oriented: ____ yes, ____ no. New confusion: ____ yes, ____ no.
Vital signs: temp ____, pulse _____, resp _____, b/p ______, 02 _____ %, ____ liters.
Glucose level: _____. Insulin: ___ yes, ___ no. Type: ____________ # of units ____.

Nurse ____________, CNA ____________, in at _____ am/pm. Left at ______ am/pm.
Wash hands and wear gloves before touching patient: ______ yes, ______ no.
Wash hands before leaving room: ___ yes, ___ no. Wear protective gear: __ yes, __ no.
Clean stethoscope: __ yes, __ no. Oral care: __ yes, __ no. Suctioned: __ yes, __ no.
Repositioned: ___ yes, ___ no. Turned to: ___ left, ___ right, ___ backside ___.
Head of bed at: _______ degrees. Incontinence/skin breakdown: ____ yes, ____ no.
Linens wet or soiled: _____ yes, _____ no. Linens changed: _____ yes, ______ no.
Dressing changed: ____ yes, ____ no. Location: ______________________.
IV site checked: _____ yes, _____ no. IV tubing labeled: _____ yes, _____no.
IV fluids at: ______________________________________.
Pain level (0-10 scale.0-no pain, 10 intolerable): ______________________.
Location of pain: ______________. Medicated for pain: _____ yes, ____ no.
Patient is alert/oriented: ____ yes, ____ no. New confusion: ____ yes, ____ no.
Vital signs: temp ____, pulse _____, resp _____, b/p ______, 02 _____ %, ____ liters.
Glucose level: _____. Insulin: ___ yes, ___ no. Type: ____________ # of units ____.

Nurse ____________, CNA ____________, in at _____ am/pm. Left at ______ am/pm.
Wash hands and wear gloves before touching patient: ______ yes, ______ no.
Wash hands before leaving room: ___ yes, ___ no. Wear protective gear: __ yes, __ no.
Clean stethoscope: __ yes, __ no. Oral care: __ yes, __ no. Suctioned: __ yes, __ no.
Repositioned: ___ yes, ___ no. Turned to: ___ left, ___ right, ___ backside ___.
Head of bed at: _______ degrees. Incontinence/skin breakdown: ____ yes, ____ no.
Linens wet or soiled: _____ yes, _____ no. Linens changed: _____ yes, ______ no.
Dressing changed: ____ yes, ____ no. Location: ______________________.
IV site checked: _____ yes, _____ no. IV tubing labeled: _____ yes, _____no.
IV fluids at: ______________________________________.
Pain level (0-10 scale.0-no pain, 10 intolerable): ______________________.
Location of pain: ______________. Medicated for pain: _____ yes, ____ no.
Patient is alert/oriented: ____ yes, ____ no. New confusion: ____ yes, ____ no.
Vital signs: temp ____, pulse _____, resp _____, b/p ______, 02 _____ %, ____ liters.
Glucose level: _____. Insulin: ___ yes, ___ no. Type: ____________ # of units ____.

NURSING CARE CONTINUED FOR ____________________
DATE ____________________, DAY NUMBER ____________________

FOLLOWING EXAMINATIONS FOR DAY SHIFT:

Nurse ____________, CNA ____________, in at _____ am/pm. Left at ______ am/pm.
Wash hands and wear gloves before touching patient: ______ yes, ______ no.
Wash hands before leaving room: ___ yes, ___ no. Wear protective gear: __ yes, __ no.
Clean stethoscope: __ yes, __ no. Oral care: __ yes, __ no. Suctioned: __ yes, __ no.
Repositioned: ___ yes, ___ no. Turned to: ___ left, ___ right, ___ backside ___.
Head of bed at: ________ degrees. Incontinence/skin breakdown: ____ yes, ____ no.
Linens wet or soiled: ____ yes, ____ no. Linens changed: ____ yes, ____ no.
Dressing changed: ____ yes, ____ no. Location: ____________________.
IV site checked: _____ yes, _____ no. IV tubing labeled: ____ yes, ____ no.
IV fluids at: ____________________.
Pain level (0-10 scale.0-no pain, 10 intolerable): ____________________.
Location of pain: ____________. Medicated for pain: ____ yes, ____ no.
Patient is alert/oriented: ____ yes, ____ no. New confusion: ____ yes, ____ no.
Vital signs: temp ____, pulse ____, resp ____, b/p _____, 02 ____ %, ____ liters.
Glucose level: _____. Insulin: ___ yes, ___ no. Type: _______ # of units ____.

Nurse ____________, CNA ____________, in at _____ am/pm. Left at ______ am/pm.
Wash hands and wear gloves before touching patient: ______ yes, ______ no.
Wash hands before leaving room: ___ yes, ___ no. Wear protective gear: __ yes, __ no.
Clean stethoscope: __ yes, __ no. Oral care: __ yes, __ no. Suctioned: __ yes, __ no.
Repositioned: ___ yes, ___ no. Turned to: ___ left, ___ right, ___ backside ___.
Head of bed at: ________ degrees. Incontinence/skin breakdown: ____ yes, ____ no.
Linens wet or soiled: ____ yes, ____ no. Linens changed: ____ yes, ____ no.
Dressing changed: ____ yes, ____ no. Location: ____________________.
IV site checked: _____ yes, _____ no. IV tubing labeled: ____ yes, ____ no.
IV fluids at: ____________________.
Pain level (0-10 scale.0-no pain, 10 intolerable): ____________________.
Location of pain: ____________. Medicated for pain: ____ yes, ____ no.
Patient is alert/oriented: ____ yes, ____ no. New confusion: ____ yes, ____ no.
Vital signs: temp ____, pulse ____, resp ____, b/p _____, 02 ____ %, ____ liters.
Glucose level: _____. Insulin: ___ yes, ___ no. Type: _______ # of units ____.

Nurse ____________, CNA ____________, in at _____ am/pm. Left at ______ am/pm.
Wash hands and wear gloves before touching patient: ______ yes, ______ no.
Wash hands before leaving room: ___ yes, ___ no. Wear protective gear: __ yes, __ no.
Clean stethoscope: __ yes, __ no. Oral care: __ yes, __ no. Suctioned: __ yes, __ no.
Repositioned: ___ yes, ___ no. Turned to: ___ left, ___ right, ___ backside ___.
Head of bed at: ________ degrees. Incontinence/skin breakdown: ____ yes, ____ no.
Linens wet or soiled: ____ yes, ____ no. Linens changed: ____ yes, ____ no.
Dressing changed: ____ yes, ____ no. Location: ____________________.
IV site checked: _____ yes, _____ no. IV tubing labeled: ____ yes, ____ no.
IV fluids at: ____________________.
Pain level (0-10 scale.0-no pain, 10 intolerable): ____________________.
Location of pain: ____________. Medicated for pain: ____ yes, ____ no.
Patient is alert/oriented: ____ yes, ____ no. New confusion: ____ yes, ____ no.
Vital signs: temp ____, pulse ____, resp ____, b/p _____, 02 ____ %, ____ liters.
Glucose level: _____. Insulin: ___ yes, ___ no. Type: _______ # of units ____.

NURSING CARE FOR ______________________________

DATE ____________________, DAY NUMBER ____________________

INITIAL NIGHT SHIFT EXAM:

My nurse has _____ # of patients. CNA ___yes, ___no. Charge nurse ______________
Nurse ______________ RN/LPN came in at _________ am/pm. Left at _________ am/pm.
Did nurse wash hands and wear gloves before touching patient: ______ yes, ______ no.
Wash hands after touching patient and before leaving the room: ______ yes, ______ no.
Don't hesitate to request staff to wash their hands. This will help decrease the risk of spreading potentially lethal germs.
Did nurse wear protective gear (isolation precautions only): ______ yes, ______ no.
Did nurse provide oral care (to be done every two hours if unable to provide for self, also decreases risk of pneumonia, infections, and aspiration): ______ yes, ______ no.
If able to provide own oral care, then supplies at bedside: ______ yes, ______ no.
Was patient repositioned (every two hours if unable to turn self): _____ yes _____ no.
Head of bed at ________ degrees. This is important for patients on ventilators or on tube feedings. Anything less than thirty degrees places patients at risk for aspiration of stomach contents into the lungs causing aspiration pneumonia.
Checked for incontinence and skin breakdown: ____ yes, _____ no.
Patient's linens wet or soiled: _____yes, ____ no. Linens changed: ____ yes, ____ no.
Time linens changed: ________ am/pm. Any skin redness or breakdown: ____ yes, ____ no.
If yes, what stage is pressure ulcer: ________. Acquired when: ______________________.
List wounds not associated with pressure ulcers and how acquired: _______________
____.
Mattress type: ____.
Specialty mattresses are important to help prevent pressure ulcers)
If patient on ventilator or has tracheostomy, suction performed: _____ yes, _____ no.
Did nurse listen to lung sounds: _____ yes, _____ no.
Does patient have chest tubes: ____ yes, ____ no. Functioning _____ yes, ______ no.
Bowel sounds: ______ yes, ______ no. Bowel sounds active: ______ yes, ______ no.
Neurological exam: ______ yes, ______ no. Follow commands: ______ yes, ______ no.
Is patient alert and oriented to person, place, time, and events: _____ yes, _____ no.
If confused, patient is not oriented to: ____ person, ___ place, ___ time, ___ event.
Confusion began (time and date): ____.
Glasgow coma scale (checks conscious scale of patient): ____________________.
Intracranial pressure monitoring: _____ yes, _____ no.
If yes, pressure is at ________ mm mercury. (Normal is one to fifteen).
Moves extremities: ___ yes, ___ no.
Paralysis: (inability to move extremities) ________ yes, ______ no.
If yes, extremities affected and when paralysis began: ______________________.
Is patient in pain: ____ yes, ____ no. Describe pain and location ____________.
Patient able to eat: ____ yes, _____ no. What type of diet? __________________.
If patient on tube feedings list type: ____________ at __________ cc/ml per hour.
Nausea ____, vomiting ____. If so, describe: ________________________________.
Patient has: Nasal gastric tube ______, Dobhoff tube _____, Peg or gastric tube _____.
When was feeding tube placed and what site: ____________________________________.
Catheter for draining urine: ____ yes, ____ no. If so, when placed: __________.
Find out policy for allowed time to remain in bladder. Too long may cause infections.)
IV site(s) where: ______________________ when placed: __________________.
IV fluids (types and rates): ____________________, ____________________,
____________________, ____________________, ____________________,
Is patient on oxygen: _____ yes, _____ no. If so, how much and route delivered (see oxygen routes): ____.
If patient on ventilator, list settings (see list on ventilator settings): _________
____.
Vital signs: temp ______, pulse ______, resp ______, b/p ______, o2 ______%,
current weight ______ pounds, _____ kg. Glucose level: ______
Insulin coverage: ____ yes, ____ no. Insulin type: ____________, # of units: ______.

NURSING CARE CONTINUED FOR ____________________
DATE ____________________, DAY NUMBER ____________________

FOLLOWING EXAMINATIONS FOR NIGHT SHIFT:

Nurse ____________, CNA ____________, in at _____ am/pm. Left at ______ am/pm.
Wash hands and wear gloves before touching patient: ______ yes, ______ no.
Wash hands before leaving room: __ yes, __ no. Wear protective gear: __ yes, __ no.
Clean stethoscope: yes, __ no. Oral care: __ yes, __ no. Suctioned: __ yes, __ no.
Repositioned: ___ yes, ___ no. Turned to: ___ left, ___ right, ___ backside ___.
Head of bed at: ______ degrees. Incontinence/skin breakdown: ____ yes, ____ no.
Linens wet or soiled: ____ yes, ____ no. Linens changed: ____ yes, ____ no.
Dressing changed: ____ yes, ____ no. Location: ____________________.
IV site checked: ____ yes, ____ no. IV tubing labeled: ____ yes, ____ no.
IV fluids at: ____.
Pain level (0-10 scale.0-no pain, 10 intolerable): ____________________.
Location of pain: ____________. Medicated for pain: ____ yes, ____ no.
Patient is alert/oriented: ____ yes, ____ no. New confusion: ____ yes, ____ no.
Vital signs: temp ____, pulse ____, resp ____, b/p ____, 02 ____ %, ____ liters.
Glucose level: _____. Insulin: ___ yes, ___ no. Type: __________ # of units ____.

Nurse ____________, CNA ____________, in at _____ am/pm. Left at ______ am/pm.
Wash hands and wear gloves before touching patient: ______ yes, ______ no.
Wash hands before leaving room: __ yes, __ no. Wear protective gear: __ yes, __ no.
Clean stethoscope: yes, __ no. Oral care: __ yes, __ no. Suctioned: __ yes, __ no.
Repositioned: ___ yes, ___ no. Turned to: ___ left, ___ right, ___ backside ___.
Head of bed at: ______ degrees. Incontinence/skin breakdown: ____ yes, ____ no.
Linens wet or soiled: ____ yes, ____ no. Linens changed: ____ yes, ____ no.
Dressing changed: ____ yes, ____ no. Location: ____________________.
IV site checked: ____ yes, ____ no. IV tubing labeled: ____ yes, ____ no.
IV fluids at: ____.
Pain level (0-10 scale.0-no pain, 10 intolerable): ____________________.
Location of pain: ____________. Medicated for pain: ____ yes, ____ no.
Patient is alert/oriented: ____ yes, ____ no. New confusion: ____ yes, ____ no.
Vital signs: temp ____, pulse ____, resp ____, b/p ____, 02 ____ %, ____ liters.
Glucose level: _____. Insulin: ___ yes, ___ no. Type: __________ # of units ____.

Nurse ____________, CNA ____________, in at _____ am/pm. Left at ______ am/pm.
Wash hands and wear gloves before touching patient: ______ yes, ______ no.
Wash hands before leaving room: __ yes, __ no. Wear protective gear: __ yes, __ no.
Clean stethoscope: yes, __ no. Oral care: __ yes, __ no. Suctioned: __ yes, __ no.
Repositioned: ___ yes, ___ no. Turned to: ___ left, ___ right, ___ backside ___.
Head of bed at: ______ degrees. Incontinence/skin breakdown: ____ yes, ____ no.
Linens wet or soiled: ____ yes, ____ no. Linens changed: ____ yes, ____ no.
Dressing changed: ____ yes, ____ no. Location: ____________________.
IV site checked: ____ yes, ____ no. IV tubing labeled: ____ yes, ____ no.
IV fluids at: ____.
Pain level (0-10 scale.0-no pain, 10 intolerable): ____________________.
Location of pain: ____________. Medicated for pain: ____ yes, ____ no.
Patient is alert/oriented: ____ yes, ____ no. New confusion: ____ yes, ____ no.
Vital signs: temp ____, pulse ____, resp ____, b/p ____, 02 ____ %, ____ liters.
Glucose level: _____. Insulin: ___ yes, ___ no. Type: __________ # of units ____.

NURSING CARE CONTINUED FOR ______________________
DATE ____________________, DAY NUMBER ________________

FOLLOWING EXAMINATIONS FOR NIGHT SHIFT:

Nurse ____________, CNA ____________, in at _____ am/pm. Left at ______ am/pm.
Wash hands and wear gloves before touching patient: ______ yes, ______ no.
Wash hands before leaving room: __ yes, __ no. Wear protective gear: __ yes, __ no.
Clean stethoscope: __ yes, __ no. Oral care: __ yes, __ no. Suctioned: __ yes, __ no.
Repositioned: ___ yes, ___ no. Turned to: ___ left, ___ right, ___ backside ___.
Head of bed at: _______ degrees. Incontinence/skin breakdown: ____ yes, ____ no.
Linens wet or soiled: _____ yes, _____ no. Linens changed: _____ yes, ______ no.
Dressing changed: ____ yes, ____ no. Location: ______________________________.
IV site checked: _____ yes, _____ no. IV tubing labeled: _____ yes, _____no.
IV fluids at: ____.
Pain level (0-10 scale.0-no pain, 10 intolerable): ___________________________.
Location of pain: ______________. Medicated for pain: ____ yes, ____ no.
Patient is alert/oriented: ____ yes, ____ no. New confusion: ____ yes, ____ no.
Vital signs: temp ____, pulse _____, resp ______, b/p ______, 02 _____%, ____ liters.
Glucose level: _____. Insulin: ___ yes, ___ no. Type: ______________ # of units ____.

Nurse ____________, CNA ____________, in at _____ am/pm. Left at ______ am/pm.
Wash hands and wear gloves before touching patient: ______ yes, ______ no.
Wash hands before leaving room: ___ yes, ___ no. Wear protective gear: __ yes, __ no.
Clean stethoscope: __ yes, __ no. Oral care: __ yes, __ no. Suctioned: __ yes, __ no.
Repositioned: ___ yes, ___ no. Turned to: ___ left, ___ right, ___ backside ___.
Head of bed at: _______ degrees. Incontinence/skin breakdown: ____ yes, ____ no.
Linens wet or soiled: _____ yes, _____ no. Linens changed: _____ yes, ______ no.
Dressing changed: ____ yes, ____ no. Location: ______________________________.
IV site checked: _____ yes, _____ no. IV tubing labeled: _____ yes, _____no.
IV fluids at: ____.
Pain level (0-10 scale.0-no pain, 10 intolerable): ___________________________.
Location of pain: ______________. Medicated for pain: ____ yes, ____ no.
Patient is alert/oriented: ____ yes, ____ no. New confusion: ____ yes, ____ no.
Vital signs: temp ____, pulse _____, resp ______, b/p ______, 02 _____%, ____ liters.
Glucose level: _____. Insulin: ___ yes, ___ no. Type: ______________ # of units ____.

Nurse ____________, CNA ____________, in at _____ am/pm. Left at ______ am/pm.
Wash hands and wear gloves before touching patient: ______ yes, ______ no.
Wash hands before leaving room: ___ yes, ___ no. Wear protective gear: __ yes, __ no.
Clean stethoscope: __ yes, __ no. Oral care: __ yes, __ no. Suctioned: __ yes, __ no.
Repositioned: ___ yes, ___ no. Turned to: ___ left, ___ right, ___ backside ___.
Head of bed at: _______ degrees. Incontinence/skin breakdown: ____ yes, ____ no.
Linens wet or soiled: _____ yes, _____ no. Linens changed: _____ yes, ______ no.
Dressing changed: ____ yes, ____ no. Location: ______________________________.
IV site checked: _____ yes, _____ no. IV tubing labeled: _____ yes, _____no.
IV fluids at: ____.
Pain level (0-10 scale.0-no pain, 10 intolerable): ___________________________.
Location of pain: ______________. Medicated for pain: ____ yes, ____ no.
Patient is alert/oriented: ____ yes, ____ no. New confusion: ____ yes, ____ no.
Vital signs: temp ____, pulse _____, resp ______, b/p ______, 02 _____%, ____ liters.
Glucose level: _____. Insulin: ___ yes, ___ no. Type: ______________ # of units ____.

MEDICATION ADMINISTRATION LIST FOR ____________________
DATE ________________ DAY NUMBER ____________________

List the medication for each day. Routes of administration: oral, thru feeding tube, intravenous (IV), intramuscular (IM), subcutaneous (SQ), epidural or a catheter in your spinal column, rectal, topical, eye drops, and ear drops.

Medication: ____________________ Route: ____________________ Time: ________________
Medication: ____________________ Route: ____________________ Time: ________________
Medication: ____________________ Route: ____________________ Time: ________________
Medication: ____________________ Route: ____________________ Time: ________________
Medication: ____________________ Route: ____________________ Time: ________________
Medication: ____________________ Route: ____________________ Time: ________________
Medication: ____________________ Route: ____________________ Time: ________________
Medication: ____________________ Route: ____________________ Time: ________________
Medication: ____________________ Route: ____________________ Time: ________________
Medication: ____________________ Route: ____________________ Time: ________________
Medication: ____________________ Route: ____________________ Time: ________________
Medication: ____________________ Route: ____________________ Time: ________________
Medication: ____________________ Route: ____________________ Time: ________________
Medication: ____________________ Route: ____________________ Time: ________________
Medication: ____________________ Route: ____________________ Time: ________________
Medication: ____________________ Route: ____________________ Time: ________________
Medication: ____________________ Route: ____________________ Time: ________________
Medication: ____________________ Route: ____________________ Time: ________________
Medication: ____________________ Route: ____________________ Time: ________________
Medication: ____________________ Route: ____________________ Time: ________________
Medication: ____________________ Route: ____________________ Time: ________________
Medication: ____________________ Route: ____________________ Time: ________________
Medication: ____________________ Route: ____________________ Time: ________________
Medication: ____________________ Route: ____________________ Time: ________________
Medication: ____________________ Route: ____________________ Time: ________________
Medication: ____________________ Route: ____________________ Time: ________________
Medication: ____________________ Route: ____________________ Time: ________________
Medication: ____________________ Route: ____________________ Time: ________________
Medication: ____________________ Route: ____________________ Time: ________________
Medication: ____________________ Route: ____________________ Time: ________________
Medication: ____________________ Route: ____________________ Time: ________________
Medication: ____________________ Route: ____________________ Time: ________________
Medication: ____________________ Route: ____________________ Time: ________________
Medication: ____________________ Route: ____________________ Time: ________________
Medication: ____________________ Route: ____________________ Time: ________________
Medication: ____________________ Route: ____________________ Time: ________________
Medication: ____________________ Route: ____________________ Time: ________________
Medication: ____________________ Route: ____________________ Time: ________________
Medication: ____________________ Route: ____________________ Time: ________________
Medication: ____________________ Route: ____________________ Time: ________________
Medication: ____________________ Route: ____________________ Time: ________________
Medication: ____________________ Route: ____________________ Time: ________________
Medication: ____________________ Route: ____________________ Time: ________________
Medication: ____________________ Route: ____________________ Time: ________________
Medication: ____________________ Route: ____________________ Time: ________________
Medication: ____________________ Route: ____________________ Time: ________________
Medication: ____________________ Route: ____________________ Time: ________________
Medication: ____________________ Route: ____________________ Time: ________________
Medication: ____________________ Route: ____________________ Time: ________________
Medication: ____________________ Route: ____________________ Time: ________________
Medication: ____________________ Route: ____________________ Time: ________________
Medication: ____________________ Route: ____________________ Time: ________________
Medication: ____________________ Route: ____________________ Time: ________________
Medication: ____________________ Route: ____________________ Time: ________________

NOTES FOR DAY NUMBER ____________________

DATE ____________________

MEDICAL JOURNAL FOR ______________________

DATE ______________, DAY NUMBER ____________

VISITS FROM MY DOCTORS TODAY

Goals for today: ______________________

____

______________________.

Things to discuss with my doctor(s): ______________________

____

______________________.

Dr.________ came in at _____ am/pm. Left at _____ am/pm.
We discussed ______________________.
Did doctor examine patient: _____ yes, _____ no.
Wash hands before touching patient: _____ yes, _____ no.
Wear gloves: ____ yes, ___ no. Clean stethoscope: ____ yes, ____ no.
Wear gown and mask (precautions only):____ yes, _____ no.
Wash hands before leaving the room: _____ yes, _____ no.

Dr.________ came in at _____ am/pm. Left at _____ am/pm.
We discussed ______________________.
Did doctor examine patient: _____ yes, _____ no.
Wash hands before touching patient: _____ yes, _____ no.
Wear gloves: ____ yes, ___ no. Clean stethoscope: ____ yes, ____ no.
Wear gown and mask (precautions only):____ yes, _____ no.
Wash hands before leaving the room: _____ yes, _____ no.

Dr.________ came in at _____ am/pm. Left at _____ am/pm.
We discussed ______________________.
Did doctor examine patient: _____ yes, _____ no.
Wash hands before touching patient: _____ yes, _____ no.
Wear gloves: ____ yes, ___ no. Clean stethoscope: ____ yes, ____ no.
Wear gown and mask (precautions only):____ yes, _____ no.
Wash hands before leaving the room: _____ yes, _____ no.

Dr.________ came in at _____ am/pm. Left at _____ am/pm.
We discussed ______________________.
Did doctor examine patient: _____ yes, _____ no.
Wash hands before touching patient: _____ yes, _____ no.
Wear gloves: ____ yes, ___ no. Clean stethoscope: ____ yes, ____ no.
Wear gown and mask (precautions only):____ yes, _____ no.
Wash hands before leaving the room: _____ yes, _____ no.

Dr.________ came in at _____ am/pm. Left at _____ am/pm.
We discussed ______________________.
Did doctor examine patient: _____ yes, _____ no.
Wash hands before touching patient: _____ yes, _____ no.
Wear gloves: ____ yes, ___ no. Clean stethoscope: ____ yes, ____ no.
Wear gown and mask (precautions only):____ yes, _____ no.
Wash hands before leaving the room: _____ yes, _____ no.

NURSING CARE FOR ________________________________

DATE ________________, DAY NUMBER ________________

INITIAL DAY SHIFT EXAM:

My nurse has ______ # of patients. CNA ___yes, ___no. Charge nurse ______________
Nurse ________________ RN/LPN came in at _________ am/pm. Left at __________ am/pm.
Did nurse wash hands and wear gloves before touching patient: _______ yes, _______ no.
Wash hands after touching patient and before leaving the room: _______ yes, _______ no.
Don't hesitate to request staff to wash their hands. This will help decrease the risk of spreading potentially lethal germs.
Did nurse wear protective gear (isolation precautions only): _______ yes, _______ no.
Did nurse provide oral care (to be done every two hours if unable to provide for self, also decreases risk of pneumonia, infections, and aspiration): _______ yes, _______ no.
If able to provide own oral care, then supplies at bedside: ________ yes, _______ no.
Was patient repositioned (every two hours if unable to turn self): _____ yes _____ no.
Head of bed at ________ degrees. This is important for patients on ventilators or on tube feedings. Anything less than thirty degrees places patients at risk for aspiration of stomach contents into the lungs causing aspiration pneumonia.
Checked for incontinence and skin breakdown: _____ yes, _____ no.
Patient's linens wet or soiled: _____ yes, ____ no. Linens changed: ____ yes, ____ no.
Time linens changed: ________ am/pm. Any skin redness or breakdown: ____ yes, ____ no.
If yes, what stage is pressure ulcer: ________. Acquired when: ________________.
List wounds not associated with pressure ulcers and how acquired: ______________
____.
Mattress type: ____.
Specialty mattresses are important to help prevent pressure ulcers)
If patient on ventilator or has tracheostomy, suction performed: _____ yes, ______ no.
Did nurse listen to lung sounds: _____ yes, _____ no.
Does patient have chest tubes: ____ yes, ____ no. Functioning _____ yes, ______ no.
Bowel sounds: _______ yes, _______ no. Bowel sounds active: ______ yes, ______ no.
Neurological exam: ______ yes, ______ no. Follow commands: ______ yes, ______ no.
Is patient alert and oriented to person, place, time, and events: _____ yes, _____ no.
If confused, patient is not oriented to: ____ person, ___ place, ___ time, ___ event.
Confusion began (time and date): ______________________________________.
Glasgow coma scale (checks conscious scale of patient): ____________________.
Intracranial pressure monitoring: ______ yes, _____ no.
If yes, pressure is at ______ mm mercury. (Normal is one to fifteen).
Moves extremities: ___ yes, ___ no.
Paralysis: (inability to move extremities) ________ yes, ________ no.
If yes, extremities affected and when paralysis began: ____________________.
Is patient in pain: ____ yes, ____ no. Describe pain and location ______________.
Patient able to eat: ____ yes, ____ no. What type of diet? ___________________.
If patient on tube feedings list type: __________ at ___________ cc/ml per hour.
Nausea ____, vomiting _____. If so, describe: ____________________________.
Patient has: Nasal gastric tube _____, Dobhoff tube _____, Peg or gastric tube _____.
When was feeding tube placed and what site: _______________________________.
Catheter for draining urine: ____ yes, ____ no. If so, when placed: ____________.
Find out policy for allowed time to remain in bladder. Too long may cause infections.)
IV site(s) where: __________________________ when placed: _______________.
IV fluids (types and rates): _________________, ________________,
_______________, _________________, ________________,
Is patient on oxygen: _____ yes, _____ no. If so, how much and route delivered (see oxygen routes): ____.
If patient on ventilator, list settings (see list on ventilator settings): ________
____.
Vital signs: temp _____, pulse _____, resp _____, b/p _____, o2 _____%,
current weight ______ pounds, ______ kg. Glucose level: ______
Insulin coverage: ____ yes, ____ no. Insulin type: __________, # of units: _____.

NURSING CARE CONTINUED FOR ____________________
DATE ____________________, DAY NUMBER ____________________

FOLLOWING EXAMINATIONS FOR DAY SHIFT:

Nurse ____________, CNA ____________, in at ______ am/pm. Left at _______ am/pm.
Wash hands and wear gloves before touching patient: _______ yes, _____ no.
Wash hands before leaving room: ___ yes, ___ no. Wear protective gear: __ yes, __ no.
Clean stethoscope: __ yes, __ no. Oral care: __ yes, __ no. Suctioned: __ yes, __ no.
Repositioned: ___ yes, ___ no. Turned to: ___ left, ___ right, ___ backside ___.
Head of bed at: ______ degrees. Incontinence/skin breakdown: ___ yes, ___ no.
Linens wet or soiled: _____ yes, _____ no. Linens changed: _____ yes, _____ no.
Dressing changed: ____ yes, ____ no. Location: ____________________.
IV site checked: _____ yes, _____ no. IV tubing labeled: _____ yes, _____ no.
IV fluids at: ____.
Pain level (0-10 scale.0-no pain, 10 intolerable): ____________________.
Location of pain: ____________. Medicated for pain: ____ yes, ____ no.
Patient is alert/oriented: _____ yes, ___ no. New confusion: ____ yes, ____ no.
Vital signs: temp ____, pulse ____, resp ____, b/p ____, 02 ____ %, ____ liters.
Glucose level: _____. Insulin: ___ yes, ___ no. Type: ___________ # of units ____.

Nurse ____________, CNA ____________, in at ______ am/pm. Left at _______ am/pm.
Wash hands and wear gloves before touching patient: _______ yes, _____ no.
Wash hands before leaving room: ___ yes, ___ no. Wear protective gear: __ yes, __ no.
Clean stethoscope: __ yes, __ no. Oral care: __ yes, __ no. Suctioned: __ yes, __ no.
Repositioned: ___ yes, ___ no. Turned to: ___ left, ___ right, ___ backside ___.
Head of bed at: ______ degrees. Incontinence/skin breakdown: ___ yes, ___ no.
Linens wet or soiled: _____ yes, _____ no. Linens changed: _____ yes, _____ no.
Dressing changed: ____ yes, ____ no. Location: ____________________.
IV site checked: _____ yes, _____ no. IV tubing labeled: _____ yes, _____ no.
IV fluids at: ____.
Pain level (0-10 scale.0-no pain, 10 intolerable): ____________________.
Location of pain: ____________. Medicated for pain: ____ yes, ____ no.
Patient is alert/oriented: _____ yes, ___ no. New confusion: ____ yes, ____ no.
Vital signs: temp ____, pulse ____, resp ____, b/p ____, 02 ____ %, ____ liters.
Glucose level: _____. Insulin: ___ yes, ___ no. Type: ___________ # of units ____.

Nurse ____________, CNA ____________, in at ______ am/pm. Left at _______ am/pm.
Wash hands and wear gloves before touching patient: _______ yes, _____ no.
Wash hands before leaving room: ___ yes, ___ no. Wear protective gear: __ yes, __ no.
Clean stethoscope: __ yes, __ no. Oral care: __ yes, __ no. Suctioned: __ yes, __ no.
Repositioned: ___ yes, ___ no. Turned to: ___ left, ___ right, ___ backside ___.
Head of bed at: ______ degrees. Incontinence/skin breakdown: ___ yes, ___ no.
Linens wet or soiled: _____ yes, _____ no. Linens changed: _____ yes, _____ no.
Dressing changed: ____ yes, ____ no. Location: ____________________.
IV site checked: _____ yes, _____ no. IV tubing labeled: _____ yes, _____ no.
IV fluids at: ____.
Pain level (0-10 scale.0-no pain, 10 intolerable): ____________________.
Location of pain: ____________. Medicated for pain: ____ yes, ____ no.
Patient is alert/oriented: _____ yes, ___ no. New confusion: ____ yes, ____ no.
Vital signs: temp ____, pulse ____, resp ____, b/p ____, 02 ____ %, ____ liters.
Glucose level: _____. Insulin: ___ yes, ___ no. Type: ___________ # of units ____.

NURSING CARE CONTINUED FOR ____________________
DATE ________________, DAY NUMBER ________________

FOLLOWING EXAMINATIONS FOR DAY SHIFT:

Nurse ____________, CNA ____________, in at _____ am/pm. Left at ______ am/pm.
Wash hands and wear gloves before touching patient: _______ yes, _______ no.
Wash hands before leaving room: ___ yes, ___ no. Wear protective gear: __ yes, __ no.
Clean stethoscope: __ yes, __ no. Oral care: __ yes, __ no. Suctioned: __ yes, __ no.
Repositioned: ___ yes, ___ no. Turned to: ___ left, ___ right, ___ backside ___.
Head of bed at: ________ degrees. Incontinence/skin breakdown: ____ yes, ____ no.
Linens wet or soiled: ____ yes, ____ no. Linens changed: ____ yes, ____ no.
Dressing changed: ____ yes, ____ no. Location: ____________________.
IV site checked: _____ yes, _____ no. IV tubing labeled: _____ yes, _____no.
IV fluids at: ________________________________.
Pain level (0-10 scale.0-no pain, 10 intolerable): ________________.
Location of pain: ____________. Medicated for pain: _____ yes, ____ no.
Patient is alert/oriented: ____ yes, ____ no. New confusion: ____ yes, ____ no.
Vital signs: temp ____, pulse ____, resp _____, b/p _____, 02 _____ %, ____ liters.
Glucose level: _____. Insulin: ___ yes, ___ no. Type: ____________ # of units ____.

Nurse ____________, CNA ____________, in at _____ am/pm. Left at ______ am/pm.
Wash hands and wear gloves before touching patient: _______ yes, _______ no.
Wash hands before leaving room: ___ yes, ___ no. Wear protective gear: __ yes, __ no.
Clean stethoscope: __ yes, __ no. Oral care: __ yes, __ no. Suctioned: __ yes, __ no.
Repositioned: ___ yes, ___ no. Turned to: ___ left, ___ right, ___ backside ___.
Head of bed at: ________ degrees. Incontinence/skin breakdown: ____ yes, ____ no.
Linens wet or soiled: ____ yes, ____ no. Linens changed: ____ yes, ____ no.
Dressing changed: ____ yes, ____ no. Location: ____________________.
IV site checked: _____ yes, _____ no. IV tubing labeled: _____ yes, _____no.
IV fluids at: ________________________________.
Pain level (0-10 scale.0-no pain, 10 intolerable): ________________.
Location of pain: ____________. Medicated for pain: _____ yes, ____ no.
Patient is alert/oriented: ____ yes, ____ no. New confusion: ____ yes, ____ no.
Vital signs: temp ____, pulse ____, resp _____, b/p _____, 02 _____ %, ____ liters.
Glucose level: _____. Insulin: ___ yes, ___ no. Type: ____________ # of units ____.

Nurse ____________, CNA ____________, in at _____ am/pm. Left at ______ am/pm.
Wash hands and wear gloves before touching patient: _______ yes, _______ no.
Wash hands before leaving room: ___ yes, ___ no. Wear protective gear: __ yes, __ no.
Clean stethoscope: __ yes, __ no. Oral care: __ yes, __ no. Suctioned: __ yes, __ no.
Repositioned: ___ yes, ___ no. Turned to: ___ left, ___ right, ___ backside ___.
Head of bed at: ________ degrees. Incontinence/skin breakdown: ____ yes, ____ no.
Linens wet or soiled: ____ yes, ____ no. Linens changed: ____ yes, ____ no.
Dressing changed: ____ yes, ____ no. Location: ____________________.
IV site checked: _____ yes, _____ no. IV tubing labeled: _____ yes, _____no.
IV fluids at: ________________________________.
Pain level (0-10 scale.0-no pain, 10 intolerable): ________________.
Location of pain: ____________. Medicated for pain: _____ yes, ____ no.
Patient is alert/oriented: ____ yes, ____ no. New confusion: ____ yes, ____ no.
Vital signs: temp ____, pulse ____, resp _____, b/p _____, 02 _____ %, ____ liters.
Glucose level: _____. Insulin: ___ yes, ___ no. Type: ____________ # of units ____.

NURSING CARE FOR ______________________________

DATE ____________________, DAY NUMBER ________________

INITIAL NIGHT SHIFT EXAM:

My nurse has _____ # of patients. CNA ___yes, ___no. Charge nurse ____________
Nurse ______________ RN/LPN came in at __________ am/pm. Left at __________ am/pm.
Did nurse wash hands and wear gloves before touching patient: _______ yes, _______ no.
Wash hands after touching patient and before leaving the room: _______ yes, _______ no.
Don't hesitate to request staff to wash their hands. This will help decrease the risk of spreading potentially lethal germs.
Did nurse wear protective gear (isolation precautions only): _______ yes, _______ no.
Did nurse provide oral care (to be done every two hours if unable to provide for self, also decreases risk of pneumonia, infections, and aspiration): _______ yes, _______ no.
If able to provide own oral care, then supplies at bedside: _______ yes, _______ no.
Was patient repositioned (every two hours if unable to turn self): _______ yes _____ no.
Head of bed at __________ degrees. This is important for patients on ventilators or on tube feedings. Anything less than thirty degrees places patients at risk for aspiration of stomach contents into the lungs causing aspiration pneumonia.
Checked for incontinence and skin breakdown: ____ yes, ____ no.
Patient's linens wet or soiled: _____ yes, ____ no. Linens changed: ____ yes, ____ no.
Time linens changed: _______ am/pm. Any skin redness or breakdown: ____ yes, ____ no.
If yes, what stage is pressure ulcer: _______. Acquired when: ______________.
List wounds not associated with pressure ulcers and how acquired: ______________
____
Mattress type: ____
Specialty mattresses are important to help prevent pressure ulcers)
If patient on ventilator or has tracheostomy, suction performed: ____ yes, _____ no.
Did nurse listen to lung sounds: _____ yes, _______ no.
Does patient have chest tubes: ____ yes, ____ no. Functioning _____ yes, _____ no.
Bowel sounds: _______ yes, _______ no. Bowel sounds active: _____ yes, _____ no.
Neurological exam: ______ yes, ______ no. Follow commands: ______ yes, ______ no.
Is patient alert and oriented to person, place, time, and events: ____ yes, ____ no.
If confused, patient is not oriented to: ___ person, ___ place, ___ time, ___ event.
Confusion began (time and date): ____.
Glasgow coma scale (checks conscious scale of patient): _______________________.
Intracranial pressure monitoring: ____ yes, ____ no.
If yes, pressure is at ________ mm mercury. (Normal is one to fifteen).
Moves extremities: ___ yes, ___ no.
Paralysis: (inability to move extremities) _______ yes, _______ no.
If yes, extremities affected and when paralysis began: ________________________.
Is patient in pain: ____ yes, ____ no. Describe pain and location ______________.
Patient able to eat: _____ yes, _____ no. What type of diet? __________________.
If patient on tube feedings list type: __________ at _________ cc/ml per hour.
Nausea ____, vomiting ____. If so, describe: __________________________________.
Patient has: Nasal gastric tube ______, Dobhoff tube _____, Peg or gastric tube _____.
When was feeding tube placed and what site: ___________________________________.
Catheter for draining urine: ____ yes, ____ no. If so, when placed: ___________.
Find out policy for allowed time to remain in bladder. Too long may cause infections.)
IV site(s) where: ____________________ when placed: ___________________________.
IV fluids (types and rates): ____,
____________________, ____________________, ____________________, ____________.
Is patient on oxygen: _____ yes, _____ no. If so, how much and route delivered (see oxygen routes): ____.
If patient on ventilator, list settings (see list on ventilator settings): ________
____.
Vital signs: temp ______, pulse ______, resp ______, b/p ______, o2 ______%,
current weight ______ pounds, ______ kg. Glucose level: ______
Insulin coverage: ____ yes, ____ no. Insulin type: ____________, # of units: ______.

NURSING CARE CONTINUED FOR ____________________
DATE ____________________, DAY NUMBER ____________________

FOLLOWING EXAMINATIONS FOR NIGHT SHIFT:

Nurse ______________, CNA ____________, in at _____ am/pm. Left at ______ am/pm.
Wash hands and wear gloves before touching patient: ______ yes, ______ no.
Wash hands before leaving room: ___ yes, ___ no. Wear protective gear: __ yes, __ no.
Clean stethoscope: __ yes, __ no. Oral care: __ yes, __ no. Suctioned: __ yes, __ no.
Repositioned: ___ yes, ___ no. Turned to: ___ left, ___ right, ___ backside ___.
Head of bed at: _______ degrees. Incontinence/skin breakdown: ____ yes, ____ no.
Linens wet or soiled: _____ yes, _____ no. Linens changed: _____ yes, ______ no.
Dressing changed: ____ yes, ____ no. Location: ____________________.
IV site checked: _____ yes, _____ no. IV tubing labeled: _____ yes, _____no.
IV fluids at: ______________________________.
Pain level (0-10 scale.0-no pain, 10 intolerable): ____________.
Location of pain: ____________. Medicated for pain: _____ yes, ____ no.
Patient is alert/oriented: ____ yes, ____ no. New confusion: ____ yes, ____ no.
Vital signs: temp ____, pulse _____, resp _____, b/p ______, 02 _____ %, ____ liters.
Glucose level: _____. Insulin: ___ yes, ___ no. Type: __________ # of units ____.

Nurse ______________, CNA ____________, in at _____ am/pm. Left at ______ am/pm.
Wash hands and wear gloves before touching patient: ______ yes, ______ no.
Wash hands before leaving room: ___ yes, ___ no. Wear protective gear: __ yes, __ no.
Clean stethoscope: __ yes, __ no. Oral care: __ yes, __ no. Suctioned: __ yes, __ no.
Repositioned: ___ yes, ___ no. Turned to: ___ left, ___ right, ___ backside ___.
Head of bed at: _______ degrees. Incontinence/skin breakdown: ____ yes, ____ no.
Linens wet or soiled: _____ yes, _____ no. Linens changed: _____ yes, ______ no.
Dressing changed: ____ yes, ____ no. Location: ____________________.
IV site checked: _____ yes, _____ no. IV tubing labeled: _____ yes, _____no.
IV fluids at: ______________________________.
Pain level (0-10 scale.0-no pain, 10 intolerable): ____________.
Location of pain: ____________. Medicated for pain: _____ yes, ____ no.
Patient is alert/oriented: ____ yes, ____ no. New confusion: ____ yes, ____ no.
Vital signs: temp ____, pulse _____, resp _____, b/p ______, 02 _____ %, ____ liters.
Glucose level: _____. Insulin: ___ yes, ___ no. Type: __________ # of units ____.

Nurse ______________, CNA ____________, in at _____ am/pm. Left at ______ am/pm.
Wash hands and wear gloves before touching patient: ______ yes, ______ no.
Wash hands before leaving room: ___ yes, ___ no. Wear protective gear: __ yes, __ no.
Clean stethoscope: __ yes, __ no. Oral care: __ yes, __ no. Suctioned: __ yes, __ no.
Repositioned: ___ yes, ___ no. Turned to: ___ left, ___ right, ___ backside ___.
Head of bed at: _______ degrees. Incontinence/skin breakdown: ____ yes, ____ no.
Linens wet or soiled: _____ yes, _____ no. Linens changed: _____ yes, ______ no.
Dressing changed: ____ yes, ____ no. Location: ____________________.
IV site checked: _____ yes, _____ no. IV tubing labeled: _____ yes, _____no.
IV fluids at: ______________________________.
Pain level (0-10 scale.0-no pain, 10 intolerable): ____________.
Location of pain: ____________. Medicated for pain: _____ yes, ____ no.
Patient is alert/oriented: ____ yes, ____ no. New confusion: ____ yes, ____ no.
Vital signs: temp ____, pulse _____, resp _____, b/p ______, 02 _____ %, ____ liters.
Glucose level: _____. Insulin: ___ yes, ___ no. Type: __________ # of units ____.

NURSING CARE CONTINUED FOR ______________________
DATE ____________________, DAY NUMBER ______________

FOLLOWING EXAMINATIONS FOR NIGHT SHIFT:

Nurse ______________, CNA ______________, in at _____ am/pm. Left at _______ am/pm.
Wash hands and wear gloves before touching patient: ________ yes, ________ no.
Wash hands before leaving room: ___ yes, ___ no. Wear protective gear: __ yes, __ no.
Clean stethoscope: __ yes, __ no. Oral care: __ yes, __ no. Suctioned: __ yes, __ no.
Repositioned: ___ yes, ___ no. Turned to: ___ left, ___ right, ___ backside ___.
Head of bed at: _______ degrees. Incontinence/skin breakdown: ____ yes, ____ no.
Linens wet or soiled: _____ yes, _____ no. Linens changed: _____ yes, _____ no.
Dressing changed: ____ yes, ____ no. Location: ______________________________.
IV site checked: _____ yes, _____ no. IV tubing labeled: _____ yes, _____no.
IV fluids at: ____.
Pain level (0-10 scale.0-no pain, 10 intolerable): ___________________________.
Location of pain: ________________. Medicated for pain: _____ yes, ____ no.
Patient is alert/oriented: ____ yes, ____ no. New confusion: ____ yes, ____ no.
Vital signs: temp ____, pulse ____, resp _____, b/p _____, 02 _____ %, ____ liters.
Glucose level: _____. Insulin: ___ yes, ___ no. Type: _____________ # of units ____.

Nurse ______________, CNA ______________, in at _____ am/pm. Left at _______ am/pm.
Wash hands and wear gloves before touching patient: ________ yes, ________ no.
Wash hands before leaving room: ___ yes, ___ no. Wear protective gear: __ yes, __ no.
Clean stethoscope: __ yes, __ no. Oral care: __ yes, __ no. Suctioned: __ yes, __ no.
Repositioned: ___ yes, ___ no. Turned to: ___ left, ___ right, ___ backside ___.
Head of bed at: _______ degrees. Incontinence/skin breakdown: ____ yes, ____ no.
Linens wet or soiled: _____ yes, _____ no. Linens changed: _____ yes, _____ no.
Dressing changed: ____ yes, ____ no. Location: ______________________________.
IV site checked: _____ yes, _____ no. IV tubing labeled: _____ yes, _____no.
IV fluids at: ____.
Pain level (0-10 scale.0-no pain, 10 intolerable): ___________________________.
Location of pain: ________________. Medicated for pain: _____ yes, ____ no.
Patient is alert/oriented: ____ yes, ____ no. New confusion: ____ yes, ____ no.
Vital signs: temp ____, pulse ____, resp _____, b/p _____, 02 _____ %, ____ liters.
Glucose level: _____. Insulin: ___ yes, ___ no. Type: _____________ # of units ____.

Nurse ______________, CNA ______________, in at _____ am/pm. Left at _______ am/pm.
Wash hands and wear gloves before touching patient: ________ yes, ________ no.
Wash hands before leaving room: ___ yes, ___ no. Wear protective gear: __ yes, __ no.
Clean stethoscope: __ yes, __ no. Oral care: __ yes, __ no. Suctioned: __ yes, __ no.
Repositioned: ___ yes, ___ no. Turned to: ___ left, ___ right, ___ backside ___.
Head of bed at: _______ degrees. Incontinence/skin breakdown: ____ yes, ____ no.
Linens wet or soiled: _____ yes, _____ no. Linens changed: _____ yes, _____ no.
Dressing changed: ____ yes, ____ no. Location: ______________________________.
IV site checked: _____ yes, _____ no. IV tubing labeled: _____ yes, _____no.
IV fluids at: ____.
Pain level (0-10 scale.0-no pain, 10 intolerable): ___________________________.
Location of pain: ________________. Medicated for pain: _____ yes, ____ no.
Patient is alert/oriented: ____ yes, ____ no. New confusion: ____ yes, ____ no.
Vital signs: temp ____, pulse ____, resp _____, b/p _____, 02 _____ %, ____ liters.
Glucose level: _____. Insulin: ___ yes, ___ no. Type: _____________ # of units ____.

MEDICATION ADMINISTRATION LIST FOR ____________________
DATE ________________ DAY NUMBER ________________

List the medication for each day. Routes of administration: oral, thru feeding tube, intravenous (IV), intramuscular (IM), subcutaneous (SQ), epidural or a catheter in your spinal column, rectal, topical, eye drops, and ear drops.

Medication: ____________ Route: ____________ Time: ____________
Medication: ____________ Route: ____________ Time: ____________
Medication: ____________ Route: ____________ Time: ____________
Medication: ____________ Route: ____________ Time: ____________
Medication: ____________ Route: ____________ Time: ____________
Medication: ____________ Route: ____________ Time: ____________
Medication: ____________ Route: ____________ Time: ____________
Medication: ____________ Route: ____________ Time: ____________
Medication: ____________ Route: ____________ Time: ____________
Medication: ____________ Route: ____________ Time: ____________
Medication: ____________ Route: ____________ Time: ____________
Medication: ____________ Route: ____________ Time: ____________
Medication: ____________ Route: ____________ Time: ____________
Medication: ____________ Route: ____________ Time: ____________
Medication: ____________ Route: ____________ Time: ____________
Medication: ____________ Route: ____________ Time: ____________
Medication: ____________ Route: ____________ Time: ____________
Medication: ____________ Route: ____________ Time: ____________
Medication: ____________ Route: ____________ Time: ____________
Medication: ____________ Route: ____________ Time: ____________
Medication: ____________ Route: ____________ Time: ____________
Medication: ____________ Route: ____________ Time: ____________
Medication: ____________ Route: ____________ Time: ____________
Medication: ____________ Route: ____________ Time: ____________
Medication: ____________ Route: ____________ Time: ____________
Medication: ____________ Route: ____________ Time: ____________
Medication: ____________ Route: ____________ Time: ____________
Medication: ____________ Route: ____________ Time: ____________
Medication: ____________ Route: ____________ Time: ____________
Medication: ____________ Route: ____________ Time: ____________
Medication: ____________ Route: ____________ Time: ____________
Medication: ____________ Route: ____________ Time: ____________
Medication: ____________ Route: ____________ Time: ____________
Medication: ____________ Route: ____________ Time: ____________
Medication: ____________ Route: ____________ Time: ____________
Medication: ____________ Route: ____________ Time: ____________
Medication: ____________ Route: ____________ Time: ____________
Medication: ____________ Route: ____________ Time: ____________
Medication: ____________ Route: ____________ Time: ____________
Medication: ____________ Route: ____________ Time: ____________
Medication: ____________ Route: ____________ Time: ____________
Medication: ____________ Route: ____________ Time: ____________
Medication: ____________ Route: ____________ Time: ____________
Medication: ____________ Route: ____________ Time: ____________
Medication: ____________ Route: ____________ Time: ____________
Medication: ____________ Route: ____________ Time: ____________
Medication: ____________ Route: ____________ Time: ____________
Medication: ____________ Route: ____________ Time: ____________
Medication: ____________ Route: ____________ Time: ____________
Medication: ____________ Route: ____________ Time: ____________
Medication: ____________ Route: ____________ Time: ____________
Medication: ____________ Route: ____________ Time: ____________
Medication: ____________ Route: ____________ Time: ____________
Medication: ____________ Route: ____________ Time: ____________

NOTES FOR DAY NUMBER ______________________

DATE ______________________________________

MEDICAL JOURNAL FOR ______________________________

DATE ____________________, DAY NUMBER ________________

VISITS FROM MY DOCTORS TODAY

Goals for today: ____

____

____.

Things to discuss with my doctor(s): _________________________________

____

____

Dr.______________ came in at _____ am/pm. Left at _____ am/pm.
We discussed ____.
Did doctor examine patient: _____ yes, _____ no.
Wash hands before touching patient: _____ yes, _____ no.
Wear gloves: ____ yes, ___ no. Clean stethoscope: ____ yes, ____ no.
Wear gown and mask (precautions only):____ yes, _____ no.
Wash hands before leaving the room: _____ yes, _____ no.

Dr.______________ came in at _____ am/pm. Left at _____ am/pm.
We discussed ____.
Did doctor examine patient: _____ yes, _____ no.
Wash hands before touching patient: _____ yes, _____ no.
Wear gloves: ____ yes, ___ no. Clean stethoscope: ____ yes, ____ no.
Wear gown and mask (precautions only):____ yes, _____ no.
Wash hands before leaving the room: _____ yes, _____ no.

Dr.______________ came in at _____ am/pm. Left at _____ am/pm.
We discussed ____.
Did doctor examine patient: _____ yes, _____ no.
Wash hands before touching patient: _____ yes, _____ no.
Wear gloves: ____ yes, ___ no. Clean stethoscope: ____ yes, ____ no.
Wear gown and mask (precautions only):____ yes, _____ no.
Wash hands before leaving the room: _____ yes, _____ no.

Dr.______________ came in at _____ am/pm. Left at _____ am/pm.
We discussed ____.
Did doctor examine patient: _____ yes, _____ no.
Wash hands before touching patient: _____ yes, _____ no.
Wear gloves: ____ yes, ___ no. Clean stethoscope: ____ yes, ____ no.
Wear gown and mask (precautions only):____ yes, _____ no.
Wash hands before leaving the room: _____ yes, _____ no.

Dr.______________ came in at _____ am/pm. Left at _____ am/pm.
We discussed ____.
Did doctor examine patient: _____ yes, _____ no.
Wash hands before touching patient: _____ yes, _____ no.
Wear gloves: ____ yes, ___ no. Clean stethoscope: ____ yes, ____ no.
Wear gown and mask (precautions only):____ yes, _____ no.
Wash hands before leaving the room: _____ yes, _____ no.

NURSING CARE FOR ________________________________

DATE ______________________, DAY NUMBER ______________________

INITIAL DAY SHIFT EXAM:

My nurse has ______ # of patients. CNA ___yes, ___no. Charge nurse ___________
Nurse _____________ RN/LPN came in at _________ am/pm. Left at _________ am/pm.
Did nurse wash hands and wear gloves before touching patient: _____ yes, _____ no.
Wash hands after touching patient and before leaving the room: _____ yes, _____ no.
Don't hesitate to request staff to wash their hands. This will help decrease the risk of spreading potentially lethal germs.
Did nurse wear protective gear (isolation precautions only): _______ yes, _____ no.
Did nurse provide oral care (to be done every two hours if unable to provide for self, also decreases risk of pneumonia, infections, and aspiration): _______ yes, _____ no.
If able to provide own oral care, then supplies at bedside: _______ yes, _____ no.
Was patient repositioned (every two hours if unable to turn self): _____ yes _____ no.
Head of bed at _________ degrees. This is important for patients on ventilators or on tube feedings. Anything less than thirty degrees places patients at risk for aspiration of stomach contents into the lungs causing aspiration pneumonia.
Checked for incontinence and skin breakdown: _____ yes, _____ no.
Patient's linens wet or soiled: _____ yes, ____ no. Linens changed: ____ yes, ____ no.
Time linens changed: ________ am/pm. Any skin redness or breakdown: ____ yes, ____ no.
If yes, what stage is pressure ulcer: ______. Acquired when: ________________.
List wounds not associated with pressure ulcers and how acquired: ______________
____.
Mattress type: ____.
Specialty mattresses are important to help prevent pressure ulcers)
If patient on ventilator or has tracheostomy, suction performed: ______ yes, _____ no.
Did nurse listen to lung sounds: _____ yes, _____ no.
Does patient have chest tubes: ____ yes, ____ no. Functioning _____ yes, _____ no.
Bowel sounds: ________ yes, ________ no. Bowel sounds active: _______ yes, _______ no.
Neurological exam: ______ yes, ______ no. Follow commands: _______ yes, _______ no.
Is patient alert and oriented to person, place, time, and events: _____ yes, _____ no.
If confused, patient is not oriented to: ___ person, ___ place, ___ time, ___ event.
Confusion began (time and date): ______________________________________.
Glasgow coma scale (checks conscious scale of patient): ________________________.
Intracranial pressure monitoring: _____ yes, _____ no.
If yes, pressure is at _________ mm mercury. (Normal is one to fifteen).
Moves extremities: ___ yes, ___ no.
Paralysis: (inability to move extremities) _______ yes, _______ no.
If yes, extremities affected and when paralysis began: _______________________.
Is patient in pain: ____ yes, ____ no. Describe pain and location _______________.
Patient able to eat: ____ yes, ____ no. What type of diet? ______________________.
If patient on tube feedings list type: ____________ at __________ cc/ml per hour.
Nausea ____, vomiting ____. If so, describe: ___________________________________.
Patient has: Nasal gastric tube _____, Dobhoff tube _____, Peg or gastric tube _____.
When was feeding tube placed and what site: ____________________________________.
Catheter for draining urine: ____ yes, ____ no. If so, when placed: _____________.
Find out policy for allowed time to remain in bladder. Too long may cause infections.)
IV site(s) where: _________________________ when placed: ________________________.
IV fluids (types and rates): _____________________________, _____________________,
_________________________, _______________________________, _____________________.
Is patient on oxygen: _____ yes, _____ no. If so, how much and route delivered (see oxygen routes): ____.
If patient on ventilator, list settings (see list on ventilator settings): ________
____.
Vital signs: temp ______, pulse ______, resp _____, b/p ______, o2 ______%,
current weight ______ pounds, ______ kg. Glucose level: ______
Insulin coverage: ____ yes, ____ no. Insulin type: ____________, # of units: _____.

NURSING CARE CONTINUED FOR ____________________________
DATE ____________________, DAY NUMBER ____________________

FOLLOWING EXAMINATIONS FOR DAY SHIFT:

Nurse ____________, CNA ____________, in at ______ am/pm. Left at ______ am/pm.
Wash hands and wear gloves before touching patient: ______ yes, ______ no.
Wash hands before leaving room: ___ yes, ___ no. Wear protective gear: __ yes, __ no.
Clean stethoscope: __ yes, __ no. Oral care: __ yes, __ no. Suctioned: __ yes, __ no.
Repositioned: ___ yes, ___ no. Turned to: ___ left, ___ right, backside ___.
Head of bed at: ______ degrees. Incontinence/skin breakdown: ____ yes, ____ no.
Linens wet or soiled: ____ yes, ____ no. Linens changed: _____ yes, ______ no.
Dressing changed: ____ yes, ____ no. Location: ______________________.
IV site checked: _____ yes, _____ no. IV tubing labeled: _____ yes, _____no.
IV fluids at: ____.
Pain level (0-10 scale.0-no pain, 10 intolerable): ____________________.
Location of pain: _______________. Medicated for pain: ____ yes, ____ no.
Patient is alert/oriented: ____ yes, ____ no. New confusion: ____ yes, ____ no.
Vital signs: temp ____, pulse ____, resp _____, b/p _____, 02 _____ %, ____ liters.
Glucose level: _____. Insulin: ___ yes, ___ no. Type: __________ # of units ___.

Nurse ____________, CNA ____________, in at ______ am/pm. Left at ______ am/pm.
Wash hands and wear gloves before touching patient: ______ yes, ______ no.
Wash hands before leaving room: ___ yes, ___ no. Wear protective gear: __ yes, __ no.
Clean stethoscope: __ yes, __ no. Oral care: __ yes, __ no. Suctioned: __ yes, __ no.
Repositioned: ___ yes, ___ no. Turned to: ___ left, ___ right, backside ___.
Head of bed at: ______ degrees. Incontinence/skin breakdown: ____ yes, ____ no.
Linens wet or soiled: ____ yes, ____ no. Linens changed: _____ yes, ______ no.
Dressing changed: ____ yes, ____ no. Location: ______________________.
IV site checked: _____ yes, _____ no. IV tubing labeled: _____ yes, _____no.
IV fluids at: ____.
Pain level (0-10 scale.0-no pain, 10 intolerable): ____________________.
Location of pain: _______________. Medicated for pain: ____ yes, ____ no.
Patient is alert/oriented: ____ yes, ____ no. New confusion: ____ yes, ____ no.
Vital signs: temp ____, pulse ____, resp _____, b/p _____, 02 _____ %, ____ liters.
Glucose level: _____. Insulin: ___ yes, ___ no. Type: __________ # of units ___.

Nurse ____________, CNA ____________, in at ______ am/pm. Left at ______ am/pm.
Wash hands and wear gloves before touching patient: ______ yes, ______ no.
Wash hands before leaving room: ___ yes, ___ no. Wear protective gear: __ yes, __ no.
Clean stethoscope: __ yes, __ no. Oral care: __ yes, __ no. Suctioned: __ yes, __ no.
Repositioned: ___ yes, ___ no. Turned to: ___ left, ___ right, backside ___.
Head of bed at: ______ degrees. Incontinence/skin breakdown: ____ yes, ____ no.
Linens wet or soiled: ____ yes, ____ no. Linens changed: _____ yes, ______ no.
Dressing changed: ____ yes, ____ no. Location: ______________________.
IV site checked: _____ yes, _____ no. IV tubing labeled: _____ yes, _____no.
IV fluids at: ____.
Pain level (0-10 scale.0-no pain, 10 intolerable): ____________________.
Location of pain: _______________. Medicated for pain: ____ yes, ____ no.
Patient is alert/oriented: ____ yes, ____ no. New confusion: ____ yes, ____ no.
Vital signs: temp ____, pulse ____, resp _____, b/p _____, 02 _____ %, ____ liters.
Glucose level: _____. Insulin: ___ yes, ___ no. Type: __________ # of units ___.

NURSING CARE CONTINUED FOR ______________________________
DATE ____________________, DAY NUMBER ____________________

FOLLOWING EXAMINATIONS FOR DAY SHIFT:

Nurse _____________, CNA _____________, in at _____ am/pm. Left at ______ am/pm.
Wash hands and wear gloves before touching patient: ______ yes, ______ no.
Wash hands before leaving room: ___ yes, ___ no. Wear protective gear: __ yes, __ no.
Clean stethoscope: __ yes, __ no. Oral care: __ yes, __ no. Suctioned: __ yes, __ no.
Repositioned: ___ yes, ___ no. Turned to: ___ left, ___ right, ___ backside ___.
Head of bed at: _______ degrees. Incontinence/skin breakdown: ____ yes, ____ no.
Linens wet or soiled: ____ yes, ____ no. Linens changed: _____ yes, _____ no.
Dressing changed: ____ yes, ____ no. Location: ____________________.
IV site checked: _____ yes, _____ no. IV tubing labeled: ____ yes, ____no.
IV fluids at: ____.
Pain level (0-10 scale.0-no pain, 10 intolerable): ____________.
Location of pain: ______________. Medicated for pain: ____ yes, ____ no.
Patient is alert/oriented: ____ yes, ____ no. New confusion: ____ yes, ____ no.
Vital signs: temp ____, pulse ____, resp ____, b/p ______, 02 _____ %, ____ liters.
Glucose level: _____. Insulin: ___ yes, ___ no. Type: __________ # of units ____.

Nurse _____________, CNA _____________, in at _____ am/pm. Left at ______ am/pm.
Wash hands and wear gloves before touching patient: ______ yes, ______ no.
Wash hands before leaving room: ___ yes, ___ no. Wear protective gear: __ yes, __ no.
Clean stethoscope: __ yes, __ no. Oral care: __ yes, __ no. Suctioned: __ yes, __ no.
Repositioned: ___ yes, ___ no. Turned to: ___ left, ___ right, ___ backside ___.
Head of bed at: _______ degrees. Incontinence/skin breakdown: ____ yes, ____ no.
Linens wet or soiled: ____ yes, ____ no. Linens changed: _____ yes, _____ no.
Dressing changed: ____ yes, ____ no. Location: ____________________.
IV site checked: _____ yes, _____ no. IV tubing labeled: _____ yes, ____no.
IV fluids at: ____.
Pain level (0-10 scale.0-no pain, 10 intolerable): ____________.
Location of pain: ______________. Medicated for pain: ____ yes, ____ no.
Patient is alert/oriented: ____ yes, ____ no. New confusion: ____ yes, ____ no.
Vital signs: temp ____, pulse ____, resp ____, b/p ______, 02 _____ %, ____ liters.
Glucose level: _____. Insulin: ___ yes, ___ no. Type: __________ # of units ____.

Nurse _____________, CNA _____________, in at _____ am/pm. Left at ______ am/pm.
Wash hands and wear gloves before touching patient: ______ yes, ______ no.
Wash hands before leaving room: ___ yes, ___ no. Wear protective gear: __ yes, __ no.
Clean stethoscope: __ yes, __ no. Oral care: __ yes, __ no. Suctioned: __ yes, __ no.
Repositioned: ___ yes, ___ no. Turned to: ___ left, ___ right, ___ backside ___.
Head of bed at: _______ degrees. Incontinence/skin breakdown: ____ yes, ____ no.
Linens wet or soiled: ____ yes, ____ no. Linens changed: _____ yes, _____ no.
Dressing changed: ____ yes, ____ no. Location: ____________________.
IV site checked: _____ yes, _____ no. IV tubing labeled: ____ yes, ____no.
IV fluids at: ____.
Pain level (0-10 scale.0-no pain, 10 intolerable): ____________.
Location of pain: ______________. Medicated for pain: ____ yes, ____ no.
Patient is alert/oriented: ____ yes, ____ no. New confusion: ____ yes, ____ no.
Vital signs: temp ____, pulse ____, resp ____, b/p ______, 02 _____ %, ____ liters.
Glucose level: _____. Insulin: ___ yes, ___ no. Type: __________ # of units ____.

NURSING CARE FOR ____________________________

DATE __________________, DAY NUMBER ____________________

INITIAL NIGHT SHIFT EXAM:

My nurse has ______ # of patients. CNA ___yes, ___no. Charge nurse _______________
Nurse _______________ RN/LPN came in at _________ am/pm. Left at __________ am/pm.
Did nurse wash hands and wear gloves before touching patient: ______ yes, ______ no.
Wash hands after touching patient and before leaving the room: ______ yes, ______ no.
Don't hesitate to request staff to wash their hands. This will help decrease the risk of spreading potentially lethal germs.
Did nurse wear protective gear (isolation precautions only): ______ yes, ______ no.
Did nurse provide oral care (to be done every two hours if unable to provide for self, also decreases risk of pneumonia, infections, and aspiration): ______ yes, ______ no.
If able to provide own oral care, then supplies at bedside: _______ yes, ________ no.
Was patient repositioned (every two hours if unable to turn self): _____ yes _____ no.
Head of bed at ________ degrees. This is important for patients on ventilators or on tube feedings. Anything less than thirty degrees places patients at risk for aspiration of stomach contents into the lungs causing aspiration pneumonia.
Checked for incontinence and skin breakdown: _____ yes, _____ no.
Patient's linens wet or soiled: _____ yes, ____ no. Linens changed: ____ yes, ____ no.
Time linens changed: ________ am/pm. Any skin redness or breakdown: ____ yes, ____ no.
If yes, what stage is pressure ulcer: ________. Acquired when: __________________.
List wounds not associated with pressure ulcers and how acquired: _______________
____.
Mattress type: ____.
Specialty mattresses are important to help prevent pressure ulcers)
If patient on ventilator or has tracheostomy, suction performed: _____ yes, ______ no.
Did nurse listen to lung sounds: _____ yes, _____ no.
Does patient have chest tubes: ____ yes, ____ no. Functioning _____ yes, ______ no.
Bowel sounds: _______ yes, _______ no. Bowel sounds active: ______ yes, _______ no.
Neurological exam: ______ yes, ______ no. Follow commands: _______ yes, _______ no.
Is patient alert and oriented to person, place, time, and events: _____ yes, _____ no.
If confused, patient is not oriented to: ____ person, ___ place, ___ time, ___ event.
Confusion began (time and date): _______________________________________.
Glasgow coma scale (checks conscious scale of patient): ____________________.
Intracranial pressure monitoring: _____ yes, ______ no.
If yes, pressure is at ________ mm mercury. (Normal is one to fifteen).
Moves extremities: ___ yes, ___ no.
Paralysis: (inability to move extremities) ________ yes, _______ no.
If yes, extremities affected and when paralysis began: ______________________
Is patient in pain: ____ yes, ____ no. Describe pain and location ______________
Patient able to eat: ____ yes, ____ no. What type of diet? ____________________
If patient on tube feedings list type: ____________ at ____________ cc/ml per hour.
Nausea ____, vomiting ____. If so, describe: ___________________________________.
Patient has: Nasal gastric tube ______, Dobhoff tube _____, Peg or gastric tube ____.
When was feeding tube placed and what site: _______________________________.
Catheter for draining urine: ____ yes, ____ no. If so, when placed: ____________.
Find out policy for allowed time to remain in bladder. Too long may cause infections.)
IV site(s) where: _____________________ when placed: ______________.
IV fluids (types and rates): ______________, ________________________,
__________________, ________________, ______________________.
Is patient on oxygen: _____ yes, _____ no. If so, how much and route delivered (see oxygen routes): ____.
If patient on ventilator, list settings (see list on ventilator settings): __________
____.
Vital signs: temp _____, pulse _____, resp _____, b/p _____, o2 _____%,
current weight _____ pounds, _____ kg. Glucose level: _____
Insulin coverage: ____ yes, ____ no. Insulin type: ___________, # of units: _____.

NURSING CARE CONTINUED FOR ______________________
DATE ____________________, DAY NUMBER ____________

FOLLOWING EXAMINATIONS FOR NIGHT SHIFT:

Nurse ____________, CNA ____________, in at ______ am/pm. Left at _______ am/pm.
Wash hands and wear gloves before touching patient: ______ yes, ______ no.
Wash hands before leaving room: ___ yes, ___ no. Wear protective gear: ___ yes, __ no.
Clean stethoscope: __ yes, __ no. Oral care: __ yes, __ no. Suctioned: __ yes, __ no.
Repositioned: ___ yes, ___ no. Turned to: ___ left, ___ right, ___ backside ___.
Head of bed at: _____ degrees. Incontinence/skin breakdown: ____ yes, ____ no.
Linens wet or soiled: ____ yes, ____ no. Linens changed: ____ yes, ____ no.
Dressing changed: ____ yes, ____ no. Location: ____________________________.
IV site checked: _____ yes, _____ no. IV tubing labeled: _____ yes, ___no.
IV fluids at: ____.
Pain level (0-10 scale.0-no pain, 10 intolerable): ________________________.
Location of pain: ______________. Medicated for pain: _____ yes, ____ no.
Patient is alert/oriented: ____ yes, ____ no. New confusion: ____ yes, ____ no.
Vital signs: temp ____, pulse ____, resp ______, b/p ______, 02 _____ %, ____ liters.
Glucose level: ____. Insulin: ___ yes, ___ no. Type: ____________ # of units ____.

Nurse ____________, CNA ____________, in at ______ am/pm. Left at _______ am/pm.
Wash hands and wear gloves before touching patient: ______ yes, ______ no.
Wash hands before leaving room: ___ yes, ___ no. Wear protective gear: ___ yes, __ no.
Clean stethoscope: __ yes, __ no. Oral care: __ yes, __ no. Suctioned: __ yes, __ no.
Repositioned: ___ yes, ___ no. Turned to: ___ left, ___ right, ___ backside ___.
Head of bed at: _____ degrees. Incontinence/skin breakdown: ____ yes, ____ no.
Linens wet or soiled: ____ yes, ____ no. Linens changed: ____ yes, ____ no.
Dressing changed: ____ yes, ____ no. Location: ____________________________.
IV site checked: _____ yes, _____ no. IV tubing labeled: _____ yes, ___ no.
IV fluids at: ____.
Pain level (0-10 scale.0-no pain, 10 intolerable): ________________________.
Location of pain: ______________. Medicated for pain: _____ yes, ____ no.
Patient is alert/oriented: ____ yes, ____ no. New confusion: ____ yes, ____ no.
Vital signs: temp ____, pulse ____, resp ______, b/p ______, 02 _____ %, ____ liters.
Glucose level: ____. Insulin: ___ yes, ___ no. Type: ____________ # of units ____.

Nurse ____________, CNA ____________, in at ______ am/pm. Left at _______ am/pm.
Wash hands and wear gloves before touching patient: ______ yes, ______ no.
Wash hands before leaving room: ___ yes, ___ no. Wear protective gear: ___ yes, __ no.
Clean stethoscope: __ yes, __ no. Oral care: __ yes, __ no. Suctioned: __ yes, __ no.
Repositioned: ___ yes, ___ no. Turned to: ___ left, ___ right, ___ backside ___.
Head of bed at: _____ degrees. Incontinence/skin breakdown: ____ yes, ____ no.
Linens wet or soiled: ____ yes, ____ no. Linens changed: ____ yes, ____ no.
Dressing changed: ____ yes, ____ no. Location: ____________________________.
IV site checked: _____ yes, _____ no. IV tubing labeled: _____ yes, ___no.
IV fluids at: ____.
Pain level (0-10 scale.0-no pain, 10 intolerable): ________________________.
Location of pain: ______________. Medicated for pain: _____ yes, ____ no.
Patient is alert/oriented: ____ yes, ____ no. New confusion: ____ yes, ____ no.
Vital signs: temp ____, pulse ____, resp ______, b/p ______, 02 _____ %, ____ liters.
Glucose level: ____. Insulin: ___ yes, ___ no. Type: ____________ # of units ____.

NURSING CARE CONTINUED FOR ____________________
DATE ____________________, DAY NUMBER ____________________

FOLLOWING EXAMINATIONS FOR NIGHT SHIFT:

Nurse ______________, CNA ______________, in at _____ am/pm. Left at _______ am/pm.
Wash hands and wear gloves before touching patient: _______ yes, _______ no.
Wash hands before leaving room: ___ yes, ___ no. Wear protective gear: __ yes, __ no.
Clean stethoscope: __ yes, __ no. Oral care: __ yes, __ no. Suctioned: __ yes, __ no.
Repositioned: ___ yes, ___ no. Turned to: ___ left, ___ right, ___ backside ___.
Head of bed at: _______ degrees. Incontinence/skin breakdown: ____ yes, ____ no.
Linens wet or soiled: _____ yes, _____ no. Linens changed: _____ yes, ______ no.
Dressing changed: ____ yes, ____ no. Location: ____________________.
IV site checked: _____ yes, _____ no. IV tubing labeled: _____ yes, _____no.
IV fluids at: ____________________.
Pain level (0-10 scale.0-no pain, 10 intolerable): ____________.
Location of pain: ____________. Medicated for pain: ____ yes, ____ no.
Patient is alert/oriented: ____ yes, ___ no. New confusion: ____ yes, ____ no.
Vital signs: temp ____, pulse ____, resp _____, b/p _____, 02 _____ %, ____ liters.
Glucose level: _____. Insulin: ___ yes, ___ no. Type: ___________ # of units ____.

Nurse ______________, CNA ______________, in at _____ am/pm. Left at _______ am/pm.
Wash hands and wear gloves before touching patient: _______ yes, _______ no.
Wash hands before leaving room: ___ yes, ___ no. Wear protective gear: __ yes, __ no.
Clean stethoscope: __ yes, __ no. Oral care: __ yes, __ no. Suctioned: __ yes, __ no.
Repositioned: ___ yes, ___ no. Turned to: ___ left, ___ right, ___ backside ___.
Head of bed at: _______ degrees. Incontinence/skin breakdown: ____ yes, ____ no.
Linens wet or soiled: _____ yes, _____ no. Linens changed: _____ yes, ______ no.
Dressing changed: ____ yes, ____ no. Location: ____________________.
IV site checked: _____ yes, _____ no. IV tubing labeled: _____ yes, _____no.
IV fluids at: ____________________.
Pain level (0-10 scale.0-no pain, 10 intolerable): ____________.
Location of pain: ____________. Medicated for pain: ____ yes, ____ no.
Patient is alert/oriented: ____ yes, ___ no. New confusion: ____ yes, ____ no.
Vital signs: temp ____, pulse ____, resp _____, b/p _____, 02 _____ %, ____ liters.
Glucose level: _____. Insulin: ___ yes, ___ no. Type: ___________ # of units ____.

Nurse ______________, CNA ______________, in at _____ am/pm. Left at _______ am/pm.
Wash hands and wear gloves before touching patient: _______ yes, _______ no.
Wash hands before leaving room: ___ yes, ___ no. Wear protective gear: __ yes, __ no.
Clean stethoscope: __ yes, __ no. Oral care: __ yes, __ no. Suctioned: __ yes, __ no.
Repositioned: ___ yes, ___ no. Turned to: ___ left, ___ right, ___ backside ___.
Head of bed at: _______ degrees. Incontinence/skin breakdown: ____ yes, ____ no.
Linens wet or soiled: _____ yes, _____ no. Linens changed: _____ yes, ______ no.
Dressing changed: ____ yes, ____ no. Location: ____________________.
IV site checked: _____ yes, _____ no. IV tubing labeled: _____ yes, _____no.
IV fluids at: ____________________.
Pain level (0-10 scale.0-no pain, 10 intolerable): ____________.
Location of pain: ____________. Medicated for pain: ____ yes, ____ no.
Patient is alert/oriented: ____ yes, ___ no. New confusion: ____ yes, ____ no.
Vital signs: temp ____, pulse ____, resp _____, b/p _____, 02 _____ %, ____ liters.
Glucose level: _____. Insulin: ___ yes, ___ no. Type: ___________ # of units ____.

MEDICATION ADMINISTRATION LIST FOR ____________________
DATE ________________ DAY NUMBER ____________________

List the medication for each day. Routes of administration: oral, thru feeding tube, intravenous (IV), intramuscular (IM), subcutaneous (SQ), epidural or a catheter in your spinal column, rectal, topical, eye drops, and ear drops.

Medication: ______________ Route: ______________ Time: ____________
Medication: ______________ Route: ______________ Time: ____________
Medication: ______________ Route: ______________ Time: ____________
Medication: ______________ Route: ______________ Time: ____________
Medication: ______________ Route: ______________ Time: ____________
Medication: ______________ Route: ______________ Time: ____________
Medication: ______________ Route: ______________ Time: ____________
Medication: ______________ Route: ______________ Time: ____________
Medication: ______________ Route: ______________ Time: ____________
Medication: ______________ Route: ______________ Time: ____________
Medication: ______________ Route: ______________ Time: ____________
Medication: ______________ Route: ______________ Time: ____________
Medication: ______________ Route: ______________ Time: ____________
Medication: ______________ Route: ______________ Time: ____________
Medication: ______________ Route: ______________ Time: ____________
Medication: ______________ Route: ______________ Time: ____________
Medication: ______________ Route: ______________ Time: ____________
Medication: ______________ Route: ______________ Time: ____________
Medication: ______________ Route: ______________ Time: ____________
Medication: ______________ Route: ______________ Time: ____________
Medication: ______________ Route: ______________ Time: ____________
Medication: ______________ Route: ______________ Time: ____________
Medication: ______________ Route: ______________ Time: ____________
Medication: ______________ Route: ______________ Time: ____________
Medication: ______________ Route: ______________ Time: ____________
Medication: ______________ Route: ______________ Time: ____________
Medication: ______________ Route: ______________ Time: ____________
Medication: ______________ Route: ______________ Time: ____________
Medication: ______________ Route: ______________ Time: ____________
Medication: ______________ Route: ______________ Time: ____________
Medication: ______________ Route: ______________ Time: ____________
Medication: ______________ Route: ______________ Time: ____________
Medication: ______________ Route: ______________ Time: ____________
Medication: ______________ Route: ______________ Time: ____________
Medication: ______________ Route: ______________ Time: ____________
Medication: ______________ Route: ______________ Time: ____________
Medication: ______________ Route: ______________ Time: ____________
Medication: ______________ Route: ______________ Time: ____________
Medication: ______________ Route: ______________ Time: ____________
Medication: ______________ Route: ______________ Time: ____________
Medication: ______________ Route: ______________ Time: ____________
Medication: ______________ Route: ______________ Time: ____________
Medication: ______________ Route: ______________ Time: ____________
Medication: ______________ Route: ______________ Time: ____________
Medication: ______________ Route: ______________ Time: ____________
Medication: ______________ Route: ______________ Time: ____________
Medication: ______________ Route: ______________ Time: ____________
Medication: ______________ Route: ______________ Time: ____________
Medication: ______________ Route: ______________ Time: ____________
Medication: ______________ Route: ______________ Time: ____________
Medication: ______________ Route: ______________ Time: ____________
Medication: ______________ Route: ______________ Time: ____________
Medication: ______________ Route: ______________ Time: ____________
Medication: ______________ Route: ______________ Time: ____________

NOTES FOR DAY NUMBER ____________________

DATE ____________________

MEDICAL JOURNAL FOR ______________________

DATE ____________________, DAY NUMBER ____________

VISITS FROM MY DOCTORS TODAY

Goals for today: ______________________________________

____

____

Things to discuss with my doctor(s): ___________________

____

____

Dr.____________ came in at _____ am/pm. Left at _____ am/pm.
We discussed ____.
Did doctor examine patient: _____ yes, _____ no.
Wash hands before touching patient: _____ yes, _____ no.
Wear gloves: ____ yes, ___ no. Clean stethoscope: ____ yes, ____ no.
Wear gown and mask (precautions only):____ yes, _____ no.
Wash hands before leaving the room: _____ yes, _____ no.

Dr.____________ came in at _____ am/pm. Left at _____ am/pm.
We discussed ____.
Did doctor examine patient: _____ yes, _____ no.
Wash hands before touching patient: _____ yes, _____ no.
Wear gloves: ____ yes, ___ no. Clean stethoscope: ____ yes, ____ no.
Wear gown and mask (precautions only):____ yes, _____ no.
Wash hands before leaving the room: _____ yes, _____ no.

Dr.____________ came in at _____ am/pm. Left at _____ am/pm.
We discussed ____.
Did doctor examine patient: _____ yes, _____ no.
Wash hands before touching patient: _____ yes, _____ no.
Wear gloves: ____ yes, ___ no. Clean stethoscope: ____ yes, ____ no.
Wear gown and mask (precautions only):____ yes, _____ no.
Wash hands before leaving the room: _____ yes, _____ no.

Dr.____________ came in at _____ am/pm. Left at _____ am/pm.
We discussed ____.
Did doctor examine patient: _____ yes, _____ no.
Wash hands before touching patient: _____ yes, _____ no.
Wear gloves: ____ yes, ___ no. Clean stethoscope: ____ yes, ____ no.
Wear gown and mask (precautions only):____ yes, _____ no.
Wash hands before leaving the room: _____ yes, _____ no.

Dr.____________ came in at _____ am/pm. Left at _____ am/pm.
We discussed ____.
Did doctor examine patient: _____ yes, _____ no.
Wash hands before touching patient: _____ yes, _____ no.
Wear gloves: ____ yes, ___ no. Clean stethoscope: ____ yes, ____ no.
Wear gown and mask (precautions only):____ yes, _____ no.
Wash hands before leaving the room: _____ yes, _____ no.

NURSING CARE FOR ______________________________

DATE ________________, DAY NUMBER ________________

INITIAL DAY SHIFT EXAM:

My nurse has _____ # of patients. CNA ___yes, ___no. Charge nurse ______________
Nurse _____________ RN/LPN came in at _________ am/pm. Left at _________ am/pm.
Did nurse wash hands and wear gloves before touching patient: ______ yes, ______ no.
Wash hands after touching patient and before leaving the room: ______ yes, ______ no.
Don't hesitate to request staff to wash their hands. This will help decrease the risk of spreading potentially lethal germs.
Did nurse wear protective gear (isolation precautions only): ______ yes, ______ no.
Did nurse provide oral care (to be done every two hours if unable to provide for self, also decreases risk of pneumonia, infections, and aspiration): ______ yes, _____ no.
If able to provide own oral care, then supplies at bedside: ______ yes, ______ no.
Was patient repositioned (every two hours if unable to turn self): _____ yes _____ no.
Head of bed at ________ degrees. This is important for patients on ventilators or on tube feedings. Anything less than thirty degrees places patients at risk for aspiration of stomach contents into the lungs causing aspiration pneumonia.
Checked for incontinence and skin breakdown: _____ yes, _____ no.
Patient's linens wet or soiled: _____ yes, _____ no. Linens changed: ____ yes, ____ no.
Time linens changed: _______ am/pm. Any skin redness or breakdown: ____ yes, ____ no.
If yes, what stage is pressure ulcer: _______. Acquired when: ______________.
List wounds not associated with pressure ulcers and how acquired: ____________
____.
Mattress type: ____.
Specialty mattresses are important to help prevent pressure ulcers)
If patient on ventilator or has tracheostomy, suction performed: _____ yes, ______ no.
Did nurse listen to lung sounds: _____ yes, _____ no.
Does patient have chest tubes: ____ yes, ____ no. Functioning _____ yes, ______ no.
Bowel sounds: _______ yes, _______ no. Bowel sounds active: ______ yes, ______ no.
Neurological exam: ______ yes, ______ no. Follow commands: ______ yes, ______ no.
Is patient alert and oriented to person, place, time, and events: _____ yes, _____ no.
If confused, patient is not oriented to: ___ person, ___ place, ___ time, ___ event.
Confusion began (time and date): ______________________________________.
Glasgow coma scale (checks conscious scale of patient): ____________________.
Intracranial pressure monitoring: ______ yes, ______ no.
If yes, pressure is at ________ mm mercury. (Normal is one to fifteen).
Moves extremities: ___ yes, ___ no.
Paralysis: (inability to move extremities) ______ yes, ______ no.
If yes, extremities affected and when paralysis began: ______________________.
Is patient in pain: ____ yes, ____ no. Describe pain and location ______________.
Patient able to eat: ____ yes, ____ no. What type of diet? ____________________.
If patient on tube feedings list type: ____________ at __________ cc/ml per hour.
Nausea ____, vomiting _____. If so, describe: ______________________________.
Patient has: Nasal gastric tube _____, Dobhoff tube _____, Peg or gastric tube _____.
When was feeding tube placed and what site: ___________________________.
Catheter for draining urine: ____ yes, ____ no. If so, when placed: ____________.
Find out policy for allowed time to remain in bladder. Too long may cause infections.)
IV site(s) where: ______________________________ when placed: ____________.
IV fluids (types and rates): ______________________, ______________________,
_________________________, _______________________, ______________________,
Is patient on oxygen: _____ yes, _____ no. If so, how much and route delivered
(see oxygen routes): ____.
If patient on ventilator, list settings (see list on ventilator settings): __________
____.
Vital signs: temp _____, pulse _____, resp _____, b/p _____, o2 _____%,
current weight _____ pounds, _____ kg. Glucose level: ___________________.
Insulin coverage: ____ yes, ____ no. Insulin type: _________, # of units: _____.

NURSING CARE CONTINUED FOR ______________________
DATE ____________________, DAY NUMBER ______________

FOLLOWING EXAMINATIONS FOR DAY SHIFT:

Nurse ______________, CNA ______________, in at _____ am/pm. Left at ______ am/pm.
Wash hands and wear gloves before touching patient: _____ yes, _____ no.
Wash hands before leaving room: __ yes, __ no. Wear protective gear: __ yes, __ no.
Clean stethoscope: __ yes, __ no. Oral care: __ yes, __ no. Suctioned: __ yes, __ no.
Repositioned: ___ yes, ___ no. Turned to: ___ left, ___ right, ___ backside ___.
Head of bed at: _______ degrees. Incontinence/skin breakdown: ____ yes, ___ no.
Linens wet or soiled: ____ yes, ____ no. Linens changed: ____ yes, ____ no.
Dressing changed: ____ yes, ____ no. Location: ______________________.
IV site checked: ____ yes, ____ no. IV tubing labeled: _____ yes, ____ no.
IV fluids at: ____.
Pain level (0-10 scale.0-no pain, 10 intolerable): _____________________.
Location of pain: ______________. Medicated for pain: ____ yes, ____ no.
Patient is alert/oriented: ____ yes, ____ no. New confusion: ____ yes, ____ no.
Vital signs: temp ____, pulse ____, resp ____, b/p ______, 02 ____ %, ____ liters.
Glucose level: _____. Insulin: ___ yes, __ no. Type: ____________ # of units ___.

Nurse ______________, CNA ______________, in at _____ am/pm. Left at ______ am/pm.
Wash hands and wear gloves before touching patient: _____ yes, _____ no.
Wash hands before leaving room: __ yes, __ no. Wear protective gear: __ yes, __ no.
Clean stethoscope: __ yes, __ no. Oral care: __ yes, __ no. Suctioned: __ yes, __ no.
Repositioned: ___ yes, ___ no. Turned to: ___ left, ___ right, ___ backside ___.
Head of bed at: _______ degrees. Incontinence/skin breakdown: ____ yes, ___ no.
Linens wet or soiled: ____ yes, ____ no. Linens changed: ____ yes, ____ no.
Dressing changed: ____ yes, ____ no. Location: ______________________.
IV site checked: ____ yes, ____ no. IV tubing labeled: _____ yes, ____ no.
IV fluids at: ____.
Pain level (0-10 scale.0-no pain, 10 intolerable): _____________________.
Location of pain: ______________. Medicated for pain: ____ yes, ____ no.
Patient is alert/oriented: ____ yes, ____ no. New confusion: ____ yes, ____ no.
Vital signs: temp ____, pulse ____, resp ____, b/p ______, 02 ____ %, ____ liters.
Glucose level: _____. Insulin: ___ yes, __ no. Type: ____________ # of units ___.

Nurse ______________, CNA ______________, in at _____ am/pm. Left at ______ am/pm.
Wash hands and wear gloves before touching patient: _____ yes, _____ no.
Wash hands before leaving room: __ yes, __ no. Wear protective gear: __ yes, __ no.
Clean stethoscope: __ yes, __ no. Oral care: __ yes, __ no. Suctioned: __ yes, __ no.
Repositioned: ___ yes, ___ no. Turned to: ___ left, ___ right, ___ backside ___.
Head of bed at: _______ degrees. Incontinence/skin breakdown: ____ yes, ___ no.
Linens wet or soiled: ____ yes, ____ no. Linens changed: ____ yes, ____ no.
Dressing changed: ____ yes, ____ no. Location: ______________________.
IV site checked: ____ yes, ____ no. IV tubing labeled: _____ yes, ____ no.
IV fluids at: ____.
Pain level (0-10 scale.0-no pain, 10 intolerable): _____________________.
Location of pain: ______________. Medicated for pain: ____ yes, ____ no.
Patient is alert/oriented: ____ yes, ____ no. New confusion: ____ yes, ____ no.
Vital signs: temp ____, pulse ____, resp ____, b/p ______, 02 ____ %, ____ liters.
Glucose level: _____. Insulin: ___ yes, __ no. Type: ____________ # of units ___.

NURSING CARE CONTINUED FOR ______________________
DATE ____________________, DAY NUMBER ____________________

FOLLOWING EXAMINATIONS FOR DAY SHIFT:

Nurse ____________, CNA ____________, in at _____ am/pm. Left at ______ am/pm.
Wash hands and wear gloves before touching patient: ______ yes, ______ no.
Wash hands before leaving room: ___ yes, ___ no. Wear protective gear: __ yes, __ no.
Clean stethoscope: __ yes, __ no. Oral care: __ yes, __ no. Suctioned: __ yes, __ no.
Repositioned: ___ yes, ___ no. Turned to: ___ left, ___ right, ___ backside ___.
Head of bed at: ______ degrees. Incontinence/skin breakdown: ____ yes, ____ no.
Linens wet or soiled: ____ yes, ____ no. Linens changed: _____ yes, _____ no.
Dressing changed: ____ yes, ____ no. Location: ______________________.
IV site checked: _____ yes, _____ no. IV tubing labeled: _____ yes, _____no.
IV fluids at: ____.
Pain level (0-10 scale.0-no pain, 10 intolerable): _____________________.
Location of pain: ______________. Medicated for pain: _____ yes, ____ no.
Patient is alert/oriented: ____ yes, ____ no. New confusion: ____ yes, ____ no.
Vital signs: temp ____, pulse ____, resp ______, b/p ______, 02 _____ %, ____ liters.
Glucose level: _____. Insulin: ___ yes, ___ no. Type: ____________ # of units ____.

Nurse ____________, CNA ____________, in at _____ am/pm. Left at ______ am/pm.
Wash hands and wear gloves before touching patient: ______ yes, ______ no.
Wash hands before leaving room: ___ yes, ___ no. Wear protective gear: __ yes, __ no.
Clean stethoscope: __ yes, __ no. Oral care: __ yes, __ no. Suctioned: __ yes, __ no.
Repositioned: ___ yes, ___ no. Turned to: ___ left, ___ right, ___ backside ___.
Head of bed at: ______ degrees. Incontinence/skin breakdown: ____ yes, ____ no.
Linens wet or soiled: ____ yes, ____ no. Linens changed: _____ yes, _____ no.
Dressing changed: ____ yes, ____ no. Location: ______________________.
IV site checked: _____ yes, _____ no. IV tubing labeled: _____ yes, _____no.
IV fluids at: ____.
Pain level (0-10 scale.0-no pain, 10 intolerable): _____________________.
Location of pain: ______________. Medicated for pain: _____ yes, ____ no.
Patient is alert/oriented: ____ yes, ____ no. New confusion: ____ yes, ____ no.
Vital signs: temp ____, pulse ____, resp ______, b/p ______, 02 _____ %, ____ liters.
Glucose level: _____. Insulin: ___ yes, ___ no. Type: ____________ # of units ____.

Nurse ____________, CNA ____________, in at _____ am/pm. Left at ______ am/pm.
Wash hands and wear gloves before touching patient: ______ yes, ______ no.
Wash hands before leaving room: ___ yes, ___ no. Wear protective gear: __ yes, __ no.
Clean stethoscope: __ yes, __ no. Oral care: __ yes, __ no. Suctioned: __ yes, __ no.
Repositioned: ___ yes, ___ no. Turned to: ___ left, ___ right, ___ backside ___.
Head of bed at: ______ degrees. Incontinence/skin breakdown: ____ yes, ____ no.
Linens wet or soiled: ____ yes, ____ no. Linens changed: _____ yes, _____ no.
Dressing changed: ____ yes, ____ no. Location: ______________________.
IV site checked: _____ yes, _____ no. IV tubing labeled: _____ yes, _____no.
IV fluids at: ____.
Pain level (0-10 scale.0-no pain, 10 intolerable): _____________________.
Location of pain: ______________. Medicated for pain: _____ yes, ____ no.
Patient is alert/oriented: ____ yes, ____ no. New confusion: ____ yes, ____ no.
Vital signs: temp ____, pulse ____, resp ______, b/p ______, 02 _____ %, ____ liters.
Glucose level: _____. Insulin: ___ yes, ___ no. Type: ____________ # of units ____.

NURSING CARE FOR ______________________________

DATE ____________________, DAY NUMBER ______________________

INITIAL NIGHT SHIFT EXAM:

My nurse has ______ # of patients. CNA ___yes, ___no. Charge nurse ________________
Nurse ____________ RN/LPN came in at ________ am/pm. Left at ________ am/pm.
Did nurse wash hands and wear gloves before touching patient: ______ yes, ______ no.
Wash hands after touching patient and before leaving the room: ______ yes, ______ no.
Don't hesitate to request staff to wash their hands. This will help decrease the risk of spreading potentially lethal germs.
Did nurse wear protective gear (isolation precautions only): ______ yes, ______ no.
Did nurse provide oral care (to be done every two hours if unable to provide for self, also decreases risk of pneumonia, infections, and aspiration): ______ yes, ______ no.
If able to provide own oral care, then supplies at bedside: ______ yes, ______ no.
Was patient repositioned (every two hours if unable to turn self): _____ yes _____ no.
Head of bed at ________ degrees. This is important for patients on ventilators or on tube feedings. Anything less than thirty degrees places patients at risk for aspiration of stomach contents into the lungs causing aspiration pneumonia.
Checked for incontinence and skin breakdown: _____ yes, _____ no.
Patient's linens wet or soiled: ____yes,____ no. Linens changed: ____ yes, ____ no.
Time linens changed: ________ am/pm. Any skin redness or breakdown: ____ yes, ____ no.
If yes, what stage is pressure ulcer: _____. Acquired when: __________________.
List wounds not associated with pressure ulcers and how acquired: _______________
____.
Mattress type: ____.
Specialty mattresses are important to help prevent pressure ulcers)
If patient on ventilator or has tracheostomy, suction performed: ______ yes, ______ no.
Did nurse listen to lung sounds: ______ yes, ______ no.
Does patient have chest tubes: ____ yes, ____ no. Functioning _____ yes, _____ no.
Bowel sounds:______ yes, ______ no. Bowel sounds active: ______ yes, ______ no.
Neurological exam: ______ yes, ______ no. Follow commands: ______ yes, ______ no.
Is patient alert and oriented to person, place, time, and events: _____ yes, _____ no.
If confused, patient is not oriented to: ____ person, ___ place, ___ time, ___ event.
Confusion began (time and date): ______________________________________.
Glasgow coma scale (checks conscious scale of patient): ______________________.
Intracranial pressure monitoring: _____ yes, _____ no.
If yes, pressure is at ________ mm mercury. (Normal is one to fifteen).
Moves extremities: ___ yes, ___ no.
Paralysis: (inability to move extremities) ______ yes, ______ no.
If yes, extremities affected and when paralysis began: _______________________.
Is patient in pain: ____ yes, ____ no. Describe pain and location ______________.
Patient able to eat: ____ yes, ____ no. What type of diet? ______________________.
If patient on tube feedings list type: ____________ at ____________ cc/ml per hour.
Nausea ____, vomiting _____. If so, describe: ___________________________.
Patient has: Nasal gastric tube ______, Dobhoff tube _____, Peg or gastric tube ______
When was feeding tube placed and what site: _________________________________.
Catheter for draining urine: ____ yes, ____ no. If so, when placed: ____________.
Find out policy for allowed time to remain in bladder. Too long may cause infections.)
IV site(s) where: ______________________ when placed: _______________________.
IV fluids (types and rates): ____,
______________________, ______________________, _____________________________.
Is patient on oxygen: _____ yes, _____ no. If so, how much and route delivered (see oxygen routes): ____.
If patient on ventilator, list settings (see list on ventilator settings): ________
____.
Vital signs: temp ______, pulse ______, resp ______, b/p ______, o2 ______%,
current weight ______ pounds, ______ kg. Glucose level: ______
Insulin coverage: ____ yes, ____ no. Insulin type: ____________, # of units: ______.

NURSING CARE CONTINUED FOR ______________________________
DATE ____________________, DAY NUMBER ______________________

FOLLOWING EXAMINATIONS FOR NIGHT SHIFT:

Nurse ______________, CNA ______________, in at ______ am/pm. Left at ______ am/pm.
Wash hands and wear gloves before touching patient: ______ yes, ______ no.
Wash hands before leaving room: ___ yes, ___ no. Wear protective gear: __ yes, __ no.
Clean stethoscope: __ yes, __ no. Oral care: __ yes, __ no. Suctioned: __ yes, __ no.
Repositioned: ___ yes, ___ no. Turned to: ___ left, ___ right, ___ backside ___.
Head of bed at: _______ degrees. Incontinence/skin breakdown: ____ yes, ____ no.
Linens wet or soiled: _____ yes, _____ no. Linens changed: _____ yes, ______ no.
Dressing changed: ____ yes, ____ no. Location: ______________________________.
IV site checked: _____ yes, _____ no. IV tubing labeled: ____ yes, _____ no.
IV fluids at: ____.
Pain level (0-10 scale.0-no pain, 10 intolerable): _____________________________.
Location of pain: ________________. Medicated for pain: _____ yes, ____ no.
Patient is alert/oriented: ____ yes, ____ no. New confusion: ____ yes, ____ no.
Vital signs: temp ____, pulse _____, resp _____, b/p ______, 02 _____ %, _____ liters.
Glucose level: _____. Insulin: ___ yes, ___ no. Type: _____________ # of units ____.

Nurse ______________, CNA ______________, in at ______ am/pm. Left at ______ am/pm.
Wash hands and wear gloves before touching patient: ______ yes, ______ no.
Wash hands before leaving room: ___ yes, ___ no. Wear protective gear: __ yes, __ no.
Clean stethoscope: __ yes, __ no. Oral care: __ yes, __ no. Suctioned: __ yes, __ no.
Repositioned: ___ yes, ___ no. Turned to: ___ left, ___ right, ___ backside ___.
Head of bed at: _______ degrees. Incontinence/skin breakdown: ____ yes, ____ no.
Linens wet or soiled: _____ yes, _____ no. Linens changed: _____ yes, ______ no.
Dressing changed: ____ yes, ____ no. Location: ______________________________.
IV site checked: _____ yes, _____ no. IV tubing labeled: ____ yes, _____ no.
IV fluids at: ____.
Pain level (0-10 scale.0-no pain, 10 intolerable): _____________________________.
Location of pain: ________________. Medicated for pain: _____ yes, ____ no.
Patient is alert/oriented: ____ yes, ____ no. New confusion: ____ yes, ____ no.
Vital signs: temp ____, pulse _____, resp _____, b/p ______, 02 _____ %, _____ liters.
Glucose level: _____. Insulin: ___ yes, ___ no. Type: _____________ # of units ____.

Nurse ______________, CNA ______________, in at ______ am/pm. Left at ______ am/pm.
Wash hands and wear gloves before touching patient: ______ yes, ______ no.
Wash hands before leaving room: ___ yes, ___ no. Wear protective gear: __ yes, __ no.
Clean stethoscope: __ yes, __ no. Oral care: __ yes, __ no. Suctioned: __ yes, __ no.
Repositioned: ___ yes, ___ no. Turned to: ___ left, ___ right, ___ backside ___.
Head of bed at: _______ degrees. Incontinence/skin breakdown: ____ yes, ____ no.
Linens wet or soiled: _____ yes, _____ no. Linens changed: _____ yes, ______ no.
Dressing changed: ____ yes, ____ no. Location: ______________________________.
IV site checked: _____ yes, _____ no. IV tubing labeled: ____ yes, _____ no.
IV fluids at: ____.
Pain level (0-10 scale.0-no pain, 10 intolerable): _____________________________.
Location of pain: ________________. Medicated for pain: _____ yes, ____ no.
Patient is alert/oriented: ____ yes, ____ no. New confusion: ____ yes, ____ no.
Vital signs: temp ____, pulse _____, resp _____, b/p ______, 02 _____ %, _____ liters.
Glucose level: _____. Insulin: ___ yes, ___ no. Type: _____________ # of units ____.

NURSING CARE CONTINUED FOR ____________________
DATE ____________________, DAY NUMBER ____________________

FOLLOWING EXAMINATIONS FOR NIGHT SHIFT:

Nurse ______________, CNA ______________, in at _____ am/pm. Left at ______ am/pm.
Wash hands and wear gloves before touching patient: _______ yes, _______ no.
Wash hands before leaving room: ___ yes, ___ no. Wear protective gear: __ yes, __ no.
Clean stethoscope: __ yes, __ no. Oral care: __ yes, __ no. Suctioned: __ yes, __ no.
Repositioned: ___ yes, ___ no. Turned to: ___ left, ___ right, ___ backside ___.
Head of bed at: ________ degrees. Incontinence/skin breakdown: ____ yes, ____ no.
Linens wet or soiled: _____ yes, _____ no. Linens changed: _____ yes, _____ no.
Dressing changed: ____ yes, ____ no. Location: ______________________________.
IV site checked: _____ yes, _____ no. IV tubing labeled: _____ yes, _____no.
IV fluids at: ____.
Pain level (0-10 scale.0-no pain, 10 intolerable): ______________________.
Location of pain: ____________________. Medicated for pain: _____ yes, _____ no.
Patient is alert/oriented: ____ yes, ____ no. New confusion: ____ yes, ____ no.
Vital signs: temp ____, pulse _____, resp ______, b/p ______, 02 _____ %, ____ liters.
Glucose level: _____. Insulin: ___ yes, ___ no. Type: ______________ # of units ____.

Nurse ______________, CNA ______________, in at _____ am/pm. Left at ______ am/pm.
Wash hands and wear gloves before touching patient: _______ yes, _______ no.
Wash hands before leaving room: ___ yes, ___ no. Wear protective gear: __ yes, __ no.
Clean stethoscope: __ yes, __ no. Oral care: __ yes, __ no. Suctioned: __ yes, __ no.
Repositioned: ___ yes, ___ no. Turned to: ___ left, ___ right, ___ backside ___.
Head of bed at: ________ degrees. Incontinence/skin breakdown: ____ yes, ____ no.
Linens wet or soiled: _____ yes, _____ no. Linens changed: _____ yes, _____ no.
Dressing changed: ____ yes, ____ no. Location: ______________________________.
IV site checked: _____ yes, _____ no. IV tubing labeled: _____ yes, _____no.
IV fluids at: ____.
Pain level (0-10 scale.0-no pain, 10 intolerable): ______________________.
Location of pain: ____________________. Medicated for pain: _____ yes, _____ no.
Patient is alert/oriented: ____ yes, ____ no. New confusion: ____ yes, ____ no.
Vital signs: temp ____, pulse _____, resp ______, b/p ______, 02 _____ %, ____ liters.
Glucose level: _____. Insulin: ___ yes, ___ no. Type: ______________ # of units ____.

Nurse ______________, CNA ______________, in at _____ am/pm. Left at ______ am/pm.
Wash hands and wear gloves before touching patient: _______ yes, _______ no.
Wash hands before leaving room: ___ yes, ___ no. Wear protective gear: __ yes, __ no.
Clean stethoscope: __ yes, __ no. Oral care: __ yes, __ no. Suctioned: __ yes, __ no.
Repositioned: ___ yes, ___ no. Turned to: ___ left, ___ right, ___ backside ___.
Head of bed at: ________ degrees. Incontinence/skin breakdown: ____ yes, ____ no.
Linens wet or soiled: _____ yes, _____ no. Linens changed: _____ yes, _____ no.
Dressing changed: ____ yes, ____ no. Location: ______________________________.
IV site checked: _____ yes, _____ no. IV tubing labeled: _____ yes, _____no.
IV fluids at: ____.
Pain level (0-10 scale.0-no pain, 10 intolerable): ______________________.
Location of pain: ____________________. Medicated for pain: _____ yes, _____ no.
Patient is alert/oriented: ____ yes, ____ no. New confusion: ____ yes, ____ no.
Vital signs: temp ____, pulse _____, resp ______, b/p ______, 02 _____ %, ____ liters.
Glucose level: _____. Insulin: ___ yes, ___ no. Type: ______________ # of units ____.

MEDICATION ADMINISTRATION LIST FOR ____________________
DATE ______________ DAY NUMBER ____________________

List the medication for each day. Routes of administration: oral, thru feeding tube, intravenous (IV), intramuscular (IM), subcutaneous (SQ), epidural or a catheter in your spinal column, rectal, topical, eye drops, and ear drops.

Medication: ______________ Route: ______________ Time: ____________
Medication: ______________ Route: ______________ Time: ____________
Medication: ______________ Route: ______________ Time: ____________
Medication: ______________ Route: ______________ Time: ____________
Medication: ______________ Route: ______________ Time: ____________
Medication: ______________ Route: ______________ Time: ____________
Medication: ______________ Route: ______________ Time: ____________
Medication: ______________ Route: ______________ Time: ____________
Medication: ______________ Route: ______________ Time: ____________
Medication: ______________ Route: ______________ Time: ____________
Medication: ______________ Route: ______________ Time: ____________
Medication: ______________ Route: ______________ Time: ____________
Medication: ______________ Route: ______________ Time: ____________
Medication: ______________ Route: ______________ Time: ____________
Medication: ______________ Route: ______________ Time: ____________
Medication: ______________ Route: ______________ Time: ____________
Medication: ______________ Route: ______________ Time: ____________
Medication: ______________ Route: ______________ Time: ____________
Medication: ______________ Route: ______________ Time: ____________
Medication: ______________ Route: ______________ Time: ____________
Medication: ______________ Route: ______________ Time: ____________
Medication: ______________ Route: ______________ Time: ____________
Medication: ______________ Route: ______________ Time: ____________
Medication: ______________ Route: ______________ Time: ____________
Medication: ______________ Route: ______________ Time: ____________
Medication: ______________ Route: ______________ Time: ____________
Medication: ______________ Route: ______________ Time: ____________
Medication: ______________ Route: ______________ Time: ____________
Medication: ______________ Route: ______________ Time: ____________
Medication: ______________ Route: ______________ Time: ____________
Medication: ______________ Route: ______________ Time: ____________
Medication: ______________ Route: ______________ Time: ____________
Medication: ______________ Route: ______________ Time: ____________
Medication: ______________ Route: ______________ Time: ____________
Medication: ______________ Route: ______________ Time: ____________
Medication: ______________ Route: ______________ Time: ____________
Medication: ______________ Route: ______________ Time: ____________
Medication: ______________ Route: ______________ Time: ____________
Medication: ______________ Route: ______________ Time: ____________
Medication: ______________ Route: ______________ Time: ____________
Medication: ______________ Route: ______________ Time: ____________
Medication: ______________ Route: ______________ Time: ____________
Medication: ______________ Route: ______________ Time: ____________
Medication: ______________ Route: ______________ Time: ____________
Medication: ______________ Route: ______________ Time: ____________
Medication: ______________ Route: ______________ Time: ____________
Medication: ______________ Route: ______________ Time: ____________
Medication: ______________ Route: ______________ Time: ____________
Medication: ______________ Route: ______________ Time: ____________
Medication: ______________ Route: ______________ Time: ____________
Medication: ______________ Route: ______________ Time: ____________
Medication: ______________ Route: ______________ Time: ____________
Medication: ______________ Route: ______________ Time: ____________
Medication: ______________ Route: ______________ Time: ____________

NOTES FOR DAY NUMBER ____________________

DATE ____________________

MEDICAL JOURNAL FOR ______________________________

DATE ________________, DAY NUMBER ______________

VISITS FROM MY DOCTORS TODAY

Goals for today: ____

____

____.

Things to discuss with my doctor(s): ___________________________

____

____

Dr.___________ came in at ____ am/pm. Left at ____ am/pm.
We discussed ____.
Did doctor examine patient: ____ yes, ____ no.
Wash hands before touching patient: ____ yes, ____ no.
Wear gloves: ___ yes, __ no. Clean stethoscope: ___ yes, ___ no.
Wear gown and mask (precautions only):___ yes, ____ no.
Wash hands before leaving the room: ____ yes, ____ no.

Dr.___________ came in at ____ am/pm. Left at ____ am/pm.
We discussed ____.
Did doctor examine patient: ____ yes, ____ no.
Wash hands before touching patient: ____ yes, ____ no.
Wear gloves: ___ yes, __ no. Clean stethoscope: ___ yes, ___ no.
Wear gown and mask (precautions only):___ yes, ____ no.
Wash hands before leaving the room: ____ yes, ____ no.

Dr.___________ came in at ____ am/pm. Left at ____ am/pm.
We discussed ____.
Did doctor examine patient: ____ yes, ____ no.
Wash hands before touching patient: ____ yes, ____ no.
Wear gloves: ___ yes, __ no. Clean stethoscope: ___ yes, ___ no.
Wear gown and mask (precautions only):___ yes, ____ no.
Wash hands before leaving the room: ____ yes, ____ no.

Dr.___________ came in at ____ am/pm. Left at ____ am/pm.
We discussed ____.
Did doctor examine patient: ____ yes, ____ no.
Wash hands before touching patient: ____ yes, ____ no.
Wear gloves: ___ yes, __ no. Clean stethoscope: ___ yes, ___ no.
Wear gown and mask (precautions only):___ yes, ____ no.
Wash hands before leaving the room: ____ yes, ____ no.

Dr.___________ came in at ____ am/pm. Left at ____ am/pm.
We discussed ____.
Did doctor examine patient: ____ yes, ____ no.
Wash hands before touching patient: ____ yes, ____ no.
Wear gloves: ___ yes, __ no. Clean stethoscope: ___ yes, ___ no.
Wear gown and mask (precautions only):___ yes, ____ no.
Wash hands before leaving the room: ____ yes, ____ no.

NURSING CARE FOR ____________________________

DATE ____________________, DAY NUMBER ____________________

INITIAL DAY SHIFT EXAM:

My nurse has ______ # of patients. CNA ___yes, ___no. Charge nurse ______________
Nurse ____________ RN/LPN came in at __________ am/pm. Left at __________ am/pm.
Did nurse wash hands and wear gloves before touching patient: ______ yes, ______ no.
Wash hands after touching patient and before leaving the room: ______ yes, ______ no.
Don't hesitate to request staff to wash their hands. This will help decrease the risk of spreading potentially lethal germs.
Did nurse wear protective gear (isolation precautions only): ______ yes, ______ no.
Did nurse provide oral care (to be done every two hours if unable to provide for self, also decreases risk of pneumonia, infections, and aspiration): ______ yes, ______ no.
If able to provide own oral care, then supplies at bedside: ______ yes, ______ no.
Was patient repositioned (every two hours if unable to turn self): ______ yes ______ no.
Head of bed at ________ degrees. This is important for patients on ventilators or on tube feedings. Anything less than thirty degrees places patients at risk for aspiration of stomach contents into the lungs causing aspiration pneumonia.
Checked for incontinence and skin breakdown: ____ yes, ____ no.
Patient's linens wet or soiled: ____ yes, ____ no. Linens changed: ____ yes, ____ no.
Time linens changed: _______ am/pm. Any skin redness or breakdown: ____ yes, ____ no.
If yes, what stage is pressure ulcer: ________. Acquired when: ________________.
List wounds not associated with pressure ulcers and how acquired: ________________
____.
Mattress type: ____.
Specialty mattresses are important to help prevent pressure ulcers)
If patient on ventilator or has tracheostomy, suction performed: _____ yes, _____ no.
Did nurse listen to lung sounds: ____ yes, ____ no.
Does patient have chest tubes: ____ yes, ____ no. Functioning _____ yes, _____ no.
Bowel sounds: ______ yes, ______ no. Bowel sounds active: ______ yes, ______ no.
Neurological exam: ______ yes, ______ no. Follow commands: ______ yes, ______ no.
Is patient alert and oriented to person, place, time, and events: _____ yes, _____ no.
If confused, patient is not oriented to: ___ person, ___ place, ___ time, ___ event.
Confusion began (time and date): ______________________________________
Glasgow coma scale (checks conscious scale of patient): ______________________
Intracranial pressure monitoring: _____ yes, _____ no.
If yes, pressure is at ________ mm mercury. (Normal is one to fifteen).
Moves extremities: ___ yes, ___ no.
Paralysis: (inability to move extremities) ______ yes, ______ no.
If yes, extremities affected and when paralysis began: ____________________.
Is patient in pain: ___ yes, ___ no. Describe pain and location ____________
Patient able to eat: ___ yes, ___ no. What type of diet? ____________________
If patient on tube feedings list type: __________ at ________ cc/ml per hour.
Nausea ____, vomiting _____. If so, describe: ______________________________
Patient has: Nasal gastric tube _____, Dobhoff tube _____, Peg or gastric tube _____.
When was feeding tube placed and what site: ________________________________.
Catheter for draining urine: ____ yes, ____ no. If so, when placed: __________.
Find out policy for allowed time to remain in bladder. Too long may cause infections.)
IV site(s) where: ____________________ when placed: ____________________.
IV fluids (types and rates): ____,
______________________, ______________________, ______________________.
Is patient on oxygen: ____ yes, ____ no. If so, how much and route delivered (see oxygen routes): ____.
If patient on ventilator, list settings (see list on ventilator settings): ________
____.
Vital signs: temp _____, pulse _____, resp _____, b/p _____, o2 _____%,
current weight _____ pounds, _____ kg. Glucose level: _____
Insulin coverage: ____ yes, ____ no. Insulin type: __________, # of units: _____.

NURSING CARE CONTINUED FOR ____________________
DATE ____________________, DAY NUMBER ____________________

FOLLOWING EXAMINATIONS FOR DAY SHIFT:

Nurse ____________, CNA ____________, in at ______ am/pm. Left at ______ am/pm.
Wash hands and wear gloves before touching patient: ______ yes, ______ no.
Wash hands before leaving room: ___ yes, ___ no. Wear protective gear: __ yes, __ no.
Clean stethoscope: __ yes, __ no. Oral care: __ yes, __ no. Suctioned: __ yes, __ no.
Repositioned: ___ yes, ___ no. Turned to: ___ left, ___ right, ___ backside ___.
Head of bed at: _______ degrees. Incontinence/skin breakdown: ___ yes, ___ no.
Linens wet or soiled: ____ yes, ____ no. Linens changed: ____ yes, ____ no.
Dressing changed: ____ yes, ____ no. Location: ____________________.
IV site checked: _____ yes, _____ no. IV tubing labeled: _____ yes, _____no.
IV fluids at: ____.
Pain level (0-10 scale.0-no pain, 10 intolerable): ____________________.
Location of pain: ________________. Medicated for pain: _____ yes, ____ no.
Patient is alert/oriented: ____ yes, ____ no. New confusion: ____ yes, ____ no.
Vital signs: temp ____, pulse ____, resp _____, b/p _____, O2 _____ %, ____ liters.
Glucose level: _____. Insulin: ___ yes, ___ no. Type: __________ # of units ____.

Nurse ____________, CNA ____________, in at ______ am/pm. Left at ______ am/pm.
Wash hands and wear gloves before touching patient: ______ yes, ______ no.
Wash hands before leaving room: ___ yes, ___ no. Wear protective gear: __ yes, __ no.
Clean stethoscope: __ yes, __ no. Oral care: __ yes, __ no. Suctioned: __ yes, __ no.
Repositioned: ___ yes, ___ no. Turned to: ___ left, ___ right, ___ backside ___.
Head of bed at: _______ degrees. Incontinence/skin breakdown: ___ yes, ___ no.
Linens wet or soiled: ____ yes, ____ no. Linens changed: ____ yes, ____ no.
Dressing changed: ____ yes, ____ no. Location: ____________________.
IV site checked: _____ yes, _____ no. IV tubing labeled: _____ yes, _____no.
IV fluids at: ____.
Pain level (0-10 scale.0-no pain, 10 intolerable): ____________________.
Location of pain: ________________. Medicated for pain: _____ yes, ____ no.
Patient is alert/oriented: ____ yes, ____ no. New confusion: ____ yes, ____ no.
Vital signs: temp ____, pulse ____, resp _____, b/p _____, O2 _____ %, ____ liters.
Glucose level: _____. Insulin: ___ yes, ___ no. Type: __________ # of units ____.

Nurse ____________, CNA ____________, in at ______ am/pm. Left at ______ am/pm.
Wash hands and wear gloves before touching patient: ______ yes, ______ no.
Wash hands before leaving room: ___ yes, ___ no. Wear protective gear: __ yes, __ no.
Clean stethoscope: __ yes, __ no. Oral care: __ yes, __ no. Suctioned: __ yes, __ no.
Repositioned: ___ yes, ___ no. Turned to: ___ left, ___ right, ___ backside ___.
Head of bed at: _______ degrees. Incontinence/skin breakdown: ___ yes, ___ no.
Linens wet or soiled: ____ yes, ____ no. Linens changed: ____ yes, ____ no.
Dressing changed: ____ yes, ____ no. Location: ____________________.
IV site checked: _____ yes, _____ no. IV tubing labeled: _____ yes, _____no.
IV fluids at: ____.
Pain level (0-10 scale.0-no pain, 10 intolerable): ____________________.
Location of pain: ________________. Medicated for pain: _____ yes, ____ no.
Patient is alert/oriented: ____ yes, ____ no. New confusion: ____ yes, ____ no.
Vital signs: temp ____, pulse ____, resp _____, b/p _____, O2 _____ %, ____ liters.
Glucose level: _____. Insulin: ___ yes, ___ no. Type: __________ # of units ____.

NURSING CARE CONTINUED FOR ______________________________
DATE ____________________, DAY NUMBER ____________________

FOLLOWING EXAMINATIONS FOR DAY SHIFT:

Nurse _______________, CNA _______________, in at ______ am/pm. Left at _______ am/pm.
Wash hands and wear gloves before touching patient: _______ yes, _______ no.
Wash hands before leaving room: ___ yes, ___ no. Wear protective gear: __ yes, __ no.
Clean stethoscope: __ yes, __ no. Oral care: __ yes, __ no. Suctioned: __ yes, __ no.
Repositioned: ___ yes, ___ no. Turned to: __ left, __ right, ___ backside ___.
Head of bed at: ________ degrees. Incontinence/skin breakdown: ___ yes, ___ no.
Linens wet or soiled: ____ yes, ____ no. Linens changed: _____ yes, _____ no.
Dressing changed: ____ yes, ____ no. Location: ___________________________.
IV site checked: _____ yes, _____ no. IV tubing labeled: _____ yes, _____no.
IV fluids at: ____.
Pain level (0-10 scale.0-no pain, 10 intolerable): _________________________.
Location of pain: _______________. Medicated for pain: ____ yes, ____ no.
Patient is alert/oriented: ____ yes, ____ no. New confusion: ____ yes, ____ no.
Vital signs: temp ____, pulse ____, resp ____, b/p ______, 02 ____ %, ____ liters.
Glucose level: _____. Insulin: ___ yes, ___ no. Type: __________ # of units ___.

Nurse _______________, CNA _______________, in at ______ am/pm. Left at _______ am/pm.
Wash hands and wear gloves before touching patient: _______ yes, _______ no.
Wash hands before leaving room: ___ yes, ___ no. Wear protective gear: __ yes, __ no.
Clean stethoscope: __ yes, __ no. Oral care: __ yes, __ no. Suctioned: __ yes, __ no.
Repositioned: ___ yes, ___ no. Turned to: __ left, __ right, ___ backside ___.
Head of bed at: ________ degrees. Incontinence/skin breakdown: ___ yes, ___ no.
Linens wet or soiled: ____ yes, ____ no. Linens changed: _____ yes, _____ no.
Dressing changed: ____ yes, ____ no. Location: ___________________________.
IV site checked: _____ yes, _____ no. IV tubing labeled: _____ yes, _____no.
IV fluids at: ____.
Pain level (0-10 scale.0-no pain, 10 intolerable): _________________________.
Location of pain: _______________. Medicated for pain: ____ yes, ____ no.
Patient is alert/oriented: ____ yes, ____ no. New confusion: ____ yes, ____ no.
Vital signs: temp ____, pulse ____, resp ____, b/p ______, 02 ____ %, ____ liters.
Glucose level: _____. Insulin: ___ yes, ___ no. Type: __________ # of units ___.

Nurse _______________, CNA _______________, in at ______ am/pm. Left at _______ am/pm.
Wash hands and wear gloves before touching patient: _______ yes, _______ no.
Wash hands before leaving room: ___ yes, ___ no. Wear protective gear: __ yes, __ no.
Clean stethoscope: __ yes, __ no. Oral care: __ yes, __ no. Suctioned: __ yes, __ no.
Repositioned: ___ yes, ___ no. Turned to: __ left, __ right, ___ backside ___.
Head of bed at: ________ degrees. Incontinence/skin breakdown: ___ yes, ___ no.
Linens wet or soiled: ____ yes, ____ no. Linens changed: _____ yes, _____ no.
Dressing changed: ____ yes, ____ no. Location: ___________________________.
IV site checked: _____ yes, _____ no. IV tubing labeled: _____ yes, _____no.
IV fluids at: ____.
Pain level (0-10 scale.0-no pain, 10 intolerable): _________________________.
Location of pain: _______________. Medicated for pain: ____ yes, ____ no.
Patient is alert/oriented: ____ yes, ____ no. New confusion: ____ yes, ____ no.
Vital signs: temp ____, pulse ____, resp ____, b/p ______, 02 ____ %, ____ liters.
Glucose level: _____. Insulin: ___ yes, ___ no. Type: __________ # of units ___.

NURSING CARE FOR ____________________________

DATE ________________, DAY NUMBER ________________

INITIAL NIGHT SHIFT EXAM:

My nurse has _____ # of patients. CNA ___yes, ___no. Charge nurse ____________
Nurse ____________ RN/LPN came in at ________ am/pm. Left at ________ am/pm.
Did nurse wash hands and wear gloves before touching patient: _____ yes, _____ no.
Wash hands after touching patient and before leaving the room: _____ yes, _____ no.
Don't hesitate to request staff to wash their hands. This will help decrease the risk of spreading potentially lethal germs.
Did nurse wear protective gear (isolation precautions only): _____ yes, _____ no.
Did nurse provide oral care (to be done every two hours if unable to provide for self, also decreases risk of pneumonia, infections, and aspiration): _____ yes, _____ no.
If able to provide own oral care, then supplies at bedside: _____ yes, _____ no.
Was patient repositioned (every two hours if unable to turn self): _____ yes _____ no.
Head of bed at ________ degrees. This is important for patients on ventilators or on tube feedings. Anything less than thirty degrees places patients at risk for aspiration of stomach contents into the lungs causing aspiration pneumonia.
Checked for incontinence and skin breakdown: _____ yes, _____ no.
Patient's linens wet or soiled: _____ yes, _____ no. Linens changed: ____ yes, ____ no.
Time linens changed: ________ am/pm. Any skin redness or breakdown: ____ yes, ____ no.
If yes, what stage is pressure ulcer: ______. Acquired when: ______________.
List wounds not associated with pressure ulcers and how acquired: ______________
____.
Mattress type: ____.
Specialty mattresses are important to help prevent pressure ulcers)
If patient on ventilator or has tracheostomy, suction performed: _____ yes, _____ no.
Did nurse listen to lung sounds: _____ yes, _____ no.
Does patient have chest tubes: _____ yes, _____ no. Functioning _____ yes, _____ no.
Bowel sounds: _____ yes, _____ no. Bowel sounds active: _____ yes, _____ no.
Neurological exam: _____ yes, _____ no. Follow commands: _____ yes, _____ no.
Is patient alert and oriented to person, place, time, and events: _____ yes, _____ no.
If confused, patient is not oriented to: ___ person, ___ place, ___ time, ___ event.
Confusion began (time and date): ______________________________.
Glasgow coma scale (checks conscious scale of patient): ______________________.
Intracranial pressure monitoring: _____ yes, _____ no.
If yes, pressure is at ________ mm mercury. (Normal is one to fifteen).
Moves extremities: ___ yes, ___ no.
Paralysis: (inability to move extremities) _____ yes, _____ no.
If yes, extremities affected and when paralysis began: ______________________.
Is patient in pain: ____ yes, ____ no. Describe pain and location ______________
Patient able to eat: ____ yes, ____ no. What type of diet? ______________
If patient on tube feedings list type: ____________ at ________ cc/ml per hour.
Nausea ____, vomiting ____. If so, describe: ______________________________.
Patient has: Nasal gastric tube _____, Dobhoff tube _____, Peg or gastric tube ____.
When was feeding tube placed and what site: ______________________________.
Catheter for draining urine: ____ yes, ____ no. If so, when placed: ____________.
Find out policy for allowed time to remain in bladder. Too long may cause infections.)
IV site(s) where: ____________ when placed: ____________.
IV fluids (types and rates): ______________, ______________, ______________,
______________, ______________, ______________,
Is patient on oxygen: _____ yes, _____ no. If so, how much and route delivered (see oxygen routes): ______________________________________.
If patient on ventilator, list settings (see list on ventilator settings): ________
____.
Vital signs: temp _____, pulse _____, resp _____, b/p _____, o2 _____%,
current weight _____ pounds, _____ kg. Glucose level: _____
Insulin coverage: ____ yes, ____ no. Insulin type: __________, # of units: _____.

NURSING CARE CONTINUED FOR ____________________
DATE ______________, DAY NUMBER ______________

FOLLOWING EXAMINATIONS FOR NIGHT SHIFT:

Nurse ________, CNA __________, in at _____ am/pm. Left at ______ am/pm.
Wash hands and wear gloves before touching patient: _____ yes, _____ no.
Wash hands before leaving room: ___ yes, ___ no. Wear protective gear: __ yes, __ no.
Clean stethoscope: __ yes, __ no. Oral care: __ yes, __ no. Suctioned: __ yes, __ no.
Repositioned: ___ yes, ___ no. Turned to: ___ left, ___ right, ___ backside ___.
Head of bed at: _______ degrees. Incontinence/skin breakdown: ____ yes, ____ no.
Linens wet or soiled: ____ yes, ____ no. Linens changed: ____ yes, ____ no.
Dressing changed: ____ yes, ____ no. Location: __________.
IV site checked: ____ yes, ____ no. IV tubing labeled: ____ yes, ____no.
IV fluids at: ____.
Pain level (0-10 scale.0-no pain, 10 intolerable): __________.
Location of pain: __________. Medicated for pain: ____ yes, ____ no.
Patient is alert/oriented: ____ yes, ____ no. New confusion: ____ yes, ____ no
Vital signs: temp ____, pulse ____, resp ____, b/p ______, 02 _____ %, ____ liters.
Glucose level: _____. Insulin: ___ yes, __ no. Type: _________ # of units ___.

Nurse ________, CNA __________, in at _____ am/pm. Left at ______ am/pm.
Wash hands and wear gloves before touching patient: _____ yes, _____ no.
Wash hands before leaving room: ___ yes, ___ no. Wear protective gear: __ yes, __ no.
Clean stethoscope: __ yes, __ no. Oral care: __ yes, __ no. Suctioned: __ yes, __ no.
Repositioned: ___ yes, ___ no. Turned to: ___ left, ___ right, ___ backside ___.
Head of bed at: _______ degrees. Incontinence/skin breakdown: ____ yes, ____ no.
Linens wet or soiled: ____ yes, ____ no. Linens changed: ____ yes, ____ no.
Dressing changed: ____ yes, ____ no. Location: __________.
IV site checked: ____ yes, ____ no. IV tubing labeled: ____ yes, ____no.
IV fluids at: ____.
Pain level (0-10 scale.0-no pain, 10 intolerable): __________.
Location of pain: __________. Medicated for pain: ____ yes, ____ no.
Patient is alert/oriented: ____ yes, ____ no. New confusion: ____ yes, ____ no.
Vital signs: temp ____, pulse ____, resp ____, b/p ______, 02 _____ %, ____ liters.
Glucose level: _____. Insulin: ___ yes, __ no. Type: _________ # of units ___.

Nurse ________, CNA __________, in at _____ am/pm. Left at ______ am/pm.
Wash hands and wear gloves before touching patient: _____ yes, _____ no.
Wash hands before leaving room: ___ yes, ___ no. Wear protective gear: __ yes, __ no.
Clean stethoscope: __ yes, __ no. Oral care: __ yes, __ no. Suctioned: __ yes, __ no.
Repositioned: ___ yes, ___ no. Turned to: ___ left, ___ right, ___ backside ___.
Head of bed at: _______ degrees. Incontinence/skin breakdown: ____ yes, ____ no.
Linens wet or soiled: ____ yes, ____ no. Linens changed: ____ yes, ____ no.
Dressing changed: ____ yes, ____ no. Location: __________.
IV site checked: ____ yes, ____ no. IV tubing labeled: ____ yes, ____ no.
IV fluids at: ____.
Pain level (0-10 scale.0-no pain, 10 intolerable): __________.
Location of pain: __________. Medicated for pain: ____ yes, ____ no.
Patient is alert/oriented: ____ yes, ____ no. New confusion: ____ yes, ____ no.
Vital signs: temp ____, pulse ____, resp ____, b/p ______, 02 _____ %, ____ liters.
Glucose level: _____. Insulin: ___ yes, __ no. Type: _________ # of units ___.

NURSING CARE CONTINUED FOR ____________________
DATE ____________________, DAY NUMBER ____________________

FOLLOWING EXAMINATIONS FOR NIGHT SHIFT:

Nurse ____________, CNA ____________, in at _____ am/pm. Left at ______ am/pm.
Wash hands and wear gloves before touching patient: ______ yes, ______ no.
Wash hands before leaving room: ___ yes, ___ no. Wear protective gear: __ yes, __ no.
Clean stethoscope: __ yes, __ no. Oral care: __ yes, __ no. Suctioned: __ yes, __ no.
Repositioned: ___ yes, ___ no. Turned to: ___ left, ___ right, ___ backside ___.
Head of bed at: ______ degrees. Incontinence/skin breakdown: ____ yes, ____ no.
Linens wet or soiled: ____ yes, ____ no. Linens changed: ____ yes, ______ no.
Dressing changed: ____ yes, ____ no. Location: ____________________.
IV site checked: _____ yes, _____ no. IV tubing labeled: _____ yes, _____no.
IV fluids at: ____.
Pain level (0-10 scale.0-no pain, 10 intolerable): ____________________.
Location of pain: ______________. Medicated for pain: ____ yes, ____ no.
Patient is alert/oriented: ___ yes, ___ no. New confusion: ____ yes, ____ no.
Vital signs: temp ____, pulse _____, resp _____, b/p _____, 02 _____ %, ____ liters.
Glucose level: _____. Insulin: ___ yes, ___ no. Type: ____________ # of units ____.

Nurse ____________, CNA ____________, in at _____ am/pm. Left at ______ am/pm.
Wash hands and wear gloves before touching patient: ______ yes, ______ no.
Wash hands before leaving room: ___ yes, ___ no. Wear protective gear: __ yes, __ no.
Clean stethoscope: __ yes, __ no. Oral care: __ yes, __ no. Suctioned: __ yes, __ no.
Repositioned: ___ yes, ___ no. Turned to: ___ left, ___ right, ___ backside ___.
Head of bed at: ______ degrees. Incontinence/skin breakdown: ____ yes, ____ no.
Linens wet or soiled: ____ yes, ____ no. Linens changed: ____ yes, ______ no.
Dressing changed: ____ yes, ____ no. Location: ____________________.
IV site checked: _____ yes, _____ no. IV tubing labeled: _____ yes, _____no.
IV fluids at: ____.
Pain level (0-10 scale.0-no pain, 10 intolerable): ____________________.
Location of pain: ______________. Medicated for pain: ____ yes, ____ no.
Patient is alert/oriented: ___ yes, ___ no. New confusion: ____ yes, ____ no.
Vital signs: temp ____, pulse _____, resp _____, b/p _____, 02 _____ %, ____ liters.
Glucose level: _____. Insulin: ___ yes, ___ no. Type: ____________ # of units ____.

Nurse ____________, CNA ____________, in at _____ am/pm. Left at ______ am/pm.
Wash hands and wear gloves before touching patient: ______ yes, ______ no.
Wash hands before leaving room: ___ yes, ___ no. Wear protective gear: __ yes, __ no.
Clean stethoscope: __ yes, __ no. Oral care: __ yes, __ no. Suctioned: __ yes, __ no.
Repositioned: ___ yes, ___ no. Turned to: ___ left, ___ right, ___ backside ___.
Head of bed at: ______ degrees. Incontinence/skin breakdown: ____ yes, ____ no.
Linens wet or soiled: ____ yes, ____ no. Linens changed: ____ yes, ______ no.
Dressing changed: ____ yes, ____ no. Location: ____________________.
IV site checked: _____ yes, _____ no. IV tubing labeled: _____ yes, _____no.
IV fluids at: ____.
Pain level (0-10 scale.0-no pain, 10 intolerable): ____________________.
Location of pain: ______________. Medicated for pain: ____ yes, ____ no.
Patient is alert/oriented: ___ yes, ___ no. New confusion: ____ yes, ____ no.
Vital signs: temp ____, pulse _____, resp _____, b/p _____, 02 _____ %, ____ liters.
Glucose level: _____. Insulin: ___ yes, ___ no. Type: ____________ # of units ____.

MEDICATION ADMINISTRATION LIST FOR ____________________
DATE ______________ DAY NUMBER ____________________

List the medication for each day. Routes of administration: oral, thru feeding tube, intravenous (IV), intramuscular (IM), subcutaneous (SQ), epidural or a catheter in your spinal column, rectal, topical, eye drops, and ear drops.

Medication: ____________ Route: ____________ Time: ____________
Medication: ____________ Route: ____________ Time: ____________
Medication: ____________ Route: ____________ Time: ____________
Medication: ____________ Route: ____________ Time: ____________
Medication: ____________ Route: ____________ Time: ____________
Medication: ____________ Route: ____________ Time: ____________
Medication: ____________ Route: ____________ Time: ____________
Medication: ____________ Route: ____________ Time: ____________
Medication: ____________ Route: ____________ Time: ____________
Medication: ____________ Route: ____________ Time: ____________
Medication: ____________ Route: ____________ Time: ____________
Medication: ____________ Route: ____________ Time: ____________
Medication: ____________ Route: ____________ Time: ____________
Medication: ____________ Route: ____________ Time: ____________
Medication: ____________ Route: ____________ Time: ____________
Medication: ____________ Route: ____________ Time: ____________
Medication: ____________ Route: ____________ Time: ____________
Medication: ____________ Route: ____________ Time: ____________
Medication: ____________ Route: ____________ Time: ____________
Medication: ____________ Route: ____________ Time: ____________
Medication: ____________ Route: ____________ Time: ____________
Medication: ____________ Route: ____________ Time: ____________
Medication: ____________ Route: ____________ Time: ____________
Medication: ____________ Route: ____________ Time: ____________
Medication: ____________ Route: ____________ Time: ____________
Medication: ____________ Route: ____________ Time: ____________
Medication: ____________ Route: ____________ Time: ____________
Medication: ____________ Route: ____________ Time: ____________
Medication: ____________ Route: ____________ Time: ____________
Medication: ____________ Route: ____________ Time: ____________
Medication: ____________ Route: ____________ Time: ____________
Medication: ____________ Route: ____________ Time: ____________
Medication: ____________ Route: ____________ Time: ____________
Medication: ____________ Route: ____________ Time: ____________
Medication: ____________ Route: ____________ Time: ____________
Medication: ____________ Route: ____________ Time: ____________
Medication: ____________ Route: ____________ Time: ____________
Medication: ____________ Route: ____________ Time: ____________
Medication: ____________ Route: ____________ Time: ____________
Medication: ____________ Route: ____________ Time: ____________
Medication: ____________ Route: ____________ Time: ____________
Medication: ____________ Route: ____________ Time: ____________
Medication: ____________ Route: ____________ Time: ____________
Medication: ____________ Route: ____________ Time: ____________
Medication: ____________ Route: ____________ Time: ____________
Medication: ____________ Route: ____________ Time: ____________
Medication: ____________ Route: ____________ Time: ____________
Medication: ____________ Route: ____________ Time: ____________
Medication: ____________ Route: ____________ Time: ____________
Medication: ____________ Route: ____________ Time: ____________
Medication: ____________ Route: ____________ Time: ____________
Medication: ____________ Route: ____________ Time: ____________
Medication: ____________ Route: ____________ Time: ____________
Medication: ____________ Route: ____________ Time: ____________

NOTES FOR DAY NUMBER ______________________________

DATE ______________________________

MEDICAL JOURNAL FOR ______________________________

DATE __________________, DAY NUMBER ______________

VISITS FROM MY DOCTORS TODAY

Goals for today: ____

____

____.

Things to discuss with my doctor(s): ______________________________

____

____

Dr.__________ came in at ____ am/pm. Left at ____ am/pm.
We discussed ____.
Did doctor examine patient: ____ yes, ____ no.
Wash hands before touching patient: ____ yes, ____ no.
Wear gloves: ____ yes, ___ no. Clean stethoscope: ____ yes, ____ no.
Wear gown and mask (precautions only):____ yes, ____ no.
Wash hands before leaving the room: ____ yes, ____ no.

Dr.__________ came in at ____ am/pm. Left at ____ am/pm.
We discussed ____.
Did doctor examine patient: ____ yes, ____ no.
Wash hands before touching patient: ____ yes, ____ no.
Wear gloves: ____ yes, ___ no. Clean stethoscope: ____ yes, ____ no.
Wear gown and mask (precautions only):____ yes, ____ no.
Wash hands before leaving the room: ____ yes, ____ no.

Dr.__________ came in at ____ am/pm. Left at ____ am/pm.
We discussed ____.
Did doctor examine patient: ____ yes, ____ no.
Wash hands before touching patient: ____ yes, ____ no.
Wear gloves: ____ yes, ___ no. Clean stethoscope: ____ yes, ____ no.
Wear gown and mask (precautions only):____ yes, ____ no.
Wash hands before leaving the room: ____ yes, ____ no.

Dr.__________ came in at ____ am/pm. Left at ____ am/pm.
We discussed ____.
Did doctor examine patient: ____ yes, ____ no.
Wash hands before touching patient: ____ yes, ____ no.
Wear gloves: ____ yes, ___ no. Clean stethoscope: ____ yes, ____ no.
Wear gown and mask (precautions only):____ yes, ____ no.
Wash hands before leaving the room: ____ yes, ____ no.

Dr.__________ came in at ____ am/pm. Left at ____ am/pm.
We discussed ____.
Did doctor examine patient: ____ yes, ____ no.
Wash hands before touching patient: ____ yes, ____ no.
Wear gloves: ____ yes, ___ no. Clean stethoscope: ____ yes, ____ no.
Wear gown and mask (precautions only):____ yes, ____ no.
Wash hands before leaving the room: ____ yes, ____ no.

NURSING CARE FOR ______________________________

DATE ____________________, DAY NUMBER ________________

INITIAL DAY SHIFT EXAM:

My nurse has ______ # of patients. CNA ___yes, ___no. Charge nurse ________
Nurse ______________ RN/LPN came in at _________ am/pm. Left at __________ am/pm.
Did nurse wash hands and wear gloves before touching patient: _______ yes, _______ no.
Wash hands after touching patient and before leaving the room: _____ yes, _______ no.
Don't hesitate to request staff to wash their hands. This will help decrease the risk of spreading potentially lethal germs.
Did nurse wear protective gear (isolation precautions only): _______ yes, _______ no.
Did nurse provide oral care (to be done every two hours if unable to provide for self, also decreases risk of pneumonia, infections, and aspiration): _______ yes, _______ no.
If able to provide own oral care, then supplies at bedside: ________ yes, _______ no.
Was patient repositioned (every two hours if unable to turn self): _____ yes _____ no.
Head of bed at _________ degrees. This is important for patients on ventilators or on tube feedings. Anything less than thirty degrees places patients at risk for aspiration of stomach contents into the lungs causing aspiration pneumonia.
Checked for incontinence and skin breakdown: _____ yes, _____ no.
Patient's linens wet or soiled: _____ yes, ____ no. Linens changed: ____ yes, _____ no.
Time linens changed: ________ am/pm. Any skin redness or breakdown: ____ yes, ____ no.
If yes, what stage is pressure ulcer: ________. Acquired when: ______________.
List wounds not associated with pressure ulcers and how acquired: _____________
____.
Mattress type: ____.
Specialty mattresses are important to help prevent pressure ulcers)
If patient on ventilator or has tracheostomy, suction performed: _____ yes, ______ no.
Did nurse listen to lung sounds: _____ yes, _____ no.
Does patient have chest tubes: ____ yes, ____ no. Functioning _____ yes, ______ no.
Bowel sounds: _______ yes, _______ no. Bowel sounds active: ______ yes, ______ no.
Neurological exam: ______ yes, ______ no. Follow commands: ______ yes, ______ no.
Is patient alert and oriented to person, place, time, and events: _____ yes, _____ no.
If confused, patient is not oriented to: ____ person, ___ place, ___ time, ___ event.
Confusion began (time and date): ______________________________________.
Glasgow coma scale (checks conscious scale of patient): ____________________.
Intracranial pressure monitoring: ______ yes, ______ no.
If yes, pressure is at _________ mm mercury. (Normal is one to fifteen).
Moves extremities: ___ yes, ___ no.
Paralysis: (inability to move extremities) ______ yes, ______ no.
If yes, extremities affected and when paralysis began: ___________________.
Is patient in pain: ____ yes, ____ no. Describe pain and location ______________.
Patient able to eat: _____ yes, ____ no. What type of diet? _________________.
If patient on tube feedings list type: _______________ at ____________ cc/ml per hour.
Nausea ____, vomiting _____. If so, describe: _______________________________.
Patient has: Nasal gastric tube ______, Dobhoff tube ______, Peg or gastric tube _____.
When was feeding tube placed and what site: ______________________________.
Catheter for draining urine: ____ yes, ____ no. If so, when placed: ____________
Find out policy for allowed time to remain in bladder. Too long may cause infections.)
IV site(s) where: ____________________________ when placed: ______________.
IV fluids (types and rates): ________________________, ______________________,
______________________, _________________________, ______________________,
Is patient on oxygen: _____ yes, ______ no. If so, how much and route delivered (see oxygen routes): ____
If patient on ventilator, list settings (see list on ventilator settings): __________
____.
Vital signs: temp ______, pulse ______, resp ______, b/p ______, o2 ______%,
current weight ______ pounds, ______ kg. Glucose level: ____________________.
Insulin coverage: ____ yes, ____ no. Insulin type: ____________, # of units: ______.

NURSING CARE CONTINUED FOR ______________________
DATE ______________________, DAY NUMBER ______________

FOLLOWING EXAMINATIONS FOR DAY SHIFT:

Nurse ____________, CNA ____________, in at _____ am/pm. Left at ______ am/pm.
Wash hands and wear gloves before touching patient: _____ yes, _____ no.
Wash hands before leaving room: ___ yes, ___ no. Wear protective gear: __ yes, __ no.
Clean stethoscope: __ yes, __ no. Oral care: __ yes, __ no. Suctioned: __ yes, __ no.
Repositioned: ___ yes, ___ no. Turned to: ___ left, ___ right, ___ backside ___.
Head of bed at: _______ degrees. Incontinence/skin breakdown: ____ yes, ____ no.
Linens wet or soiled: _____ yes, _____ no. Linens changed: _____ yes, _____ no.
Dressing changed: ____ yes, ____ no. Location: ______________________.
IV site checked: _____ yes, _____ no. IV tubing labeled: _____ yes, ____ no.
IV fluids at: ____.
Pain level (0-10 scale.0-no pain, 10 intolerable): ________________________.
Location of pain: ____________. Medicated for pain: _____ yes, _____ no.
Patient is alert/oriented: ___ yes, ____ no. New confusion: ___ yes, ____ no.
Vital signs: temp ___, pulse ____, resp _____, b/p _____, 02 _____ %, ____ liters.
Glucose level: _____. Insulin: ___ yes, ___ no. Type: __________ # of units ____.

Nurse ____________, CNA ____________, in at _____ am/pm. Left at ______ am/pm.
Wash hands and wear gloves before touching patient: _____ yes, _____ no.
Wash hands before leaving room: ___ yes, ___ no. Wear protective gear: __ yes, __ no.
Clean stethoscope: __ yes, __ no. Oral care: __ yes, __ no. Suctioned: __ yes, __ no.
Repositioned: ___ yes, ___ no. Turned to: ___ left, ___ right, ___ backside ___.
Head of bed at: _______ degrees. Incontinence/skin breakdown: ____ yes, ____ no.
Linens wet or soiled: _____ yes, _____ no. Linens changed: _____ yes, _____ no.
Dressing changed: ____ yes, ____ no. Location: ______________________.
IV site checked: _____ yes, _____ no. IV tubing labeled: _____ yes, ____ no.
IV fluids at: ____.
Pain level (0-10 scale.0-no pain, 10 intolerable): ________________________.
Location of pain: ____________. Medicated for pain: _____ yes, _____ no.
Patient is alert/oriented: ___ yes, ____ no. New confusion: ___ yes, ____ no.
Vital signs: temp ___, pulse ____, resp _____, b/p _____, 02 _____ %, ____ liters.
Glucose level: _____. Insulin: ___ yes, ___ no. Type: __________ # of units ____.

Nurse ____________, CNA ____________, in at _____ am/pm. Left at ______ am/pm.
Wash hands and wear gloves before touching patient: _____ yes, _____ no.
Wash hands before leaving room: ___ yes, ___ no. Wear protective gear: __ yes, __ no.
Clean stethoscope: __ yes, __ no. Oral care: __ yes, __ no. Suctioned: __ yes, __ no.
Repositioned: ___ yes, ___ no. Turned to: ___ left, ___ right, ___ backside ___.
Head of bed at: _______ degrees. Incontinence/skin breakdown: ____ yes, ____ no.
Linens wet or soiled: _____ yes, _____ no. Linens changed: _____ yes, _____ no.
Dressing changed: ____ yes, ____ no. Location: ______________________.
IV site checked: _____ yes, _____ no. IV tubing labeled: _____ yes, ____ no.
IV fluids at: ____.
Pain level (0-10 scale.0-no pain, 10 intolerable): ________________________.
Location of pain: ____________. Medicated for pain: _____ yes, _____ no.
Patient is alert/oriented: ___ yes, ____ no. New confusion: ___ yes, ____ no.
Vital signs: temp ___, pulse ____, resp _____, b/p _____, 02 _____ %, ____ liters.
Glucose level: _____. Insulin: ___ yes, ___ no. Type: __________ # of units ____.

NURSING CARE CONTINUED FOR ______________________
DATE ____________________, DAY NUMBER ______________________

FOLLOWING EXAMINATIONS FOR DAY SHIFT:

Nurse ____________, CNA ____________, in at _____ am/pm. Left at ______ am/pm.
Wash hands and wear gloves before touching patient: ______ yes, ______ no.
Wash hands before leaving room: ___ yes, ___ no. Wear protective gear: __ yes, __ no.
Clean stethoscope: __ yes, __ no. Oral care: __ yes, __ no. Suctioned: __ yes, __ no.
Repositioned: ___ yes, ___ no. Turned to: ___ left, ___ right, ___ backside ___.
Head of bed at: ______ degrees. Incontinence/skin breakdown: ____ yes, ____ no.
Linens wet or soiled: ____ yes, ____ no. Linens changed: ____ yes, _____ no.
Dressing changed: ____ yes, ____ no. Location: ______________________.
IV site checked: _____ yes, _____ no. IV tubing labeled: _____ yes, _____ no.
IV fluids at: ____.
Pain level (0-10 scale.0-no pain, 10 intolerable): ______________________.
Location of pain: ______________. Medicated for pain: _____ yes, ____ no.
Patient is alert/oriented: ____ yes, ____ no. New confusion: ____ yes, ____ no.
Vital signs: temp ____, pulse _____, resp ______, b/p ______, 02 _____ %, ____ liters.
Glucose level: _____. Insulin: ___ yes, ___ no. Type: ______________ # of units ____.

Nurse ____________, CNA ____________, in at _____ am/pm. Left at ______ am/pm.
Wash hands and wear gloves before touching patient: ______ yes, ______ no.
Wash hands before leaving room: ___ yes, ___ no. Wear protective gear: __ yes, __ no.
Clean stethoscope: __ yes, __ no. Oral care: __ yes, __ no. Suctioned: __ yes, __ no.
Repositioned: ___ yes, ___ no. Turned to: ___ left, ___ right, ___ backside ___.
Head of bed at: ______ degrees. Incontinence/skin breakdown: ____ yes, ____ no.
Linens wet or soiled: ____ yes, ____ no. Linens changed: ____ yes, _____ no.
Dressing changed: ____ yes, ____ no. Location: ______________________.
IV site checked: _____ yes, _____ no. IV tubing labeled: _____ yes, _____ no.
IV fluids at: ____.
Pain level (0-10 scale.0-no pain, 10 intolerable): ______________________.
Location of pain: ______________. Medicated for pain: _____ yes, ____ no.
Patient is alert/oriented: ____ yes, ____ no. New confusion: ____ yes, ____ no.
Vital signs: temp ____, pulse _____, resp ______, b/p ______, 02 _____ %, ____ liters.
Glucose level: _____. Insulin: ___ yes, ___ no. Type: ______________ # of units ____.

Nurse ____________, CNA ____________, in at _____ am/pm. Left at ______ am/pm.
Wash hands and wear gloves before touching patient: ______ yes, ______ no.
Wash hands before leaving room: ___ yes, ___ no. Wear protective gear: __ yes, __ no.
Clean stethoscope: __ yes, __ no. Oral care: __ yes, __ no. Suctioned: __ yes, __ no.
Repositioned: ___ yes, ___ no. Turned to: ___ left, ___ right, ___ backside ___.
Head of bed at: ______ degrees. Incontinence/skin breakdown: ____ yes, ____ no.
Linens wet or soiled: ____ yes, ____ no. Linens changed: ____ yes, _____ no.
Dressing changed: ____ yes, ____ no. Location: ______________________.
IV site checked: _____ yes, _____ no. IV tubing labeled: _____ yes, _____ no.
IV fluids at: ____.
Pain level (0-10 scale.0-no pain, 10 intolerable): ______________________.
Location of pain: ______________. Medicated for pain: _____ yes, ____ no.
Patient is alert/oriented: ____ yes, ____ no. New confusion: ____ yes, ____ no.
Vital signs: temp ____, pulse _____, resp ______, b/p ______, 02 _____ %, ____ liters.
Glucose level: _____. Insulin: ___ yes, ___ no. Type: ______________ # of units ____.

NURSING CARE FOR ______________________________

DATE ____________________, DAY NUMBER ____________________

INITIAL NIGHT SHIFT EXAM:

My nurse has ______ # of patients. CNA ___yes, ___no. Charge nurse ______________
Nurse ____________ RN/LPN came in at ___________ am/pm. Left at __________ am/pm.
Did nurse wash hands and wear gloves before touching patient: ______ yes, ______ no.
Wash hands after touching patient and before leaving the room: ______ yes, ______ no.
Don't hesitate to request staff to wash their hands. This will help decrease the risk of spreading potentially lethal germs.
Did nurse wear protective gear (isolation precautions only): ______ yes, ______ no.
Did nurse provide oral care (to be done every two hours if unable to provide for self, also decreases risk of pneumonia, infections, and aspiration): ______ yes, ______ no.
If able to provide own oral care, then supplies at bedside: ______ yes, ______ no.
Was patient repositioned (every two hours if unable to turn self): ______ yes ______ no.
Head of bed at ________ degrees. This is important for patients on ventilators or on tube feedings. Anything less than thirty degrees places patients at risk for aspiration of stomach contents into the lungs causing aspiration pneumonia.
Checked for incontinence and skin breakdown: ______ yes, ______ no.
Patient's linens wet or soiled: ______ yes, ______ no. Linens changed: ____ yes, ____ no.
Time linens changed: ________ am/pm. Any skin redness or breakdown: ____ yes, ____ no.
If yes, what stage is pressure ulcer: ________. Acquired when: ________________.
List wounds not associated with pressure ulcers and how acquired: ________________
____.
Mattress type: ____.
Specialty mattresses are important to help prevent pressure ulcers)
If patient on ventilator or has tracheostomy, suction performed: _____ yes, _____ no.
Did nurse listen to lung sounds: _____ yes, _____ no.
Does patient have chest tubes: ____ yes, ____ no. Functioning ______ yes, ______ no.
Bowel sounds: _______ yes, _______ no. Bowel sounds active: ______ yes, ______ no.
Neurological exam: ______ yes, ______ no. Follow commands: ______ yes, ______ no.
Is patient alert and oriented to person, place, time, and events: ______ yes, ______ no.
If confused, patient is not oriented to: ___ person, ___ place, ___ time, ___ event.
Confusion began (time and date): ____.
Glasgow coma scale (checks conscious scale of patient): ____________________________.
Intracranial pressure monitoring: ______ yes, ______ no.
If yes, pressure is at __________ mm mercury. (Normal is one to fifteen).
Moves extremities: _____ yes, _____ no.
Paralysis: (inability to move extremities) ______ yes, ______ no.
If yes, extremities affected and when paralysis began: ____________________________.
Is patient in pain: ____ yes, ____ no. Describe pain and location ____________________.
Patient able to eat: ____ yes, ____ no. What type of diet? ________________________.
If patient on tube feedings list type: ____________ at ____________ cc/ml per hour.
Nausea ____, vomiting ______. If so, describe: ____________________________________.
Patient has: Nasal gastric tube ______, Dobhoff tube ____, Peg or gastric tube ____.
When was feeding tube placed and what site: ____.
Catheter for draining urine: ____ yes, ____ no. If so, when placed: ______________.
Find out policy for allowed time to remain in bladder. Too long may cause infections.)
IV site(s) where: ______________________ when placed: ____________________________.
IV fluids (types and rates): ______________, ______________, ______________,
______________, ______________, ______________.
Is patient on oxygen: ______ yes, ______ no. If so, how much and route delivered (see oxygen routes): ____.
If patient on ventilator, list settings (see list on ventilator settings): __________
____.
Vital signs: temp ______, pulse ______, resp ______, b/p ______, o2 ______%,
current weight ______ pounds, ______ kg. Glucose level: ______
Insulin coverage: ____ yes, ____ no. Insulin type: ____________, # of units: ______.

NURSING CARE CONTINUED FOR ______________________
DATE ____________________, DAY NUMBER ____________________

FOLLOWING EXAMINATIONS FOR NIGHT SHIFT:

Nurse ______________, CNA _____________, in at _____ am/pm. Left at ______ am/pm.
Wash hands and wear gloves before touching patient: _____ yes, _____ no.
Wash hands before leaving room: ___ yes, ___ no. Wear protective gear: __ yes, __ no.
Clean stethoscope:__ yes, __ no. Oral care: __ yes, __ no. Suctioned: __ yes, __ no.
Repositioned: ___ yes, ___ no. Turned to: ___ left, ___ right, ___ backside ___.
Head of bed at: _______ degrees. Incontinence/skin breakdown: ____ yes, ____ no.
Linens wet or soiled: _____ yes, _____ no. Linens changed: _____ yes, _____ no.
Dressing changed: ____ yes, ____ no. Location: ______________________.
IV site checked: _____ yes, _____ no. IV tubing labeled: _____ yes, _____no.
IV fluids at: ______________________________________.
Pain level (0-10 scale.0-no pain, 10 intolerable): ______________________.
Location of pain: _____________. Medicated for pain: ____ yes, ____ no.
Patient is alert/oriented: ____ yes, ____ no. New confusion: ____ yes, ____ no.
Vital signs: temp ____, pulse _____, resp ______, b/p ______, 02 _____ %, ____ liters.
Glucose level:_____. Insulin: ___ yes, ___ no. Type: _____________ # of units ____.

Nurse ______________, CNA _____________, in at _____ am/pm. Left at ______ am/pm.
Wash hands and wear gloves before touching patient: _____ yes, _____ no.
Wash hands before leaving room: ___ yes, ___ no. Wear protective gear: __ yes, __ no.
Clean stethoscope: __ yes, __ no. Oral care: __ yes, __ no. Suctioned: __ yes, __ no.
Repositioned: ___ yes, ___ no. Turned to: ___ left, ___ right, ___ backside ___.
Head of bed at: _______ degrees. Incontinence/skin breakdown: ____ yes, ____ no.
Linens wet or soiled: _____ yes, _____ no. Linens changed: _____ yes, _____ no.
Dressing changed: ____ yes, ____ no. Location: ______________________.
IV site checked: _____ yes, _____ no. IV tubing labeled: _____ yes, _____no.
IV fluids at: ______________________________________.
Pain level (0-10 scale.0-no pain, 10 intolerable): ______________________.
Location of pain: _____________. Medicated for pain: ____ yes, ____ no.
Patient is alert/oriented: ____ yes, ____ no. New confusion: ____ yes, ____ no.
Vital signs: temp ____, pulse _____, resp ______, b/p ______, 02 _____ %, ____ liters.
Glucose level: _____. Insulin: ___ yes, ___ no. Type: _____________ # of units ____.

Nurse ______________, CNA _____________, in at _____ am/pm. Left at ______ am/pm.
Wash hands and wear gloves before touching patient: _____ yes, _____ no.
Wash hands before leaving room: ___ yes, ___ no. Wear protective gear: __ yes, __ no.
Clean stethoscope: __ yes, __ no. Oral care: __ yes, __ no. Suctioned: __ yes, __ no.
Repositioned: ___ yes, ___ no. Turned to: ___ left, ___ right, ___ backside ___.
Head of bed at: _______ degrees. Incontinence/skin breakdown: ____ yes, ____ no.
Linens wet or soiled: _____ yes, _____ no. Linens changed: _____ yes, _____ no.
Dressing changed: ____ yes, ____ no. Location: ______________________.
IV site checked: _____ yes, _____ no. IV tubing labeled: _____ yes, _____no.
IV fluids at: ______________________________________.
Pain level (0-10 scale.0-no pain, 10 intolerable): ______________________.
Location of pain: _____________. Medicated for pain: ____ yes, ____ no.
Patient is alert/oriented: ____ yes, ____ no. New confusion: ____ yes, ____ no.
Vital signs: temp ____, pulse _____, resp ______, b/p ______, 02 _____ %, ____ liters.
Glucose level: ____. Insulin: ___ yes, ___ no. Type: _____________ # of units ____.

NURSING CARE CONTINUED FOR ____________________
DATE ____________________, DAY NUMBER ____________________

FOLLOWING EXAMINATIONS FOR NIGHT SHIFT:

Nurse ______________, CNA ______________, in at ______ am/pm. Left at _______ am/pm.
Wash hands and wear gloves before touching patient: _______ yes, _______ no.
Wash hands before leaving room: ___ yes, ___ no. Wear protective gear: __ yes, __ no.
Clean stethoscope: __ yes, __ no. Oral care: __ yes, __ no. Suctioned: __ yes, __ no.
Repositioned: ___ yes, ___ no. Turned to: ___ left, ___ right, ___ backside ___.
Head of bed at: _______ degrees. Incontinence/skin breakdown: ____ yes, ____ no.
Linens wet or soiled: _____ yes, _____ no. Linens changed: _____ yes, _____ no.
Dressing changed: ____ yes, _____ no. Location: ____________________.
IV site checked: _____ yes, _____ no. IV tubing labeled: _____ yes, _____no.
IV fluids at: ____.
Pain level (0-10 scale.0-no pain, 10 intolerable): ____________________.
Location of pain: ______________. Medicated for pain: _____ yes, ____ no.
Patient is alert/oriented: ____ yes, ____ no. New confusion: ____ yes, ____ no
Vital signs: temp ____, pulse _____, resp ______, b/p ______, 02 ____ %, ____ liters.
Glucose level: _____. Insulin: ___ yes, ___ no. Type: ______________ # of units ___.

Nurse ______________, CNA ______________, in at ______ am/pm. Left at _______ am/pm.
Wash hands and wear gloves before touching patient: _______ yes, _______ no.
Wash hands before leaving room: ___ yes, ___ no. Wear protective gear: __ yes, __ no.
Clean stethoscope: __ yes, __ no. Oral care: __ yes, __ no. Suctioned: __ yes, __ no.
Repositioned: ___ yes, ___ no. Turned to: ___ left, ___ right, ___ backside ___.
Head of bed at: _______ degrees. Incontinence/skin breakdown: ____ yes, ____ no.
Linens wet or soiled: _____ yes, _____ no. Linens changed: _____ yes, _____ no.
Dressing changed: ____ yes, _____ no. Location: ____________________.
IV site checked: _____ yes, _____ no. IV tubing labeled: _____ yes, _____no.
IV fluids at: ____.
Pain level (0-10 scale.0-no pain, 10 intolerable): ____________________.
Location of pain: ______________. Medicated for pain: _____ yes, ____ no.
Patient is alert/oriented: ____ yes, ____ no. New confusion: ____ yes, ____ no.
Vital signs: temp ____, pulse _____, resp ______, b/p ______, 02 ____ %, ____ liters.
Glucose level: _____. Insulin: ___ yes, ___ no. Type: ______________ # of units ___.

Nurse ______________, CNA ______________, in at ______ am/pm. Left at _______ am/pm.
Wash hands and wear gloves before touching patient: _______ yes, _______ no.
Wash hands before leaving room: ___ yes, ___ no. Wear protective gear: __ yes, __ no.
Clean stethoscope: __ yes, __ no. Oral care: __ yes, __ no. Suctioned: __ yes, __ no.
Repositioned: ___ yes, ___ no. Turned to: ___ left, ___ right, ___ backside ___.
Head of bed at: _______ degrees. Incontinence/skin breakdown: ____ yes, ____ no.
Linens wet or soiled: _____ yes, _____ no. Linens changed: _____ yes, _____ no.
Dressing changed: ____ yes, _____ no. Location: ____________________.
IV site checked: _____ yes, _____ no. IV tubing labeled: _____ yes, _____no.
IV fluids at: ____.
Pain level (0-10 scale.0-no pain, 10 intolerable): ____________________.
Location of pain: ______________. Medicated for pain: _____ yes, ____ no.
Patient is alert/oriented: ____ yes, ____ no. New confusion: ____ yes, ____ no.
Vital signs: temp ____, pulse _____, resp ______, b/p ______, 02 ____ %, ____ liters.
Glucose level: _____. Insulin: ___ yes, ___ no. Type: ______________ # of units ___.

MEDICATION ADMINISTRATION LIST FOR ____________________
DATE ________________ DAY NUMBER ________________________

List the medication for each day. Routes of administration: oral, thru feeding tube, intravenous (IV), intramuscular (IM), subcutaneous (SQ), epidural or a catheter in your spinal column, rectal, topical, eye drops, and ear drops.

Medication: ______________ Route: ______________ Time: ______________
Medication: ______________ Route: ______________ Time: ______________
Medication: ______________ Route: ______________ Time: ______________
Medication: ______________ Route: ______________ Time: ______________
Medication: ______________ Route: ______________ Time: ______________
Medication: ______________ Route: ______________ Time: ______________
Medication: ______________ Route: ______________ Time: ______________
Medication: ______________ Route: ______________ Time: ______________
Medication: ______________ Route: ______________ Time: ______________
Medication: ______________ Route: ______________ Time: ______________
Medication: ______________ Route: ______________ Time: ______________
Medication: ______________ Route: ______________ Time: ______________
Medication: ______________ Route: ______________ Time: ______________
Medication: ______________ Route: ______________ Time: ______________
Medication: ______________ Route: ______________ Time: ______________
Medication: ______________ Route: ______________ Time: ______________
Medication: ______________ Route: ______________ Time: ______________
Medication: ______________ Route: ______________ Time: ______________
Medication: ______________ Route: ______________ Time: ______________
Medication: ______________ Route: ______________ Time: ______________
Medication: ______________ Route: ______________ Time: ______________
Medication: ______________ Route: ______________ Time: ______________
Medication: ______________ Route: ______________ Time: ______________
Medication: ______________ Route: ______________ Time: ______________
Medication: ______________ Route: ______________ Time: ______________
Medication: ______________ Route: ______________ Time: ______________
Medication: ______________ Route: ______________ Time: ______________
Medication: ______________ Route: ______________ Time: ______________
Medication: ______________ Route: ______________ Time: ______________
Medication: ______________ Route: ______________ Time: ______________
Medication: ______________ Route: ______________ Time: ______________
Medication: ______________ Route: ______________ Time: ______________
Medication: ______________ Route: ______________ Time: ______________
Medication: ______________ Route: ______________ Time: ______________
Medication: ______________ Route: ______________ Time: ______________
Medication: ______________ Route: ______________ Time: ______________
Medication: ______________ Route: ______________ Time: ______________
Medication: ______________ Route: ______________ Time: ______________
Medication: ______________ Route: ______________ Time: ______________
Medication: ______________ Route: ______________ Time: ______________
Medication: ______________ Route: ______________ Time: ______________
Medication: ______________ Route: ______________ Time: ______________
Medication: ______________ Route: ______________ Time: ______________
Medication: ______________ Route: ______________ Time: ______________
Medication: ______________ Route: ______________ Time: ______________
Medication: ______________ Route: ______________ Time: ______________
Medication: ______________ Route: ______________ Time: ______________
Medication: ______________ Route: ______________ Time: ______________
Medication: ______________ Route: ______________ Time: ______________
Medication: ______________ Route: ______________ Time: ______________
Medication: ______________ Route: ______________ Time: ______________
Medication: ______________ Route: ______________ Time: ______________
Medication: ______________ Route: ______________ Time: ______________
Medication: ______________ Route: ______________ Time: ______________

NOTES FOR DAY NUMBER ______________________

DATE ______________________________

MEDICAL JOURNAL FOR ______________________________

DATE ____________________, DAY NUMBER ________________

VISITS FROM MY DOCTORS TODAY

Goals for today: ____

____

____.

Things to discuss with my doctor(s): ________________________________

____

____

Dr.____________ came in at ____ am/pm. Left at ____ am/pm.
We discussed ____.
Did doctor examine patient: _____ yes, _____ no.
Wash hands before touching patient: _____ yes, _____ no.
Wear gloves: ____ yes, ___ no. Clean stethoscope: ____ yes, ____ no.
Wear gown and mask (precautions only):____ yes, _____ no.
Wash hands before leaving the room: _____ yes, _____ no.

Dr.____________ came in at ____ am/pm. Left at ____ am/pm.
We discussed ____.
Did doctor examine patient: _____ yes, _____ no.
Wash hands before touching patient: _____ yes, _____ no.
Wear gloves: ____ yes, ___ no. Clean stethoscope: ____ yes, ____ no.
Wear gown and mask (precautions only):____ yes, _____ no.
Wash hands before leaving the room: _____ yes, _____ no.

Dr.____________ came in at ____ am/pm. Left at ____ am/pm.
We discussed ____.
Did doctor examine patient: _____ yes, _____ no.
Wash hands before touching patient: _____ yes, _____ no.
Wear gloves: ____ yes, ___ no. Clean stethoscope: ____ yes, ____ no.
Wear gown and mask (precautions only):____ yes, _____ no.
Wash hands before leaving the room: _____ yes, _____ no.

Dr.____________ came in at ____ am/pm. Left at ____ am/pm.
We discussed ____.
Did doctor examine patient: _____ yes, _____ no.
Wash hands before touching patient: _____ yes, _____ no.
Wear gloves: ____ yes, ___ no. Clean stethoscope: ____ yes, ____ no.
Wear gown and mask (precautions only):____ yes, _____ no.
Wash hands before leaving the room: _____ yes, _____ no.

Dr.____________ came in at ____ am/pm. Left at ____ am/pm.
We discussed ____.
Did doctor examine patient: _____ yes, _____ no.
Wash hands before touching patient: _____ yes, _____ no.
Wear gloves: ____ yes, ___ no. Clean stethoscope: ____ yes, ____ no.
Wear gown and mask (precautions only):____ yes, _____ no.
Wash hands before leaving the room: _____ yes, _____ no.

NURSING CARE FOR ______________________________

DATE ____________________, DAY NUMBER ____________________

INITIAL DAY SHIFT EXAM:

My nurse has ______ # of patients. CNA ___yes, ___no. Charge nurse ______________
Nurse ______________ RN/LPN came in at __________ am/pm. Left at ____________ am/pm.
Did nurse wash hands and wear gloves before touching patient: ______ yes, ______ no.
Wash hands after touching patient and before leaving the room: ______ yes, ______ no.
Don't hesitate to request staff to wash their hands. This will help decrease the risk of spreading potentially lethal germs.
Did nurse wear protective gear (isolation precautions only): ______ yes, ______ no.
Did nurse provide oral care (to be done every two hours if unable to provide for self, also decreases risk of pneumonia, infections, and aspiration): ______ yes, ______ no.
If able to provide own oral care, then supplies at bedside: ______ yes, ______ no.
Was patient repositioned (every two hours if unable to turn self): ______ yes ______ no.
Head of bed at ________ degrees. This is important for patients on ventilators or on tube feedings. Anything less than thirty degrees places patients at risk for aspiration of stomach contents into the lungs causing aspiration pneumonia.
Checked for incontinence and skin breakdown: ______ yes, ______ no.
Patient's linens wet or soiled: ______ yes, ______ no. Linens changed: ____ yes, ____ no.
Time linens changed: ________ am/pm. Any skin redness or breakdown: ____ yes, ____ no.
If yes, what stage is pressure ulcer: ______. Acquired when: ______________________.
List wounds not associated with pressure ulcers and how acquired: ___________________
____.
Mattress type: ____
Specialty mattresses are important to help prevent pressure ulcers)
If patient on ventilator or has tracheostomy, suction performed: ______ yes, ______ no.
Did nurse listen to lung sounds: ______ yes, ______ no.
Does patient have chest tubes: ____ yes, ____ no. Functioning ______ yes, ______ no.
Bowel sounds: ______ yes, ______ no. Bowel sounds active: ______ yes, ______ no.
Neurological exam: ______ yes, ______ no. Follow commands: ______ yes, ______ no.
Is patient alert and oriented to person, place, time, and events: ______ yes, ______ no.
If confused, patient is not oriented to: ____ person, ___ place, ___ time, ___ event.
Confusion began (time and date): ____.
Glasgow coma scale (checks conscious scale of patient): ______________________.
Intracranial pressure monitoring: ______ yes, ______ no.
If yes, pressure is at ________ mm mercury. (Normal is one to fifteen).
Moves extremities: ___ yes, ___ no.
Paralysis: (inability to move extremities) ________ yes, ________ no.
If yes, extremities affected and when paralysis began: _________________________.
Is patient in pain: ______ yes, ______ no. Describe pain and location ______________.
Patient able to eat: ______ yes, ______ no. What type of diet? ____________________.
If patient on tube feedings list type: ____________ at ____________ cc/ml per hour.
Nausea ____, vomiting ____. If so, describe: __________________________________.
Patient has: Nasal gastric tube ______, Dobhoff tube _____, Peg or gastric tube ____.
When was feeding tube placed and what site: ____________________________________.
Catheter for draining urine: ____ yes, ____ no. If so, when placed: ______________.
Find out policy for allowed time to remain in bladder. Too long may cause infections.)
IV site(s) where: ____________________ when placed: ____________________________.
IV fluids (types and rates): ______________, ______________, ______________,
______________, ______________, ______________, ______________, ______________.
Is patient on oxygen: _____ yes, _____ no. If so, how much and route delivered (see oxygen routes): ____.
If patient on ventilator, list settings (see list on ventilator settings): __________
____.
Vital signs: temp ______, pulse ______, resp ______, b/p ______, o2 ______%, current weight ______ pounds, ______ kg. Glucose level: ______
Insulin coverage: ____ yes, ____ no. Insulin type: ______________, # of units: ______.

NURSING CARE CONTINUED FOR ______________________
DATE ________________, DAY NUMBER ________________

FOLLOWING EXAMINATIONS FOR DAY SHIFT:

Nurse ____________, CNA ____________, in at _____ am/pm. Left at _______ am/pm.
Wash hands and wear gloves before touching patient: _______ yes, _______ no.
Wash hands before leaving room: ___ yes, ___ no. Wear protective gear: __ yes, __ no.
Clean stethoscope: __ yes, __ no. Oral care: __ yes, __ no. Suctioned: __ yes, __ no.
Repositioned: ___ yes, ___ no. Turned to: ___ left, ___ right, ___ backside ___.
Head of bed at: _______ degrees. Incontinence/skin breakdown: ___ yes, ___ no.
Linens wet or soiled: ____ yes, ____ no. Linens changed: _____ yes, _____ no.
Dressing changed: ____ yes, ____ no. Location: ________________.
IV site checked: _____ yes, _____ no. IV tubing labeled: _____ yes, _____no.
IV fluids at: ______________________________.
Pain level (0-10 scale.0-no pain, 10 intolerable): ______________.
Location of pain: ______________. Medicated for pain: _____ yes, _____ no.
Patient is alert/oriented: ____ yes, ____ no. New confusion: ____ yes, ____ no.
Vital signs: temp ____, pulse ____, resp ____, b/p _____, 02 _____ %, ____ liters.
Glucose level: _____. Insulin: ___ yes, ___ no. Type: _________ # of units ____.

Nurse ____________, CNA ____________, in at _____ am/pm. Left at _______ am/pm.
Wash hands and wear gloves before touching patient: _______ yes, _______ no.
Wash hands before leaving room: ___ yes, ___ no. Wear protective gear: __ yes, __ no.
Clean stethoscope: __ yes, __ no. Oral care: __ yes, __ no. Suctioned: __ yes, __ no.
Repositioned: ___ yes, ___ no. Turned to: ___ left, ___ right, ___ backside ___.
Head of bed at: _______ degrees. Incontinence/skin breakdown: ___ yes, ___ no.
Linens wet or soiled: ____ yes, ____ no. Linens changed: _____ yes, _____ no.
Dressing changed: ____ yes, ____ no. Location: ________________.
IV site checked: _____ yes, _____ no. IV tubing labeled: _____ yes, _____no.
IV fluids at: ______________________________.
Pain level (0-10 scale.0-no pain, 10 intolerable): ______________.
Location of pain: ______________. Medicated for pain: _____ yes, _____ no.
Patient is alert/oriented: ____ yes, ____ no. New confusion: ____ yes, ____ no.
Vital signs: temp ____, pulse ____, resp ____, b/p _____, 02 _____ %, ____ liters.
Glucose level: _____. Insulin: ___ yes, ___ no. Type: _________ # of units ____.

Nurse ____________, CNA ____________, in at _____ am/pm. Left at _______ am/pm.
Wash hands and wear gloves before touching patient: _______ yes, _______ no.
Wash hands before leaving room: ___ yes, ___ no. Wear protective gear: __ yes, __ no.
Clean stethoscope: __ yes, __ no. Oral care: __ yes, __ no. Suctioned: __ yes, __ no.
Repositioned: ___ yes, ___ no. Turned to: ___ left, ___ right, ___ backside ___.
Head of bed at: _______ degrees. Incontinence/skin breakdown: ___ yes, ___ no.
Linens wet or soiled: ____ yes, ____ no. Linens changed: _____ yes, _____ no.
Dressing changed: ____ yes, ____ no. Location: ________________.
IV site checked: _____ yes, _____ no. IV tubing labeled: _____ yes, _____no.
IV fluids at: ______________________________.
Pain level (0-10 scale.0-no pain, 10 intolerable): ______________.
Location of pain: ______________. Medicated for pain: _____ yes, _____ no.
Patient is alert/oriented: ____ yes, ____ no. New confusion: ____ yes, ____ no.
Vital signs: temp ____, pulse ____, resp ____, b/p _____, 02 _____ %, ____ liters.
Glucose level: _____. Insulin: ___ yes, ___ no. Type: _________ # of units ____.

NURSING CARE CONTINUED FOR ______________________
DATE ____________________, DAY NUMBER ________________

FOLLOWING EXAMINATIONS FOR DAY SHIFT:

Nurse ______________, CNA ______________, in at ______ am/pm. Left at ______ am/pm.
Wash hands and wear gloves before touching patient: ______ yes, ___ no.
Wash hands before leaving room: ___ yes, ___ no. Wear protective gear: __ yes, __ no.
Clean stethoscope: __ yes, __ no. Oral care: __ yes, __ no. Suctioned: __ yes, __ no.
Repositioned: ___ yes, ___ no. Turned to: ___ left, ___ right, ___ backside ___.
Head of bed at: _______ degrees. Incontinence/skin breakdown: ___ yes, ___ no.
Linens wet or soiled: ____ yes, ____ no. Linens changed: ____ yes, ___ no.
Dressing changed: ____ yes, ____ no. Location: ______________________________
IV site checked: _____ yes, _____ no. IV tubing labeled: _____ yes, _____no.
IV fluids at: ____.
Pain level (0-10 scale.0-no pain, 10 intolerable): ____________________________.
Location of pain: ____________. Medicated for pain: ____ yes, ___ no.
Patient is alert/oriented: ____ yes, ___ no. New confusion: ___ yes, ___ no.
Vital signs: temp ____, pulse ____, resp ______, b/p _____, 02 _____ %, ____ liters.
Glucose level: _____. Insulin: ___ yes, ___ no. Type: ___________ # of units ____.

Nurse ______________, CNA ______________, in at ______ am/pm. Left at ______ am/pm.
Wash hands and wear gloves before touching patient: ______ yes, ___ no.
Wash hands before leaving room: ___ yes, ___ no. Wear protective gear: __ yes, __ no.
Clean stethoscope: __ yes, __ no. Oral care: __ yes, __ no. Suctioned: __ yes, __ no.
Repositioned: ___ yes, ___ no. Turned to: ___ left, ___ right, ___ backside ___.
Head of bed at: _______ degrees. Incontinence/skin breakdown: ___ yes, ___ no.
Linens wet or soiled: ____ yes, ____ no. Linens changed: ____ yes, ___ no.
Dressing changed: ____ yes, ____ no. Location: ______________________________
IV site checked: _____ yes, _____ no. IV tubing labeled: _____ yes, _____no.
IV fluids at: ____.
Pain level (0-10 scale.0-no pain, 10 intolerable): ____________________________.
Location of pain: ____________. Medicated for pain: ____ yes, ___ no.
Patient is alert/oriented: ____ yes, ___ no. New confusion: ___ yes, ___ no.
Vital signs: temp ____, pulse ____, resp ______, b/p _____, 02 _____ %, ____ liters.
Glucose level: _____. Insulin: ___ yes, ___ no. Type: ___________ # of units ____.

Nurse ______________, CNA ______________, in at ______ am/pm. Left at ______ am/pm.
Wash hands and wear gloves before touching patient: ______ yes, ___ no.
Wash hands before leaving room: ___ yes, ___ no. Wear protective gear: __ yes, __ no.
Clean stethoscope: __ yes, __ no. Oral care: __ yes, __ no. Suctioned: __ yes, __ no.
Repositioned: ___ yes, ___ no. Turned to: ___ left, ___ right, ___ backside ___.
Head of bed at: _______ degrees. Incontinence/skin breakdown: ___ yes, ___ no.
Linens wet or soiled: ____ yes, ____ no. Linens changed: ____ yes, ___ no.
Dressing changed: ____ yes, ____ no. Location: ______________________________
IV site checked: _____ yes, _____ no. IV tubing labeled: _____ yes, _____no.
IV fluids at: ____.
Pain level (0-10 scale.0-no pain, 10 intolerable): ____________________________.
Location of pain: ____________. Medicated for pain: ____ yes, ___ no.
Patient is alert/oriented: ____ yes, ___ no. New confusion: ___ yes, ___ no.
Vital signs: temp ____, pulse ____, resp ______, b/p _____, 02 _____ %, ____ liters.
Glucose level: _____. Insulin: ___ yes, ___ no. Type: ___________ # of units ____.

NURSING CARE FOR ________________________

DATE ____________________, DAY NUMBER ______________________

INITIAL NIGHT SHIFT EXAM:

My nurse has ______ # of patients. CNA ___yes, ___no. Charge nurse ________________
Nurse ________________ RN/LPN came in at __________ am/pm. Left at ___________ am/pm.
Did nurse wash hands and wear gloves before touching patient: ________ yes, _____ no.
Wash hands after touching patient and before leaving the room: _______ yes, _____ no.
Don't hesitate to request staff to wash their hands. This will help decrease the risk of spreading potentially lethal germs.
Did nurse wear protective gear (isolation precautions only): _______ yes, _______ no.
Did nurse provide oral care (to be done every two hours if unable to provide for self, also decreases risk of pneumonia, infections, and aspiration): ______ yes, ______ no.
If able to provide own oral care, then supplies at bedside: _______ yes, ______ no.
Was patient repositioned (every two hours if unable to turn self): _____ yes _____ no.
Head of bed at ________ degrees. This is important for patients on ventilators or on tube feedings. Anything less than thirty degrees places patients at risk for aspiration of stomach contents into the lungs causing aspiration pneumonia.
Checked for incontinence and skin breakdown: ____ yes, _____ no.
Patient's linens wet or soiled: ____ yes,____ no. Linens changed: ____ yes, ____ no.
Time linens changed: ________ am/pm. Any skin redness or breakdown: ____ yes, ____ no.
If yes, what stage is pressure ulcer: _______. Acquired when: ______________________.
List wounds not associated with pressure ulcers and how acquired: ________________
____.
Mattress type: ____.
Specialty mattresses are important to help prevent pressure ulcers)
If patient on ventilator or has tracheostomy, suction performed: _____ yes, ______ no.
Did nurse listen to lung sounds: _____ yes, _____ no.
Does patient have chest tubes: ____ yes, ____ no. Functioning _____ yes, ______ no.
Bowel sounds: ______ yes, _______ no. Bowel sounds active: ______ yes, ______ no.
Neurological exam: _____ yes, ______ no. Follow commands: _______ yes, ______ no.
Is patient alert and oriented to person, place, time, and events: _____ yes, _____ no.
If confused, patient is not oriented to: ____ person, ___ place, ___ time, ___ event.
Confusion began (time and date): ____.
Glasgow coma scale (checks conscious scale of patient): ________________________.
Intracranial pressure monitoring: _____ yes, _____ no.
If yes, pressure is at ________ mm mercury. (Normal is one to fifteen).
Moves extremities: ___ yes, ___ no.
Paralysis: (inability to move extremities) ______ yes, ______ no.
If yes, extremities affected and when paralysis began: ___________________________.
Is patient in pain: ____ yes, _____ no. Describe pain and location ______________.
Patient able to eat: ____ yes, ____ no. What type of diet? _____________________.
If patient on tube feedings list type: ______________ at ___________ cc/ml per hour.
Nausea ____, vomiting _____. If so, describe: ___________________________________.
Patient has: Nasal gastric tube ______, Dobhoff tube _____, Peg or gastric tube ____.
When was feeding tube placed and what site: ______________________________________.
Catheter for draining urine: ____ yes, ____ no. If so, when placed: ______________.
Find out policy for allowed time to remain in bladder. Too long may cause infections.)
IV site(s) where: __________________________ when placed: ______________________.
IV fluids (types and rates): ____,
_____________________, ___________________________, ____________________________,
Is patient on oxygen: _____ yes, _____ no. If so, how much and route delivered (see oxygen routes): ____.
If patient on ventilator, list settings (see list on ventilator settings): __________
____.
Vital signs: temp ______, pulse ______, resp ______, b/p ______, o2 ______%,
current weight ______ pounds, ______ kg. Glucose level: ______
Insulin coverage: ____ yes, ____ no. Insulin type: ____________, # of units: ______.

NURSING CARE CONTINUED FOR ______________________
DATE ________________, DAY NUMBER ______________

FOLLOWING EXAMINATIONS FOR NIGHT SHIFT:

Nurse ____________, CNA ____________, in at _____ am/pm. Left at _____ am/pm.
Wash hands and wear gloves before touching patient: ___ yes, ___ no.
Wash hands before leaving room: ___ yes, ___ no. Wear protective gear: ___ yes, ___ no.
Clean stethoscope: ___ yes, ___ no. Oral care: ___ yes, ___ no. Suctioned: ___ yes, ___ no.
Repositioned: ___ yes, ___ no. Turned to: ___ left, ___ right, ___ backside ___.
Head of bed at: ___ degrees. Incontinence/skin breakdown: ___ yes, ___ no.
Linens wet or soiled: ___ yes, ___ no. Linens changed: ___ yes, ___ no.
Dressing changed: ___ yes, ___ no. Location: ______________.
IV site checked: ___ yes, ___ no. IV tubing labeled: ___ yes, ___ no.
IV fluids at: ______________________.
Pain level (0-10 scale.0-no pain, 10 intolerable): ______________.
Location of pain: ____________. Medicated for pain: ___ yes, ___ no.
Patient is alert/oriented: ___ yes, ___ no. New confusion: ___ yes, ___ no.
Vital signs: temp ___, pulse ___, resp ___, b/p ___, 02 ___ %, ___ liters.
Glucose level: ___. Insulin: ___ yes, ___ no. Type: ________ # of units ___.

Nurse ____________, CNA ____________, in at _____ am/pm. Left at _____ am/pm.
Wash hands and wear gloves before touching patient: ___ yes, ___ no.
Wash hands before leaving room: ___ yes, ___ no. Wear protective gear: ___ yes, ___ no.
Clean stethoscope: ___ yes, ___ no. Oral care: ___ yes, ___ no. Suctioned: ___ yes, ___ no.
Repositioned: ___ yes, ___ no. Turned to: ___ left, ___ right, ___ backside ___.
Head of bed at: ___ degrees. Incontinence/skin breakdown: ___ yes, ___ no.
Linens wet or soiled: ___ yes, ___ no. Linens changed: ___ yes, ___ no.
Dressing changed: ___ yes, ___ no. Location: ______________.
IV site checked: ___ yes, ___ no. IV tubing labeled: ___ yes, ___ no.
IV fluids at: ______________________.
Pain level (0-10 scale.0-no pain, 10 intolerable): ______________.
Location of pain: ____________. Medicated for pain: ___ yes, ___ no.
Patient is alert/oriented: ___ yes, ___ no. New confusion: ___ yes, ___ no.
Vital signs: temp ___, pulse ___, resp ___, b/p ___, 02 ___ %, ___ liters.
Glucose level: ___. Insulin: ___ yes, ___ no. Type: ________ # of units ___.

Nurse ____________, CNA ____________, in at _____ am/pm. Left at _____ am/pm.
Wash hands and wear gloves before touching patient: ___ yes, ___ no.
Wash hands before leaving room: ___ yes, ___ no. Wear protective gear: ___ yes, ___ no.
Clean stethoscope: ___ yes, ___ no. Oral care: ___ yes, ___ no. Suctioned: ___ yes, ___ no.
Repositioned: ___ yes, ___ no. Turned to: ___ left, ___ right, ___ backside ___.
Head of bed at: ___ degrees. Incontinence/skin breakdown: ___ yes, ___ no.
Linens wet or soiled: ___ yes, ___ no. Linens changed: ___ yes, ___ no.
Dressing changed: ___ yes, ___ no. Location: ______________.
IV site checked: ___ yes, ___ no. IV tubing labeled: ___ yes, ___ no.
IV fluids at: ______________________.
Pain level (0-10 scale.0-no pain, 10 intolerable): ______________.
Location of pain: ____________. Medicated for pain: ___ yes, ___ no.
Patient is alert/oriented: ___ yes, ___ no. New confusion: ___ yes, ___ no.
Vital signs: temp ___, pulse ___, resp ___, b/p ___, 02 ___ %, ___ liters.
Glucose level: ___. Insulin: ___ yes, ___ no. Type: ________ # of units ___.

NURSING CARE CONTINUED FOR ______________________________

DATE ____________________, DAY NUMBER ____________________

FOLLOWING EXAMINATIONS FOR NIGHT SHIFT:

Nurse ____________, CNA ____________, in at _____ am/pm. Left at _____ am/pm.
Wash hands and wear gloves before touching patient: _____ yes, _____ no.
Wash hands before leaving room: ___ yes, ___ no. Wear protective gear: __ yes, __ no.
Clean stethoscope: __ yes, __ no. Oral care: __ yes, __ no. Suctioned: __ yes, __ no.
Repositioned: ___ yes, ___ no. Turned to: ___ left, ___ right, ___ backside ___.
Head of bed at: ________ degrees. Incontinence/skin breakdown: ____ yes, ____ no.
Linens wet or soiled: _____ yes, _____ no. Linens changed: _____ yes, ______ no.
Dressing changed: ____ yes, ____ no. Location: ____________________.
IV site checked: _____ yes, _____ no. IV tubing labeled: _____ yes, _____no.
IV fluids at: ____.
Pain level (0-10 scale.0-no pain, 10 intolerable): ____________________.
Location of pain: ______________. Medicated for pain: ____ yes, ____ no.
Patient is alert/oriented: ____ yes, ____ no. New confusion: ____ yes, ____ no.
Vital signs: temp ____, pulse _____, resp _____, b/p _____, 02 _____ %, ____ liters.
Glucose level: _____. Insulin: ___ yes, ___ no. Type: ______________ # of units ____.

Nurse ____________, CNA ____________, in at _____ am/pm. Left at _____ am/pm.
Wash hands and wear gloves before touching patient: _____ yes, _____ no.
Wash hands before leaving room: ___ yes, ___ no. Wear protective gear: __ yes, __ no.
Clean stethoscope: __ yes, __ no. Oral care: __ yes, __ no. Suctioned: __ yes, __ no.
Repositioned: ___ yes, ___ no. Turned to: ___ left, ___ right, ___ backside ___.
Head of bed at: ________ degrees. Incontinence/skin breakdown: ____ yes, ____ no.
Linens wet or soiled: _____ yes, _____ no. Linens changed: _____ yes, ______ no.
Dressing changed: ____ yes, ____ no. Location: ____________________.
IV site checked: _____ yes, _____ no. IV tubing labeled: _____ yes, _____no.
IV fluids at: ____.
Pain level (0-10 scale.0-no pain, 10 intolerable): ____________________.
Location of pain: ______________. Medicated for pain: ____ yes, ____ no.
Patient is alert/oriented: ____ yes, ____ no. New confusion: ____ yes, ____ no.
Vital signs: temp ____, pulse _____, resp _____, b/p _____, 02 _____ %, ____ liters.
Glucose level: _____. Insulin: ___ yes, ___ no. Type: ______________ # of units ____.

Nurse ____________, CNA ____________, in at _____ am/pm. Left at _____ am/pm.
Wash hands and wear gloves before touching patient: _____ yes, _____ no.
Wash hands before leaving room: ___ yes, ___ no. Wear protective gear: __ yes, __ no.
Clean stethoscope: __ yes, __ no. Oral care: __ yes, __ no. Suctioned: __ yes, __ no.
Repositioned: ___ yes, ___ no. Turned to: ___ left, ___ right, ___ backside ___.
Head of bed at: ________ degrees. Incontinence/skin breakdown: ____ yes, ____ no.
Linens wet or soiled: _____ yes, _____ no. Linens changed: _____ yes, ______ no.
Dressing changed: ____ yes, ____ no. Location: ____________________.
IV site checked: _____ yes, _____ no. IV tubing labeled: _____ yes, _____no.
IV fluids at: ____.
Pain level (0-10 scale.0-no pain, 10 intolerable): ____________________.
Location of pain: ______________. Medicated for pain: ____ yes, ____ no.
Patient is alert/oriented: ____ yes, ____ no. New confusion: ____ yes, ____ no.
Vital signs: temp ____, pulse _____, resp _____, b/p _____, 02 _____ %, ____ liters.
Glucose level: _____. Insulin: ___ yes, ___ no. Type: ______________ # of units ____.

MEDICATION ADMINISTRATION LIST FOR ______________
DATE ______________ DAY NUMBER ______________

List the medication for each day. Routes of administration: oral, thru feeding tube, intravenous (IV), intramuscular (IM), subcutaneous (SQ), epidural or a catheter in your spinal column, rectal, topical, eye drops, and ear drops.

Medication: ______________ Route: ______________ Time: ______________
Medication: ______________ Route: ______________ Time: ______________
Medication: ______________ Route: ______________ Time: ______________
Medication: ______________ Route: ______________ Time: ______________
Medication: ______________ Route: ______________ Time: ______________
Medication: ______________ Route: ______________ Time: ______________
Medication: ______________ Route: ______________ Time: ______________
Medication: ______________ Route: ______________ Time: ______________
Medication: ______________ Route: ______________ Time: ______________
Medication: ______________ Route: ______________ Time: ______________
Medication: ______________ Route: ______________ Time: ______________
Medication: ______________ Route: ______________ Time: ______________
Medication: ______________ Route: ______________ Time: ______________
Medication: ______________ Route: ______________ Time: ______________
Medication: ______________ Route: ______________ Time: ______________
Medication: ______________ Route: ______________ Time: ______________
Medication: ______________ Route: ______________ Time: ______________
Medication: ______________ Route: ______________ Time: ______________
Medication: ______________ Route: ______________ Time: ______________
Medication: ______________ Route: ______________ Time: ______________
Medication: ______________ Route: ______________ Time: ______________
Medication: ______________ Route: ______________ Time: ______________
Medication: ______________ Route: ______________ Time: ______________
Medication: ______________ Route: ______________ Time: ______________
Medication: ______________ Route: ______________ Time: ______________
Medication: ______________ Route: ______________ Time: ______________
Medication: ______________ Route: ______________ Time: ______________
Medication: ______________ Route: ______________ Time: ______________
Medication: ______________ Route: ______________ Time: ______________
Medication: ______________ Route: ______________ Time: ______________
Medication: ______________ Route: ______________ Time: ______________
Medication: ______________ Route: ______________ Time: ______________
Medication: ______________ Route: ______________ Time: ______________
Medication: ______________ Route: ______________ Time: ______________
Medication: ______________ Route: ______________ Time: ______________
Medication: ______________ Route: ______________ Time: ______________
Medication: ______________ Route: ______________ Time: ______________
Medication: ______________ Route: ______________ Time: ______________
Medication: ______________ Route: ______________ Time: ______________
Medication: ______________ Route: ______________ Time: ______________
Medication: ______________ Route: ______________ Time: ______________
Medication: ______________ Route: ______________ Time: ______________
Medication: ______________ Route: ______________ Time: ______________
Medication: ______________ Route: ______________ Time: ______________
Medication: ______________ Route: ______________ Time: ______________
Medication: ______________ Route: ______________ Time: ______________
Medication: ______________ Route: ______________ Time: ______________
Medication: ______________ Route: ______________ Time: ______________
Medication: ______________ Route: ______________ Time: ______________
Medication: ______________ Route: ______________ Time: ______________
Medication: ______________ Route: ______________ Time: ______________
Medication: ______________ Route: ______________ Time: ______________
Medication: ______________ Route: ______________ Time: ______________
Medication: ______________ Route: ______________ Time: ______________

NOTES FOR DAY NUMBER ______________________

DATE ______________________

MEDICAL JOURNAL FOR ______________________________

DATE ____________________, DAY NUMBER ______________

VISITS FROM MY DOCTORS TODAY

Goals for today: ____
____
____.

Things to discuss with my doctor(s): ________________________
____
____

Dr.__________ came in at ____ am/pm. Left at ____ am/pm.
We discussed ____.
Did doctor examine patient: ____ yes, ____ no.
Wash hands before touching patient: ____ yes, ____ no.
Wear gloves: ___ yes, ___ no. Clean stethoscope: ___ yes, ___ no.
Wear gown and mask (precautions only):____ yes, _____ no.
Wash hands before leaving the room: ____ yes, ____ no.

Dr.__________ came in at ____ am/pm. Left at ____ am/pm.
We discussed ____.
Did doctor examine patient: ____ yes, ____ no.
Wash hands before touching patient: ____ yes, ____ no.
Wear gloves: ___ yes, ___ no. Clean stethoscope: ___ yes, ___ no.
Wear gown and mask (precautions only):____ yes, _____ no.
Wash hands before leaving the room: ____ yes, ____ no.

Dr.__________ came in at ____ am/pm. Left at ____ am/pm.
We discussed ____.
Did doctor examine patient: ____ yes, ____ no.
Wash hands before touching patient: ____ yes, ____ no.
Wear gloves: ___ yes, ___ no. Clean stethoscope: ___ yes, ___ no.
Wear gown and mask (precautions only):____ yes, _____ no.
Wash hands before leaving the room: ____ yes, ____ no.

Dr.__________ came in at ____ am/pm. Left at ____ am/pm.
We discussed ____.
Did doctor examine patient: ____ yes, ____ no.
Wash hands before touching patient: ____ yes, ____ no.
Wear gloves: ___ yes, ___ no. Clean stethoscope: ___ yes, ___ no.
Wear gown and mask (precautions only):____ yes, _____ no.
Wash hands before leaving the room: ____ yes, ____ no.

Dr.__________ came in at ____ am/pm. Left at ____ am/pm.
We discussed ____.
Did doctor examine patient: ____ yes, ____ no.
Wash hands before touching patient: ____ yes, ____ no.
Wear gloves: ___ yes, ___ no. Clean stethoscope: ___ yes, ___ no.
Wear gown and mask (precautions only):____ yes, _____ no.
Wash hands before leaving the room: ____ yes, ____ no.

NURSING CARE FOR ____________________________________

DATE ________________, DAY NUMBER ___________________

INITIAL DAY SHIFT EXAM:

My nurse has ______ # of patients. CNA ___yes, ___no. Charge nurse ___________
Nurse _______________ RN/LPN came in at __________ am/pm. Left at __________ am/pm.
Did nurse wash hands and wear gloves before touching patient: _______ yes, _______ no.
Wash hands after touching patient and before leaving the room: ______ yes, _______ no.
Don't hesitate to request staff to wash their hands. This will help decrease the risk of spreading potentially lethal germs.
Did nurse wear protective gear (isolation precautions only): _______ yes, _______ no.
Did nurse provide oral care (to be done every two hours if unable to provide for self, also decreases risk of pneumonia, infections, and aspiration): _______ yes, _______ no.
If able to provide own oral care, then supplies at bedside: ________ yes, _______ no.
Was patient repositioned (every two hours if unable to turn self): _____ yes _____ no.
Head of bed at ________ degrees. This is important for patients on ventilators or on tube feedings. Anything less than thirty degrees places patients at risk for aspiration of stomach contents into the lungs causing aspiration pneumonia.
Checked for incontinence and skin breakdown: _____ yes, _____ no.
Patient's linens wet or soiled: _____ yes, _____ no. Linens changed: ____ yes, ____ no.
Time linens changed: _______ am/pm. Any skin redness or breakdown: ____ yes, ____ no.
If yes, what stage is pressure ulcer: _______. Acquired when: ____________________.
List wounds not associated with pressure ulcers and how acquired: _________________
____.
Mattress type: ____.
Specialty mattresses are important to help prevent pressure ulcers)
If patient on ventilator or has tracheostomy, suction performed: _____ yes, ______ no.
Did nurse listen to lung sounds: _____ yes, _____ no.
Does patient have chest tubes: ____ yes, ____ no. Functioning _____ yes, _____ no.
Bowel sounds: _______ yes, _______ no. Bowel sounds active: _____ yes, _____ no.
Neurological exam: _____ yes, ______ no. Follow commands: ______ yes, ______ no.
Is patient alert and oriented to person, place, time, and events: _____ yes, _____ no.
If confused, patient is not oriented to: ____ person, ___ place, ___ time, ___ event.
Confusion began (time and date): ____.
Glasgow coma scale (checks conscious scale of patient): ______________________.
Intracranial pressure monitoring: ______ yes, ______ no.
If yes, pressure is at ________ mm mercury. (Normal is one to fifteen).
Moves extremities: ___ yes, ___ no.
Paralysis: (inability to move extremities) ________ yes, _______ no.
If yes, extremities affected and when paralysis began: _________________________.
Is patient in pain: ____ yes, ____ no. Describe pain and location _______________
Patient able to eat: ____ yes, ____ no. What type of diet? _______________________.
If patient on tube feedings list type: ____________ at ___________ cc/ml per hour.
Nausea ____, vomiting _____. If so, describe: ___________________________________.
Patient has: Nasal gastric tube ______, Dobhoff tube _____, Peg or gastric tube _____.
When was feeding tube placed and what site: ____________________________________.
Catheter for draining urine: ___ yes, ____ no. If so, when placed: ______________.
Find out policy for allowed time to remain in bladder. Too long may cause infections.)
IV site(s) where: ________________________ when placed: _________________________.
IV fluids (types and rates): ____________________, ______________________________,
____________________, ____________________, ____________________________________,
Is patient on oxygen: _____ yes, _____ no. If so, how much and route delivered (see oxygen routes): ____.
If patient on ventilator, list settings (see list on ventilator settings): ________
____.
Vital signs: temp ______, pulse ______, resp ______, b/p ______, o2 ______%,
current weight ______ pounds, ______ kg. Glucose level: ______________
Insulin coverage: ____ yes, ____ no. Insulin type: ___________, # of units: ______.

NURSING CARE CONTINUED FOR ______________________
DATE ____________________, DAY NUMBER ____________________

FOLLOWING EXAMINATIONS FOR DAY SHIFT:

Nurse ___________, CNA ___________, in at _____ am/pm. Left at ______ am/pm.
Wash hands and wear gloves before touching patient: _____ yes, ____ no.
Wash hands before leaving room: ___ yes, __ no. Wear protective gear: __ yes, __ no.
Clean stethoscope: __ yes, __ no. Oral care: __ yes, __ no. Suctioned: __ yes, __ no.
Repositioned: __ yes, __ no. Turned to: ___ left, ___ right, ___ backside ___.
Head of bed at: ______ degrees. Incontinence/skin breakdown: ___ yes, ___ no.
Linens wet or soiled: _____ yes, ___ no. Linens changed: ____ yes, ____ no.
Dressing changed: ____ yes, ____ no. Location: ______________________.
IV site checked: _____ yes, ____ no. IV tubing labeled: ___ yes, ___ no.
IV fluids at: ____.
Pain level (0-10 scale.0-no pain, 10 intolerable): _____________________.
Location of pain: __________. Medicated for pain: ____ yes, ____ no.
Patient is alert/oriented: ____ yes, ____ no. New confusion: ___ yes, ___ no.
Vital signs: temp ____, pulse ____, resp _____, b/p _____, 02 _____%, ____ liters.
Glucose level: _____. Insulin: ___ yes, ___ no. Type: ___________ # of units ____.

Nurse ___________, CNA ___________, in at _____ am/pm. Left at ______ am/pm.
Wash hands and wear gloves before touching patient: _____ yes, ____ no.
Wash hands before leaving room: ___ yes, __ no. Wear protective gear: __ yes, __ no.
Clean stethoscope: __ yes, __ no. Oral care: __ yes, __ no. Suctioned: __ yes, __ no.
Repositioned: __ yes, __ no. Turned to: ___ left, ___ right, ___ backside ___.
Head of bed at: ______ degrees. Incontinence/skin breakdown: ___ yes, ___ no.
Linens wet or soiled: _____ yes, ___ no. Linens changed: ____ yes, ____ no.
Dressing changed: ____ yes, ____ no. Location: ______________________.
IV site checked: _____ yes, ____ no. IV tubing labeled: ___ yes, ___ no.
IV fluids at: ____.
Pain level (0-10 scale.0-no pain, 10 intolerable): _____________________.
Location of pain: __________. Medicated for pain: ____ yes, ____ no.
Patient is alert/oriented: ____ yes, ____ no. New confusion: ___ yes, ___ no.
Vital signs: temp ____, pulse ____, resp _____, b/p _____, 02 _____%, ____ liters.
Glucose level: _____. Insulin: ___ yes, ___ no. Type: ___________ # of units ____.

Nurse ___________, CNA ___________, in at _____ am/pm. Left at ______ am/pm.
Wash hands and wear gloves before touching patient: _____ yes, ____ no.
Wash hands before leaving room: ___ yes, __ no. Wear protective gear: __ yes, __ no.
Clean stethoscope: __ yes, __ no. Oral care: __ yes, __ no. Suctioned: __ yes, __ no.
Repositioned: __ yes, __ no. Turned to: ___ left, ___ right, ___ backside ___.
Head of bed at: ______ degrees. Incontinence/skin breakdown: ___ yes, ___ no.
Linens wet or soiled: _____ yes, ___ no. Linens changed: ____ yes, ____ no.
Dressing changed: ____ yes, ____ no. Location: ______________________.
IV site checked: _____ yes, ____ no. IV tubing labeled: ___ yes, ___ no.
IV fluids at: ____.
Pain level (0-10 scale.0-no pain, 10 intolerable): _____________________.
Location of pain: __________. Medicated for pain: ____ yes, ____ no.
Patient is alert/oriented: ____ yes, ____ no. New confusion: ___ yes, ___ no.
Vital signs: temp ____, pulse ____, resp _____, b/p _____, 02 _____%, ____ liters.
Glucose level: _____. Insulin: ___ yes, ___ no. Type: ___________ # of units ____.

NURSING CARE CONTINUED FOR ______________________
DATE ____________________, DAY NUMBER ______________

FOLLOWING EXAMINATIONS FOR DAY SHIFT:

Nurse ______________, CNA ______________, in at _____ am/pm. Left at ______ am/pm.
Wash hands and wear gloves before touching patient: ______ yes, ______ no.
Wash hands before leaving room: ___ yes, ___ no. Wear protective gear: __ yes, __ no.
Clean stethoscope: __ yes, __ no. Oral care: __ yes, __ no. Suctioned: __ yes, __ no.
Repositioned: ___ yes, ___ no. Turned to: ___ left, ___ right, ___ backside ___.
Head of bed at: _______ degrees. Incontinence/skin breakdown: _____ yes, ___ no.
Linens wet or soiled: _____ yes, _____ no. Linens changed: _____ yes, _____ no.
Dressing changed: ____ yes, ____ no. Location: ______________________________.
IV site checked: _____ yes, _____ no. IV tubing labeled: _____ yes, _____ no.
IV fluids at: ____.
Pain level (0-10 scale.0-no pain, 10 intolerable): __________________________.
Location of pain: ________________. Medicated for pain: _____ yes, _____ no.
Patient is alert/oriented: ____ yes, ____ no. New confusion: ____ yes, ____ no.
Vital signs: temp ____, pulse _____, resp _____, b/p _____, 02 _____ %, ___ liters.
Glucose level: _____. Insulin: ___ yes, ___ no. Type: ___________ # of units ____.

Nurse ______________, CNA ______________, in at _____ am/pm. Left at ______ am/pm.
Wash hands and wear gloves before touching patient: ______ yes, ______ no.
Wash hands before leaving room: ___ yes, ___ no. Wear protective gear: __ yes, __ no.
Clean stethoscope: __ yes, __ no. Oral care: __ yes, __ no. Suctioned: __ yes, __ no.
Repositioned: ___ yes, ___ no. Turned to: ___ left, ___ right, ___ backside ___.
Head of bed at: _______ degrees. Incontinence/skin breakdown: _____ yes, ___ no.
Linens wet or soiled: _____ yes, _____ no. Linens changed: _____ yes, _____ no.
Dressing changed: ____ yes, ____ no. Location: ______________________________.
IV site checked: _____ yes, _____ no. IV tubing labeled: _____ yes, _____ no.
IV fluids at: ____.
Pain level (0-10 scale.0-no pain, 10 intolerable): __________________________.
Location of pain: ________________. Medicated for pain: _____ yes, _____ no.
Patient is alert/oriented: ____ yes, ____ no. New confusion: ____ yes, ____ no.
Vital signs: temp ____, pulse _____, resp _____, b/p _____, 02 _____ %, ___ liters.
Glucose level: _____. Insulin: ___ yes, ___ no. Type: ___________ # of units ____.

Nurse ______________, CNA ______________, in at _____ am/pm. Left at ______ am/pm.
Wash hands and wear gloves before touching patient: ______ yes, ______ no.
Wash hands before leaving room: ___ yes, ___ no. Wear protective gear: __ yes, __ no.
Clean stethoscope: __ yes, __ no. Oral care: __ yes, __ no. Suctioned: __ yes, __ no.
Repositioned: ___ yes, ___ no. Turned to: ___ left, ___ right, ___ backside ___.
Head of bed at: _______ degrees. Incontinence/skin breakdown: _____ yes, ___ no.
Linens wet or soiled: _____ yes, _____ no. Linens changed: _____ yes, _____ no.
Dressing changed: ____ yes, ____ no. Location: ______________________________.
IV site checked: _____ yes, _____ no. IV tubing labeled: _____ yes, _____ no.
IV fluids at: ____.
Pain level (0-10 scale.0-no pain, 10 intolerable): __________________________.
Location of pain: ________________. Medicated for pain: _____ yes, _____ no.
Patient is alert/oriented: ____ yes, ____ no. New confusion: ____ yes, ____ no.
Vital signs: temp ____, pulse _____, resp _____, b/p _____, 02 _____ %, ___ liters.
Glucose level: _____. Insulin: ___ yes, ___ no. Type: ___________ # of units ____.

NURSING CARE FOR ____________________

DATE ______________, DAY NUMBER ______________

INITIAL NIGHT SHIFT EXAM:

My nurse has ______ # of patients. CNA ___yes, ___no. Charge nurse ______________
Nurse ______________ RN/LPN came in at __________ am/pm. Left at __________ am/pm.
Did nurse wash hands and wear gloves before touching patient: ______ yes, ______ no.
Wash hands after touching patient and before leaving the room: ______ yes, ______ no.
Don't hesitate to request staff to wash their hands. This will help decrease the risk of spreading potentially lethal germs.
Did nurse wear protective gear (isolation precautions only): ______ yes, ______ no.
Did nurse provide oral care (to be done every two hours if unable to provide for self, also decreases risk of pneumonia, infections, and aspiration): ______ yes, ______ no.
If able to provide own oral care, then supplies at bedside: ______ yes, ______ no.
Was patient repositioned (every two hours if unable to turn self): ______ yes ______ no.
Head of bed at ________ degrees. This is important for patients on ventilators or on tube feedings. Anything less than thirty degrees places patients at risk for aspiration of stomach contents into the lungs causing aspiration pneumonia.
Checked for incontinence and skin breakdown: ____ yes, ____ no.
Patient's linens wet or soiled: ____ yes, ____ no. Linens changed: ____ yes, ____ no.
Time linens changed: ________ am/pm. Any skin redness or breakdown: ____ yes, ____ no.
If yes, what stage is pressure ulcer: ______. Acquired when: ______________
List wounds not associated with pressure ulcers and how acquired: ______________
____.
Mattress type: ____.
Specialty mattresses are important to help prevent pressure ulcers)
If patient on ventilator or has tracheostomy, suction performed: ______ yes, ______ no.
Did nurse listen to lung sounds: ____ yes, ____ no.
Does patient have chest tubes: ____ yes, ____ no. Functioning ______ yes, ______ no.
Bowel sounds: ______ yes, ______ no. Bowel sounds active: ______ yes, ______ no.
Neurological exam: ______ yes, ______ no. Follow commands: ______ yes, ______ no.
Is patient alert and oriented to person, place, time, and events: ____ yes, ____ no.
If confused, patient is not oriented to: ___ person, ___ place, ___ time, ___ event.
Confusion began (time and date): ____
Glasgow coma scale (checks conscious scale of patient): ______________________
Intracranial pressure monitoring: ____ yes, ____ no.
If yes, pressure is at ________ mm mercury. (Normal is one to fifteen).
Moves extremities: ____ yes, ____ no.
Paralysis: (inability to move extremities) ______ yes, ______ no.
If yes, extremities affected and when paralysis began: ______________________
Is patient in pain: ____ yes, ____ no. Describe pain and location ______________
Patient able to eat: ____ yes, ____ no. What type of diet? ______________
If patient on tube feedings list type: ______________ at ______________ cc/ml per hour.
Nausea ____, vomiting ____. If so, describe: ______________________________
Patient has: Nasal gastric tube ____, Dobhoff tube ____, Peg or gastric tube ____
When was feeding tube placed and what site: ______________________________
Catheter for draining urine: ____ yes, ____ no. If so, when placed: ______________.
Find out policy for allowed time to remain in bladder. Too long may cause infections.)
IV site(s) where: ______________________ when placed: ______________
IV fluids (types and rates): ______________, ______________, ______________,
______________, ______________, ______________.
Is patient on oxygen: ______ yes, ______ no. If so, how much and route delivered (see oxygen routes): ____.
If patient on ventilator, list settings (see list on ventilator settings): ______________
____.
Vital signs: temp ______, pulse ______, resp ______, b/p ______, o2 ______%,
current weight ______ pounds, ______ kg. Glucose level: ______
Insulin coverage: ____ yes, ____ no. Insulin type: ______________, # of units: ______.

NURSING CARE CONTINUED FOR ______________________________
DATE ____________________, DAY NUMBER ______________________

FOLLOWING EXAMINATIONS FOR NIGHT SHIFT:

Nurse ______________, CNA ______________, in at _____ am/pm. Left at _______ am/pm.
Wash hands and wear gloves before touching patient: _______ yes, _______ no.
Wash hands before leaving room: ___ yes, ___ no. Wear protective gear: __ yes, __ no.
Clean stethoscope: __ yes, __ no. Oral care: __ yes, __ no. Suctioned: __ yes, __ no.
Repositioned: ___ yes, ___ no. Turned to: ___ left, ___ right, ___ backside ___.
Head of bed at: _______ degrees. Incontinence/skin breakdown: ____ yes, ____ no.
Linens wet or soiled: _____ yes, _____ no. Linens changed: _____ yes, ______ no.
Dressing changed: ____ yes, ____ no. Location: ________________.
IV site checked: _____ yes, _____ no. IV tubing labeled: _____ yes, _____no.
IV fluids at: ______________________________________.
Pain level (0-10 scale.0-no pain, 10 intolerable): ___________________.
Location of pain: _______________. Medicated for pain: _______ yes, ___ no.
Patient is alert/oriented: ____ yes, ____ no. New confusion: ____ yes, ____ no.
Vital signs: temp ____, pulse _____, resp _____, b/p _____, 02 ____ %, ____ liters.
Glucose level: _____. Insulin: ___ yes, ___ no. Type: ____________ # of units ___.

Nurse ______________, CNA ______________, in at _____ am/pm. Left at _______ am/pm.
Wash hands and wear gloves before touching patient: _______ yes, _______ no.
Wash hands before leaving room: ___ yes, ___ no. Wear protective gear: __ yes, __ no.
Clean stethoscope: __ yes, __ no. Oral care: __ yes, __ no. Suctioned: __ yes, __ no.
Repositioned: ___ yes, ___ no. Turned to: ___ left, ___ right, ___ backside ___.
Head of bed at: _______ degrees. Incontinence/skin breakdown: ____ yes, ____ no.
Linens wet or soiled: _____ yes, _____ no. Linens changed: _____ yes, ______ no.
Dressing changed: ____ yes, ____ no. Location: ________________.
IV site checked: _____ yes, _____ no. IV tubing labeled: _____ yes, _____no.
IV fluids at: ______________________________________.
Pain level (0-10 scale.0-no pain, 10 intolerable): ___________________.
Location of pain: _______________. Medicated for pain: _______ yes, ___ no.
Patient is alert/oriented: ____ yes, ____ no. New confusion: ____ yes, ____ no.
Vital signs: temp ____, pulse _____, resp _____, b/p _____, 02 ____ %, ____ liters.
Glucose level: _____. Insulin: ___ yes, ___ no. Type: ____________ # of units ___.

Nurse ______________, CNA ______________, in at _____ am/pm. Left at _______ am/pm.
Wash hands and wear gloves before touching patient: _______ yes, _______ no.
Wash hands before leaving room: ___ yes, ___ no. Wear protective gear: __ yes, __ no.
Clean stethoscope: __ yes, __ no. Oral care: __ yes, __ no. Suctioned: __ yes, __ no.
Repositioned: ___ yes, ___ no. Turned to: ___ left, ___ right, ___ backside ___.
Head of bed at: _______ degrees. Incontinence/skin breakdown: ____ yes, ____ no.
Linens wet or soiled: _____ yes, _____ no. Linens changed: _____ yes, ______ no.
Dressing changed: ____ yes, ____ no. Location: ________________.
IV site checked: _____ yes, _____ no. IV tubing labeled: _____ yes, _____no.
IV fluids at: ______________________________________.
Pain level (0-10 scale.0-no pain, 10 intolerable): ___________________.
Location of pain: _______________. Medicated for pain: _______ yes, ___ no.
Patient is alert/oriented: ____ yes, ____ no. New confusion: ____ yes, ____ no.
Vital signs: temp ____, pulse _____, resp _____, b/p _____, 02 ____ %, ____ liters.
Glucose level: _____. Insulin: ___ yes, ___ no. Type: ____________ # of units ___.

NURSING CARE CONTINUED FOR ____________________
DATE ____________________, DAY NUMBER ____________________

FOLLOWING EXAMINATIONS FOR NIGHT SHIFT:

Nurse ______________, CNA ______________, in at _____ am/pm. Left at ______ am/pm.
Wash hands and wear gloves before touching patient: ______ yes, ______ no.
Wash hands before leaving room: ___ yes, ___ no. Wear protective gear: __ yes, __ no.
Clean stethoscope: __ yes, __ no. Oral care: __ yes, __ no. Suctioned: __ yes, __ no.
Repositioned: ___ yes, ___ no. Turned to: ___ left, ___ right, ___ backside ___.
Head of bed at: ______ degrees. Incontinence/skin breakdown: ____ yes, ____ no.
Linens wet or soiled: ______ yes, ______ no. Linens changed: _____ yes, _____ no.
Dressing changed: ____ yes, ____ no. Location: ______________________________.
IV site checked: _____ yes, _____ no. IV tubing labeled: _____ yes, _____ no.
IV fluids at: ____.
Pain level (0-10 scale.0-no pain, 10 intolerable): ____________________.
Location of pain: ________________. Medicated for pain: _____ yes, ____ no.
Patient is alert/oriented: ____ yes, ____ no. New confusion: ____ yes, ____ no.
Vital signs: temp ____, pulse _____, resp ______, b/p ______, 02 _____ %, ____ liters.
Glucose level: ______. Insulin: ___ yes, ___ no. Type: _______________ # of units ____.

Nurse ______________, CNA ______________, in at _____ am/pm. Left at ______ am/pm.
Wash hands and wear gloves before touching patient: ______ yes, ______ no.
Wash hands before leaving room: ___ yes, ___ no. Wear protective gear: __ yes, __ no.
Clean stethoscope: __ yes, __ no. Oral care: __ yes, __ no. Suctioned: __ yes, __ no.
Repositioned: ___ yes, ___ no. Turned to: ___ left, ___ right, ___ backside ___.
Head of bed at: ______ degrees. Incontinence/skin breakdown: ____ yes, ____ no.
Linens wet or soiled: ______ yes, ______ no. Linens changed: _____ yes, _____ no.
Dressing changed: ____ yes, ____ no. Location: ______________________________.
IV site checked: _____ yes, _____ no. IV tubing labeled: _____ yes, _____ no.
IV fluids at: ____.
Pain level (0-10 scale.0-no pain, 10 intolerable): ____________________.
Location of pain: ________________. Medicated for pain: _____ yes, ____ no.
Patient is alert/oriented: ____ yes, ____ no. New confusion: ____ yes, ____ no.
Vital signs: temp ____, pulse _____, resp ______, b/p ______, 02 _____ %, ____ liters.
Glucose level: ______. Insulin: ___ yes, ___ no. Type: _______________ # of units ____.

Nurse ______________, CNA ______________, in at _____ am/pm. Left at ______ am/pm.
Wash hands and wear gloves before touching patient: ______ yes, ______ no.
Wash hands before leaving room: ___ yes, ___ no. Wear protective gear: __ yes, __ no.
Clean stethoscope: __ yes, __ no. Oral care: __ yes, __ no. Suctioned: __ yes, __ no.
Repositioned: ___ yes, ___ no. Turned to: ___ left, ___ right, ___ backside ___.
Head of bed at: ______ degrees. Incontinence/skin breakdown: ____ yes, ____ no.
Linens wet or soiled: ______ yes, ______ no. Linens changed: _____ yes, _____ no.
Dressing changed: ____ yes, ____ no. Location: ______________________________.
IV site checked: _____ yes, _____ no. IV tubing labeled: _____ yes, _____ no.
IV fluids at: ____.
Pain level (0-10 scale.0-no pain, 10 intolerable): ____________________.
Location of pain: ________________. Medicated for pain: _____ yes, ____ no.
Patient is alert/oriented: ____ yes, ____ no. New confusion: ____ yes, ____ no.
Vital signs: temp ____, pulse _____, resp ______, b/p ______, 02 _____ %, ____ liters.
Glucose level: ______. Insulin: ___ yes, ___ no. Type: _______________ # of units ____.

MEDICATION ADMINISTRATION LIST FOR ____________________
DATE ______________ DAY NUMBER ____________________

List the medication for each day. Routes of administration: oral, thru feeding tube, intravenous (IV), intramuscular (IM), subcutaneous (SQ), epidural or a catheter in your spinal column, rectal, topical, eye drops, and ear drops.

Medication:	Route:	Time:
______________	______________	__________
______________	______________	__________
______________	______________	__________
______________	______________	__________
______________	______________	__________
______________	______________	__________
______________	______________	__________
______________	______________	__________
______________	______________	__________
______________	______________	__________
______________	______________	__________
______________	______________	__________
______________	______________	__________
______________	______________	__________
______________	______________	__________
______________	______________	__________
______________	______________	__________
______________	______________	__________
______________	______________	__________
______________	______________	__________
______________	______________	__________
______________	______________	__________
______________	______________	__________
______________	______________	__________
______________	______________	__________
______________	______________	__________
______________	______________	__________
______________	______________	__________
______________	______________	__________
______________	______________	__________
______________	______________	__________
______________	______________	__________
______________	______________	__________
______________	______________	__________
______________	______________	__________
______________	______________	__________
______________	______________	__________
______________	______________	__________
______________	______________	__________
______________	______________	__________
______________	______________	__________
______________	______________	__________
______________	______________	__________
______________	______________	__________
______________	______________	__________
______________	______________	__________
______________	______________	__________
______________	______________	__________
______________	______________	__________
______________	______________	__________
______________	______________	__________
______________	______________	__________
______________	______________	__________
______________	______________	__________

NOTES FOR DAY NUMBER ____________________

DATE ____________________

MEDICAL JOURNAL FOR ____________________________

DATE ________________, DAY NUMBER ______________

VISITS FROM MY DOCTORS TODAY

Goals for today: ____

____

____.

Things to discuss with my doctor(s): ______________________________________

____

____

Dr.______________ came in at _____ am/pm. Left at _____ am/pm.
We discussed ____.
Did doctor examine patient: _____ yes, _____ no.
Wash hands before touching patient: _____ yes, _____ no.
Wear gloves: ____ yes, ___ no. Clean stethoscope: ____ yes, ____ no.
Wear gown and mask (precautions only):____ yes, _____ no.
Wash hands before leaving the room: _____ yes, _____ no.

Dr.______________ came in at _____ am/pm. Left at _____ am/pm.
We discussed ____.
Did doctor examine patient: _____ yes, _____ no.
Wash hands before touching patient: _____ yes, _____ no.
Wear gloves: ____ yes, ___ no. Clean stethoscope: ____ yes, ____ no.
Wear gown and mask (precautions only):____ yes, _____ no.
Wash hands before leaving the room: _____ yes, _____ no.

Dr.______________ came in at _____ am/pm. Left at _____ am/pm.
We discussed ____.
Did doctor examine patient: _____ yes, _____ no.
Wash hands before touching patient: _____ yes, _____ no.
Wear gloves: ____ yes, ___ no. Clean stethoscope: ____ yes, ____ no.
Wear gown and mask (precautions only):____ yes, _____ no.
Wash hands before leaving the room: _____ yes, _____ no.

Dr.______________ came in at _____ am/pm. Left at _____ am/pm.
We discussed ____.
Did doctor examine patient: _____ yes, _____ no.
Wash hands before touching patient: _____ yes, _____ no.
Wear gloves: ____ yes, ___ no. Clean stethoscope: ____ yes, ____ no.
Wear gown and mask (precautions only):____ yes, _____ no.
Wash hands before leaving the room: _____ yes, _____ no.

Dr.______________ came in at _____ am/pm. Left at _____ am/pm.
We discussed ____.
Did doctor examine patient: _____ yes, _____ no.
Wash hands before touching patient: _____ yes, _____ no.
Wear gloves: ____ yes, ___ no. Clean stethoscope: ____ yes, ____ no.
Wear gown and mask (precautions only):____ yes, _____ no.
Wash hands before leaving the room: _____ yes, _____ no.

NURSING CARE FOR ______________________________

DATE ____________________, DAY NUMBER ____________________

INITIAL DAY SHIFT EXAM:

My nurse has _____ # of patients. CNA ___yes, ___no. Charge nurse ____________
Nurse ____________ RN/LPN came in at ________ am/pm. Left at ________ am/pm.
Did nurse wash hands and wear gloves before touching patient: ______ yes, ______ no.
Wash hands after touching patient and before leaving the room: ______ yes, ______ no.
Don't hesitate to request staff to wash their hands. This will help decrease the risk of spreading potentially lethal germs.
Did nurse wear protective gear (isolation precautions only): ______ yes, ______ no.
Did nurse provide oral care (to be done every two hours if unable to provide for self, also decreases risk of pneumonia, infections, and aspiration): ______ yes, ______ no.
If able to provide own oral care, then supplies at bedside: ______ yes, ______ no.
Was patient repositioned (every two hours if unable to turn self): ______ yes ______ no.
Head of bed at ________ degrees. This is important for patients on ventilators or on tube feedings. Anything less than thirty degrees places patients at risk for aspiration of stomach contents into the lungs causing aspiration pneumonia.
Checked for incontinence and skin breakdown: ____ yes, ____ no.
Patient's linens wet or soiled: ____ yes, ____ no. Linens changed: ____ yes, ____ no.
Time linens changed: ______ am/pm. Any skin redness or breakdown: ____ yes, ____ no.
If yes, what stage is pressure ulcer: ______. Acquired when: ______________________.
List wounds not associated with pressure ulcers and how acquired: ________________
____.
Mattress type: ____ (Specialty mattresses are important to help prevent pressure ulcers)
If patient on ventilator or has tracheostomy, suction performed: ____ yes, ____ no.
Did nurse listen to lung sounds: ____ yes, ____ no.
Does patient have chest tubes: ____ yes, ____ no. Functioning ____ yes, ____ no.
Bowel sounds: ______ yes, ______ no. Bowel sounds active: ______ yes, ______ no.
Neurological exam: ______ yes, ______ no. Follow commands: ______ yes, ______ no.
Is patient alert and oriented to person, place, time, and events: ____ yes, ____ no.
If confused, patient is not oriented to: ___ person, ___ place, ___ time, ___ event.
Confusion began (time and date): ____.
Glasgow coma scale (checks conscious scale of patient): ______________________.
Intracranial pressure monitoring: ____ yes, ____ no.
If yes, pressure is at ________ mm mercury. (Normal is one to fifteen).
Moves extremities: ___ yes, ___ no.
Paralysis: (inability to move extremities) ____ yes, ____ no.
If yes, extremities affected and when paralysis began: ______________________.
Is patient in pain: ___ yes, ___ no. Describe pain and location ______________
Patient able to eat: ___ yes, ___ no. What type of diet? ______________________
If patient on tube feedings list type: ____________ at ________ cc/ml per hour.
Nausea ______, vomiting ______. If so, describe: ______________________________
Patient has: Nasal gastric tube ______, Dobhoff tube ______, Peg or gastric tube ______
When was feeding tube placed and what site: ______________________________.
Catheter for draining urine: ____ yes, ____ no. If so, when placed: __________.
Find out policy for allowed time to remain in bladder. Too long may cause infections.)
IV site(s) where: ____________________________ when placed: ________________.
IV fluids (types and rates): ____________________, ____________________, ____________________, ____________________, ____________________.
Is patient on oxygen: _____ yes, _____ no. If so, how much and route delivered (see oxygen routes): ____.
If patient on ventilator, list settings (see list on ventilator settings): __________
____.
Vital signs: temp _____, pulse _____, resp _____, b/p _____, o2 _____%, current weight _____ pounds, _____ kg. Glucose level: _____
Insulin coverage: ____ yes, ____ no. Insulin type: ____________, # of units: _____.

NURSING CARE CONTINUED FOR ______________________
DATE ____________________, DAY NUMBER ________________

FOLLOWING EXAMINATIONS FOR DAY SHIFT:

Nurse ______________, CNA ______________, in at ______ am/pm. Left at ______ am/pm.
Wash hands and wear gloves before touching patient: ____ yes, ____ no.
Wash hands before leaving room: ___ yes, ___ no. Wear protective gear: __ yes, __ no.
Clean stethoscope: __ yes, __ no. Oral care: __ yes, __ no. Suctioned: __ yes, __ no.
Repositioned: ___ yes, ___ no. Turned to: ___ left, ___ right, ___ backside ___.
Head of bed at: ______ degrees. Incontinence/skin breakdown: ____ yes, ____ no.
Linens wet or soiled: ____ yes, ____ no. Linens changed: ____ yes, ____ no.
Dressing changed: ____ yes, ____ no. Location: ______________________.
IV site checked: _____ yes, _____ no. IV tubing labeled: ____ yes, ____no.
IV fluids at: ______________________.
Pain level (0-10 scale.0-no pain, 10 intolerable): ______________________.
Location of pain: ______________. Medicated for pain: ____ yes, ____ no.
Patient is alert/oriented: ____ yes, ____ no. New confusion: ____ yes, ____ no.
Vital signs: temp ____, pulse ____, resp ______, b/p ______, 02 ______ %, ____ liters.
Glucose level: _____. Insulin: __ yes, __ no. Type: ________ # of units ____.

Nurse ______________, CNA ______________, in at ______ am/pm. Left at ______ am/pm.
Wash hands and wear gloves before touching patient: ____ yes, ____ no.
Wash hands before leaving room: ___ yes, ___ no. Wear protective gear: __ yes, __ no.
Clean stethoscope: __ yes, __ no. Oral care: __ yes, __ no. Suctioned: __ yes, __ no.
Repositioned: ___ yes, ___ no. Turned to: ___ left, ___ right, ___ backside ___.
Head of bed at: ______ degrees. Incontinence/skin breakdown: ____ yes, ____ no.
Linens wet or soiled: ____ yes, ____ no. Linens changed: ____ yes, ____ no.
Dressing changed: ____ yes, ____ no. Location: ______________________.
IV site checked: _____ yes, _____ no. IV tubing labeled: ____ yes, ____no.
IV fluids at: ______________________.
Pain level (0-10 scale.0-no pain, 10 intolerable): ______________________.
Location of pain: ______________. Medicated for pain: ____ yes, ____ no.
Patient is alert/oriented: ____ yes, ____ no. New confusion: ____ yes, ____ no.
Vital signs: temp ____, pulse ____, resp ______, b/p ______, 02 ______ %, ____ liters.
Glucose level: _____. Insulin: __ yes, __ no. Type: ________ # of units ____.

Nurse ______________, CNA ______________, in at ______ am/pm. Left at ______ am/pm.
Wash hands and wear gloves before touching patient: ____ yes, ____ no.
Wash hands before leaving room: ___ yes, ___ no. Wear protective gear: __ yes, __ no.
Clean stethoscope: __ yes, __ no. Oral care: __ yes, __ no. Suctioned: __ yes, __ no.
Repositioned: ___ yes, ___ no. Turned to: ___ left, ___ right, ___ backside ___.
Head of bed at: ______ degrees. Incontinence/skin breakdown: ____ yes, ____ no.
Linens wet or soiled: ____ yes, ____ no. Linens changed: ____ yes, ____ no.
Dressing changed: ____ yes, ____ no. Location: ______________________.
IV site checked: _____ yes, _____ no. IV tubing labeled: ____ yes, ____no.
IV fluids at: ______________________.
Pain level (0-10 scale.0-no pain, 10 intolerable): ______________________.
Location of pain: ______________. Medicated for pain: ____ yes, ____ no.
Patient is alert/oriented: ____ yes, ____ no. New confusion: ____ yes, ____ no.
Vital signs: temp ____, pulse ____, resp ______, b/p ______, 02 ______ %, ____ liters.
Glucose level: _____. Insulin: __ yes, __ no. Type: ________ # of units ____.

NURSING CARE CONTINUED FOR ______________________________
DATE ____________________, DAY NUMBER ____________

FOLLOWING EXAMINATIONS FOR DAY SHIFT:

Nurse ____________, CNA ____________, in at ____ am/pm. Left at ______ am/pm.
Wash hands and wear gloves before touching patient: ___ yes, ___ no.
Wash hands before leaving room: ___ yes, ___ no. Wear protective gear: __ yes, __ no.
Clean stethoscope: __ yes, __ no. Oral care: __ yes, __ no. Suctioned: __ yes, __ no.
Repositioned: ___ yes, ___ no. Turned to: ___ left, ___ right, ___ backside ___.
Head of bed at: ______ degrees. Incontinence/skin breakdown: ___ yes, ___ no.
Linens wet or soiled: ___ yes, ___ no. Linens changed: ___ yes, ___ no.
Dressing changed: ____ yes, ____ no. Location: ____________________.
IV site checked: ____ yes, ____ no. IV tubing labeled: ____ yes, ____ no.
IV fluids at: ____.
Pain level (0-10 scale.0-no pain, 10 intolerable): ____________________.
Location of pain: ____________. Medicated for pain: ____ yes, ____ no.
Patient is alert/oriented: ____ yes, ____ no. New confusion: ____ yes, ____ no.
Vital signs: temp ____, pulse ____, resp _____, b/p ______, 02 ____ %, ____ liters.
Glucose level: ____. Insulin: ____ yes, ____ no. Type: __________ # of units ____

Nurse ____________, CNA ____________, in at ____ am/pm. Left at ______ am/pm.
Wash hands and wear gloves before touching patient: ___ yes, ___ no.
Wash hands before leaving room: ___ yes, ___ no. Wear protective gear: __ yes, __ no.
Clean stethoscope: __ yes, __ no. Oral care: __ yes, __ no. Suctioned: __ yes, __ no.
Repositioned: ___ yes, ___ no. Turned to: ___ left, ___ right, ___ backside ___.
Head of bed at: ______ degrees. Incontinence/skin breakdown: ___ yes, ___ no.
Linens wet or soiled: ___ yes, ___ no. Linens changed: ___ yes, ___ no.
Dressing changed: ____ yes, ____ no. Location: ____________________.
IV site checked: ____ yes, ____ no. IV tubing labeled: ____ yes, ____ no.
IV fluids at: ____.
Pain level (0-10 scale.0-no pain, 10 intolerable): ____________________.
Location of pain: ____________. Medicated for pain: ____ yes, ____ no.
Patient is alert/oriented: ____ yes, ____ no. New confusion: ____ yes, ____ no.
Vital signs: temp ____, pulse ____, resp _____, b/p ______, 02 ____ %, ____ liters.
Glucose level: ____. Insulin: ____ yes, ____ no. Type: __________ # of units ____

Nurse ____________, CNA ____________, in at ____ am/pm. Left at ______ am/pm.
Wash hands and wear gloves before touching patient: ___ yes, ___ no.
Wash hands before leaving room: ___ yes, ___ no. Wear protective gear: __ yes, __ no.
Clean stethoscope: __ yes, __ no. Oral care: __ yes, __ no. Suctioned: __ yes, __ no.
Repositioned: ___ yes, ___ no. Turned to: ___ left, ___ right, ___ backside ___.
Head of bed at: ______ degrees. Incontinence/skin breakdown: ___ yes, ___ no.
Linens wet or soiled: ___ yes, ___ no. Linens changed: ___ yes, ___ no.
Dressing changed: ____ yes, ____ no. Location: ____________________.
IV site checked: ____ yes, ____ no. IV tubing labeled: ____ yes, ____ no.
IV fluids at: ____.
Pain level (0-10 scale.0-no pain, 10 intolerable): ____________________.
Location of pain: ____________. Medicated for pain: ____ yes, ____ no.
Patient is alert/oriented: ____ yes, ____ no. New confusion: ____ yes, ____ no.
Vital signs: temp ____, pulse ____, resp _____, b/p ______, 02 ____ %, ____ liters.
Glucose level: ____. Insulin: ____ yes, ____ no. Type: __________ # of units ____

NURSING CARE FOR ________________________________

DATE ____________________, DAY NUMBER ____________________

INITIAL NIGHT SHIFT EXAM:

My nurse has ______ # of patients. CNA ___yes, ___no. Charge nurse ________________
Nurse ________________ RN/LPN came in at __________ am/pm. Left at __________ am/pm.
Did nurse wash hands and wear gloves before touching patient: _______ yes, _______ no.
Wash hands after touching patient and before leaving the room: _______ yes, _______ no.
Don't hesitate to request staff to wash their hands. This will help decrease the risk of spreading potentially lethal germs.
Did nurse wear protective gear (isolation precautions only): _______ yes, _______ no.
Did nurse provide oral care (to be done every two hours if unable to provide for self, also decreases risk of pneumonia, infections, and aspiration): _______ yes, _______ no.
If able to provide own oral care, then supplies at bedside: _______ yes, _______ no.
Was patient repositioned (every two hours if unable to turn self): _____ yes _____ no.
Head of bed at _________ degrees. This is important for patients on ventilators or on tube feedings. Anything less than thirty degrees places patients at risk for aspiration of stomach contents into the lungs causing aspiration pneumonia.
Checked for incontinence and skin breakdown: _____ yes, _____ no.
Patient's linens wet or soiled: _____ yes, _____ no. Linens changed: ____ yes, ____ no.
Time linens changed: ________ am/pm. Any skin redness or breakdown: ____ yes, ____ no.
If yes, what stage is pressure ulcer: ________. Acquired when: ____________________.
List wounds not associated with pressure ulcers and how acquired: _________________
____.
Mattress type: ____
Specialty mattresses are important to help prevent pressure ulcers)
If patient on ventilator or has tracheostomy, suction performed: _____ yes, _____ no.
Did nurse listen to lung sounds: _____ yes, _____ no.
Does patient have chest tubes: ____ yes, ____ no. Functioning _____ yes, _____ no.
Bowel sounds: _______ yes, _______ no. Bowel sounds active: _______ yes, _______ no.
Neurological exam: ______ yes, ______ no. Follow commands: _______ yes, _______ no.
Is patient alert and oriented to person, place, time, and events: _____ yes, _____ no.
If confused, patient is not oriented to: ___ person, ___ place, ___ time, ___ event.
Confusion began (time and date): ____.
Glasgow coma scale (checks conscious scale of patient): ___________________________
Intracranial pressure monitoring: _____ yes, _____ no.
If yes, pressure is at ________ mm mercury. (Normal is one to fifteen).
Moves extremities: ___ yes, ___ no.
Paralysis: (inability to move extremities) _________ yes, _________ no.
If yes, extremities affected and when paralysis began: ___________________________.
Is patient in pain: ___ yes, ___ no. Describe pain and location __________________.
Patient able to eat: ___ yes, ___ no. What type of diet? __________________________.
If patient on tube feedings list type: __________ at __________ cc/ml per hour.
Nausea ____, vomiting ____. If so, describe: _____________________________________.
Patient has: Nasal gastric tube ______, Dobhoff tube _____, Peg or gastric tube ____.
When was feeding tube placed and what site: ______________________________________.
Catheter for draining urine: ____ yes, ____ no. If so, when placed: ______________.
Find out policy for allowed time to remain in bladder. Too long may cause infections.)
IV site(s) where: ______________________ when placed: ____________________________.
IV fluids (types and rates): _______________________, ____________________________,
_____________________, _____________________, ____________________________________,
Is patient on oxygen: _____ yes, _____ no. If so, how much and route delivered (see oxygen routes): ____.
If patient on ventilator, list settings (see list on ventilator settings): ________
____.
Vital signs: temp _____, pulse _____, resp ______, b/p _____, o2 _____%,
current weight ______ pounds, ______ kg. Glucose level: ______
Insulin coverage: ____ yes, ____ no. Insulin type: _____________, # of units: _____.

NURSING CARE CONTINUED FOR ______________________
DATE ____________________, DAY NUMBER ______________

FOLLOWING EXAMINATIONS FOR NIGHT SHIFT:

Nurse ___________, CNA ___________, in at ______ am/pm. Left at ______ am/pm.
Wash hands and wear gloves before touching patient: ____ yes, ____ no.
Wash hands before leaving room: ___ yes, ___ no. Wear protective gear: __ yes, __ no.
Clean stethoscope: __ yes, __ no. Oral care: __ yes, __ no. Suctioned: __ yes, __ no.
Repositioned: ___ yes, ___ no. Turned to: ___ left, ___ right, ___ backside ___.
Head of bed at: _____ degrees. Incontinence/skin breakdown: ___ yes, ___ no.
Linens wet or soiled: _____ yes, _____ no. Linens changed: _____ yes, _____ no.
Dressing changed: ____ yes, _____ no. Location: ______________.
IV site checked: _____ yes, _____ no. IV tubing labeled: _____ yes, ____no.
IV fluids at: ____.
Pain level (0-10 scale.0-no pain, 10 intolerable): ______________.
Location of pain: ____________. Medicated for pain: _____ yes, _____ no.
Patient is alert/oriented: ____ yes, ____ no. New confusion: ____yes, ____ no.
Vital signs: temp ____, pulse ____, resp ____, b/p _____, 02 _____ %, ____ liters.
Glucose level: _____. Insulin: ___ yes, ___ no. Type: __________ # of units ____.

Nurse ___________, CNA ___________, in at ______ am/pm. Left at ______ am/pm.
Wash hands and wear gloves before touching patient: ____ yes, ____ no.
Wash hands before leaving room: ___ yes, ___ no. Wear protective gear: __ yes, __ no.
Clean stethoscope: __ yes, __ no. Oral care: __ yes, __ no. Suctioned: __ yes, __ no.
Repositioned: ___ yes, ___ no. Turned to: ___ left, ___ right, ___ backside ___.
Head of bed at: _____ degrees. Incontinence/skin breakdown: ___ yes, ___ no.
Linens wet or soiled: _____ yes, _____ no. Linens changed: _____ yes, _____ no.
Dressing changed: ____ yes, _____ no. Location: ______________.
IV site checked: _____ yes, _____ no. IV tubing labeled: _____ yes, ____no.
IV fluids at: ____.
Pain level (0-10 scale.0-no pain, 10 intolerable): ______________.
Location of pain: ____________. Medicated for pain: _____ yes, _____ no.
Patient is alert/oriented: ____ yes, ____ no. New confusion: ____yes, ____ no.
Vital signs: temp ____, pulse ____, resp ____, b/p _____, 02 _____ %, ____ liters.
Glucose level: _____. Insulin: ___ yes, ___ no. Type: __________ # of units ____.

Nurse ___________, CNA ___________, in at ______ am/pm. Left at ______ am/pm.
Wash hands and wear gloves before touching patient: ____ yes, ____ no.
Wash hands before leaving room: ___ yes, ___ no. Wear protective gear: __ yes, __ no.
Clean stethoscope: __ yes, __ no. Oral care: __ yes, __ no. Suctioned: __ yes, __ no.
Repositioned: ___ yes, ___ no. Turned to: ___ left, ___ right, ___ backside ___.
Head of bed at: _____ degrees. Incontinence/skin breakdown: ___ yes, ___ no.
Linens wet or soiled: _____ yes, _____ no. Linens changed: _____ yes, _____ no.
Dressing changed: ____ yes, _____ no. Location: ______________.
IV site checked: _____ yes, _____ no. IV tubing labeled: _____ yes, ____no.
IV fluids at: ____.
Pain level (0-10 scale.0-no pain, 10 intolerable): ______________.
Location of pain: ____________. Medicated for pain: _____ yes, _____ no.
Patient is alert/oriented: ____ yes, ____ no. New confusion: ____yes, ____ no.
Vital signs: temp ____, pulse ____, resp ____, b/p _____, 02 _____ %, ____ liters.
Glucose level: _____. Insulin: ___ yes, ___ no. Type: __________ # of units ____.

NURSING CARE CONTINUED FOR ____________________
DATE ____________________, DAY NUMBER ____________________

FOLLOWING EXAMINATIONS FOR NIGHT SHIFT:

Nurse ______________, CNA ______________, in at _____ am/pm. Left at _______ am/pm.
Wash hands and wear gloves before touching patient: _______ yes, _______ no.
Wash hands before leaving room: __ yes, __ no. Wear protective gear: __ yes, __ no.
Clean stethoscope: yes, __ no. Oral care: __ yes, __ no. Suctioned: __ yes, __ no.
Repositioned: ___ yes, ___ no. Turned to: ___ left, ___ right, ___ backside ___.
Head of bed at: ________ degrees. Incontinence/skin breakdown: ____ yes, ____ no.
Linens wet or soiled: _____ yes, _____ no. Linens changed: _____ yes, _____ no.
Dressing changed: ____ yes, ____ no. Location: ____________________.
IV site checked: _____ yes, _____ no. IV tubing labeled: _____ yes, _____ no.
IV fluids at: ____.
Pain level (0-10 scale.0-no pain, 10 intolerable): ____________________.
Location of pain: ____________. Medicated for pain: _____ yes, ____ no.
Patient is alert/oriented: ____ yes, ____ no. New confusion: ____ yes, ____ no.
Vital signs: temp ____, pulse _____, resp ______, b/p ______, 02 _____ %, ____ liters.
Glucose level: _____. Insulin: ___ yes, ___ no. Type: ______________ # of units ____.

Nurse ______________, CNA ______________, in at _____ am/pm. Left at _______ am/pm.
Wash hands and wear gloves before touching patient: _______ yes, _______ no.
Wash hands before leaving room: __ yes, ___ no. Wear protective gear: __ yes, __ no.
Clean stethoscope: __ yes, __ no. Oral care: __ yes, __ no. Suctioned: __ yes, __ no.
Repositioned: ___ yes, ___ no. Turned to: ___ left, ___ right, ___ backside ___.
Head of bed at: ________ degrees. Incontinence/skin breakdown: ____ yes, ____ no.
Linens wet or soiled: _____ yes, _____ no. Linens changed: _____ yes, _____ no.
Dressing changed: ____ yes, ____ no. Location: ____________________.
IV site checked: _____ yes, _____ no. IV tubing labeled: _____ yes, _____ no.
IV fluids at: ____.
Pain level (0-10 scale.0-no pain, 10 intolerable): ____________________.
Location of pain: ____________. Medicated for pain: _____ yes, ____ no.
Patient is alert/oriented: ____ yes, ____ no. New confusion: ____ yes, ____ no.
Vital signs: temp ____, pulse _____, resp ______, b/p ______, 02 _____ %, ____ liters.
Glucose level: _____. Insulin: ___ yes, ___ no. Type: ______________ # of units ____.

Nurse ______________, CNA ______________, in at _____ am/pm. Left at _______ am/pm.
Wash hands and wear gloves before touching patient: _______ yes, _______ no.
Wash hands before leaving room: ___ yes, ___ no. Wear protective gear: __ yes, __ no.
Clean stethoscope: __ yes, __ no. Oral care: __ yes, __ no. Suctioned: __ yes, __ no.
Repositioned: ___ yes, ___ no. Turned to: ___ left, ___ right, ___ backside ___.
Head of bed at: ________ degrees. Incontinence/skin breakdown: ____ yes, ____ no.
Linens wet or soiled: _____ yes, _____ no. Linens changed: _____ yes, _____ no.
Dressing changed: ____ yes, ____ no. Location: ____________________.
IV site checked: _____ yes, _____ no. IV tubing labeled: _____ yes, _____ no.
IV fluids at: ____.
Pain level (0-10 scale.0-no pain, 10 intolerable): ____________________.
Location of pain: ____________. Medicated for pain: _____ yes, ____ no.
Patient is alert/oriented: ____ yes, ____ no. New confusion: ____ yes, ____ no.
Vital signs: temp ____, pulse _____, resp ______, b/p ______, 02 _____ %, ____ liters.
Glucose level: _____. Insulin: ___ yes, ___ no. Type: ______________ # of units ____.

MEDICATION ADMINISTRATION LIST FOR ____________
DATE ____________ DAY NUMBER ____________

List the medication for each day. Routes of administration: oral, thru feeding tube, intravenous (IV), intramuscular (IM), subcutaneous (SQ), epidural or a catheter in your spinal column, rectal, topical, eye drops, and ear drops.

Medication: ____________ Route: ____________ Time: ____________
Medication: ____________ Route: ____________ Time: ____________
Medication: ____________ Route: ____________ Time: ____________
Medication: ____________ Route: ____________ Time: ____________
Medication: ____________ Route: ____________ Time: ____________
Medication: ____________ Route: ____________ Time: ____________
Medication: ____________ Route: ____________ Time: ____________
Medication: ____________ Route: ____________ Time: ____________
Medication: ____________ Route: ____________ Time: ____________
Medication: ____________ Route: ____________ Time: ____________
Medication: ____________ Route: ____________ Time: ____________
Medication: ____________ Route: ____________ Time: ____________
Medication: ____________ Route: ____________ Time: ____________
Medication: ____________ Route: ____________ Time: ____________
Medication: ____________ Route: ____________ Time: ____________
Medication: ____________ Route: ____________ Time: ____________
Medication: ____________ Route: ____________ Time: ____________
Medication: ____________ Route: ____________ Time: ____________
Medication: ____________ Route: ____________ Time: ____________
Medication: ____________ Route: ____________ Time: ____________
Medication: ____________ Route: ____________ Time: ____________
Medication: ____________ Route: ____________ Time: ____________
Medication: ____________ Route: ____________ Time: ____________
Medication: ____________ Route: ____________ Time: ____________
Medication: ____________ Route: ____________ Time: ____________
Medication: ____________ Route: ____________ Time: ____________
Medication: ____________ Route: ____________ Time: ____________
Medication: ____________ Route: ____________ Time: ____________
Medication: ____________ Route: ____________ Time: ____________
Medication: ____________ Route: ____________ Time: ____________
Medication: ____________ Route: ____________ Time: ____________
Medication: ____________ Route: ____________ Time: ____________
Medication: ____________ Route: ____________ Time: ____________
Medication: ____________ Route: ____________ Time: ____________
Medication: ____________ Route: ____________ Time: ____________
Medication: ____________ Route: ____________ Time: ____________
Medication: ____________ Route: ____________ Time: ____________
Medication: ____________ Route: ____________ Time: ____________
Medication: ____________ Route: ____________ Time: ____________
Medication: ____________ Route: ____________ Time: ____________
Medication: ____________ Route: ____________ Time: ____________
Medication: ____________ Route: ____________ Time: ____________
Medication: ____________ Route: ____________ Time: ____________
Medication: ____________ Route: ____________ Time: ____________
Medication: ____________ Route: ____________ Time: ____________
Medication: ____________ Route: ____________ Time: ____________
Medication: ____________ Route: ____________ Time: ____________
Medication: ____________ Route: ____________ Time: ____________
Medication: ____________ Route: ____________ Time: ____________
Medication: ____________ Route: ____________ Time: ____________
Medication: ____________ Route: ____________ Time: ____________
Medication: ____________ Route: ____________ Time: ____________
Medication: ____________ Route: ____________ Time: ____________
Medication: ____________ Route: ____________ Time: ____________
Medication: ____________ Route: ____________ Time: ____________

NOTES FOR DAY NUMBER ______________________________

DATE ____

MEDICAL JOURNAL FOR ______________________________

DATE ____________________, DAY NUMBER ______________

VISITS FROM MY DOCTORS TODAY

Goals for today: ______________________________

____

____

Things to discuss with my doctor(s): ______________________________

____

____

Dr.______________ came in at ____ am/pm. Left at ____ am/pm.
We discussed ______________________________.
Did doctor examine patient: ____ yes, ____ no.
Wash hands before touching patient: ____ yes, ____ no.
Wear gloves: ____ yes, ___ no. Clean stethoscope: ____ yes, ____ no.
Wear gown and mask (precautions only):____ yes, ____ no.
Wash hands before leaving the room: ____ yes, ____ no.

Dr.______________ came in at ____ am/pm. Left at ____ am/pm.
We discussed ______________________________.
Did doctor examine patient: ____ yes, ____ no.
Wash hands before touching patient: ____ yes, ____ no.
Wear gloves: ____ yes, ___ no. Clean stethoscope: ____ yes, ____ no.
Wear gown and mask (precautions only):____ yes, ____ no.
Wash hands before leaving the room: ____ yes, ____ no.

Dr.______________ came in at ____ am/pm. Left at ____ am/pm.
We discussed ______________________________.
Did doctor examine patient: ____ yes, ____ no.
Wash hands before touching patient: ____ yes, ____ no.
Wear gloves: ____ yes, ___ no. Clean stethoscope: ____ yes, ____ no.
Wear gown and mask (precautions only):____ yes, ____ no.
Wash hands before leaving the room: ____ yes, ____ no.

Dr.______________ came in at ____ am/pm. Left at ____ am/pm.
We discussed ______________________________.
Did doctor examine patient: ____ yes, ____ no.
Wash hands before touching patient: ____ yes, ____ no.
Wear gloves: ____ yes, ___ no. Clean stethoscope: ____ yes, ____ no.
Wear gown and mask (precautions only):____ yes, ____ no.
Wash hands before leaving the room: ____ yes, ____ no.

Dr.______________ came in at ____ am/pm. Left at ____ am/pm.
We discussed ______________________________.
Did doctor examine patient: ____ yes, ____ no.
Wash hands before touching patient: ____ yes, ____ no.
Wear gloves: ____ yes, ___ no. Clean stethoscope: ____ yes, ____ no.
Wear gown and mask (precautions only):____ yes, ____ no.
Wash hands before leaving the room: ____ yes, ____ no.

NURSING CARE FOR ____

DATE ____________________, DAY NUMBER ______________________

INITIAL DAY SHIFT EXAM:

My nurse has ______ # of patients. CNA ___yes, ___no. Charge nurse ______________
Nurse _______________ RN/LPN came in at _________ am/pm. Left at __________ am/pm.
Did nurse wash hands and wear gloves before touching patient: ______ yes, _______ no.
Wash hands after touching patient and before leaving the room: ______ yes, _______ no.
Don't hesitate to request staff to wash their hands. This will help decrease the risk of spreading potentially lethal germs.
Did nurse wear protective gear (isolation precautions only): _______ yes, _______ no.
Did nurse provide oral care (to be done every two hours if unable to provide for self, also decreases risk of pneumonia, infections, and aspiration): _______ yes, ______ no.
If able to provide own oral care, then supplies at bedside: ________ yes, ________ no.
Was patient repositioned (every two hours if unable to turn self): _____ yes _____ no.
Head of bed at _________ degrees. This is important for patients on ventilators or on tube feedings. Anything less than thirty degrees places patients at risk for aspiration of stomach contents into the lungs causing aspiration pneumonia.
Checked for incontinence and skin breakdown: _____ yes, _____ no.
Patient's linens wet or soiled: _____ yes, ____ no. Linens changed: ____ yes, ____ no.
Time linens changed: _______ am/pm. Any skin redness or breakdown: ____ yes, ____ no.
If yes, what stage is pressure ulcer: ________. Acquired when: ___________________.
List wounds not associated with pressure ulcers and how acquired: ________________
____.
Mattress type: ____.
Specialty mattresses are important to help prevent pressure ulcers)
If patient on ventilator or has tracheostomy, suction performed: _____ yes, ______ no.
Did nurse listen to lung sounds: _____ yes, _____ no.
Does patient have chest tubes: ____ yes, ____ no. Functioning _____ yes, ______ no.
Bowel sounds: _______ yes, _______ no. Bowel sounds active: _______ yes, ______ no.
Neurological exam: ______ yes, ______ no. Follow commands: _______ yes, ______ no.
Is patient alert and oriented to person, place, time, and events: _____ yes, _____ no.
If confused, patient is not oriented to: ___ person, ___ place, ___ time, ___ event.
Confusion began (time and date): ____.
Glasgow coma scale (checks conscious scale of patient): ____________________.
Intracranial pressure monitoring: _____ yes, _____ no.
If yes, pressure is at ________ mm mercury. (Normal is one to fifteen).
Moves extremities: ___ yes, ___ no.
Paralysis: (inability to move extremities) _______ yes, _______ no.
If yes, extremities affected and when paralysis began: _______________________.
Is patient in pain: ____ yes, ____ no. Describe pain and location _______________.
Patient able to eat: ____ yes, ____ no. What type of diet? ______________________.
If patient on tube feedings list type: _____________ at ____________ cc/ml per hour.
Nausea ____, vomiting ____. If so, describe: ___________________________________.
Patient has: Nasal gastric tube ______, Dobhoff tube _____, Peg or gastric tube _____.
When was feeding tube placed and what site: ___________________________________.
Catheter for draining urine: ____ yes, ____ no. If so, when placed: ______________.
Find out policy for allowed time to remain in bladder. Too long may cause infections.)
IV site(s) where: _____________________________ when placed: _______________.
IV fluids (types and rates): ______________________, ______________________,
________________________, _______________________, ______________________,
Is patient on oxygen: _____ yes, _____ no. If so, how much and route delivered (see oxygen routes): ____.
If patient on ventilator, list settings (see list on ventilator settings): __________
____.
Vital signs: temp ______, pulse _____, resp ______, b/p _____, o2 ____%,
current weight ______ pounds, ______ kg. Glucose level: _______
Insulin coverage: ____ yes, ____ no. Insulin type: __________, # of units: ______.

NURSING CARE CONTINUED FOR ______________________
DATE ______________________, DAY NUMBER ______________________

FOLLOWING EXAMINATIONS FOR DAY SHIFT:

Nurse __________, CNA __________, in at _____ am/pm. Left at ______ am/pm.
Wash hands and wear gloves before touching patient: ______ yes, ______ no.
Wash hands before leaving room: __ yes, __ no. Wear protective gear: __ yes, __ no.
Clean stethoscope: __ yes, __ no. Oral care: __ yes, __ no. Suctioned: __ yes, __ no.
Repositioned: ___ yes, ___ no. Turned to: ___ left, ___ right, ___ backside ___.
Head of bed at: ________ degrees. Incontinence/skin breakdown: ____ yes, ___ no.
Linens wet or soiled: _____ yes, ____ no. Linens changed: _____ yes, _____ no.
Dressing changed: ____ yes, ____ no. Location: ______________________.
IV site checked: ____ yes, _____ no. IV tubing labeled: _____ yes, _____ no.
IV fluids at: ____.
Pain level (0-10 scale.0-no pain, 10 intolerable): ________________________.
Location of pain: ______________. Medicated for pain: ____ yes, _____ no.
Patient is alert/oriented: _____ yes, ____ no. New confusion: ____ yes, ____ no.
Vital signs: temp ____, pulse ____, resp ____, b/p ____, 02 ____ %, ____ liters.
Glucose level: _____. Insulin: ___ yes, ___ no. Type: __________ # of units ____.

Nurse __________, CNA __________, in at _____ am/pm. Left at ______ am/pm.
Wash hands and wear gloves before touching patient: ______ yes, ______ no.
Wash hands before leaving room: __ yes, __ no. Wear protective gear: __ yes, __ no.
Clean stethoscope: __ yes, __ no. Oral care: __ yes, __ no. Suctioned: __ yes, __ no.
Repositioned: ___ yes, ___ no. Turned to: ___ left, ___ right, ___ backside ___.
Head of bed at: ________ degrees. Incontinence/skin breakdown: ____ yes, ___ no.
Linens wet or soiled: _____ yes, ____ no. Linens changed: _____ yes, _____ no.
Dressing changed: ____ yes, ____ no. Location: ______________________.
IV site checked: ____ yes, _____ no. IV tubing labeled: _____ yes, _____ no.
IV fluids at: ____.
Pain level (0-10 scale.0-no pain, 10 intolerable): ________________________.
Location of pain: ______________. Medicated for pain: ____ yes, _____ no.
Patient is alert/oriented: _____ yes, ____ no. New confusion: ____ yes, ____ no.
Vital signs: temp ____, pulse ____, resp ____, b/p ____, 02 ____ %, ____ liters.
Glucose level: _____. Insulin: ___ yes, ___ no. Type: __________ # of units ____.

Nurse __________, CNA __________, in at _____ am/pm. Left at ______ am/pm.
Wash hands and wear gloves before touching patient: ______ yes, ______ no.
Wash hands before leaving room: __ yes, __ no. Wear protective gear: __ yes, __ no.
Clean stethoscope: __ yes, __ no. Oral care: __ yes, __ no. Suctioned: __ yes, __ no.
Repositioned: ___ yes, ___ no. Turned to: ___ left, ___ right, ___ backside ___.
Head of bed at: ________ degrees. Incontinence/skin breakdown: ____ yes, ___ no.
Linens wet or soiled: _____ yes, ____ no. Linens changed: _____ yes, _____ no.
Dressing changed: ____ yes, ____ no. Location: ______________________.
IV site checked: ____ yes, _____ no. IV tubing labeled: _____ yes, _____ no.
IV fluids at: ____.
Pain level (0-10 scale.0-no pain, 10 intolerable): ________________________.
Location of pain: ______________. Medicated for pain: ____ yes, _____ no.
Patient is alert/oriented: _____ yes, ____ no. New confusion: ____ yes, ____ no.
Vital signs: temp ____, pulse ____, resp ____, b/p ____, 02 ____ %, ____ liters.
Glucose level: _____. Insulin: ___ yes, ___ no. Type: __________ # of units ____.

NURSING CARE CONTINUED FOR ____________________
DATE ____________________, DAY NUMBER ____________________

FOLLOWING EXAMINATIONS FOR DAY SHIFT:

Nurse ____________, CNA ____________, in at _____ am/pm. Left at ______ am/pm.
Wash hands and wear gloves before touching patient: ______ yes, ______ no.
Wash hands before leaving room: ___ yes, ___ no. Wear protective gear: __ yes, __ no.
Clean stethoscope: __ yes, __ no. Oral care: __ yes, __ no. Suctioned: __ yes, __ no.
Repositioned: ___ yes, ___ no. Turned to: ___ left, ___ right, ___ backside ___.
Head of bed at: ______ degrees. Incontinence/skin breakdown: ____ yes, ____ no.
Linens wet or soiled: _____ yes, _____ no. Linens changed: _____ yes, _____ no.
Dressing changed: ____ yes, ____ no. Location: ____________________.
IV site checked: _____ yes, _____ no. IV tubing labeled: _____ yes, _____no.
IV fluids at: ____________________.
Pain level (0-10 scale.0-no pain, 10 intolerable): ____________.
Location of pain: ____________. Medicated for pain: ____ yes, ____ no.
Patient is alert/oriented: ____ yes, ____ no. New confusion: ____ yes, ____ no.
Vital signs: temp ____, pulse _____, resp ______, b/p ______, 02 _____ %, ____ liters.
Glucose level: _____. Insulin: ___ yes, ___ no. Type: __________ # of units ____.

Nurse ____________, CNA ____________, in at _____ am/pm. Left at ______ am/pm.
Wash hands and wear gloves before touching patient: ______ yes, ______ no.
Wash hands before leaving room: ___ yes, ___ no. Wear protective gear: __ yes, __ no.
Clean stethoscope: __ yes, __ no. Oral care: __ yes, __ no. Suctioned: __ yes, __ no.
Repositioned: ___ yes, ___ no. Turned to: ___ left, ___ right, ___ backside ___.
Head of bed at: ______ degrees. Incontinence/skin breakdown: ____ yes, ____ no.
Linens wet or soiled: _____ yes, _____ no. Linens changed: _____ yes, _____ no.
Dressing changed: ____ yes, ____ no. Location: ____________________.
IV site checked: _____ yes, _____ no. IV tubing labeled: _____ yes, _____no.
IV fluids at: ____________________.
Pain level (0-10 scale.0-no pain, 10 intolerable): ____________.
Location of pain: ____________. Medicated for pain: ____ yes, ____ no.
Patient is alert/oriented: ____ yes, ____ no. New confusion: ____ yes, ____ no.
Vital signs: temp ____, pulse _____, resp ______, b/p ______, 02 _____ %, ____ liters.
Glucose level: _____. Insulin: ___ yes, ___ no. Type: __________ # of units ____.

Nurse ____________, CNA ____________, in at _____ am/pm. Left at ______ am/pm.
Wash hands and wear gloves before touching patient: ______ yes, ______ no.
Wash hands before leaving room: ___ yes, ___ no. Wear protective gear: __ yes, __ no.
Clean stethoscope: __ yes, __ no. Oral care: __ yes, __ no. Suctioned: __ yes, __ no.
Repositioned: ___ yes, ___ no. Turned to: ___ left, ___ right, ___ backside ___.
Head of bed at: ______ degrees. Incontinence/skin breakdown: ____ yes, ____ no.
Linens wet or soiled: _____ yes, _____ no. Linens changed: _____ yes, _____ no.
Dressing changed: ____ yes, ____ no. Location: ____________________.
IV site checked: _____ yes, _____ no. IV tubing labeled: _____ yes, _____no.
IV fluids at: ____________________.
Pain level (0-10 scale.0-no pain, 10 intolerable): ____________.
Location of pain: ____________. Medicated for pain: ____ yes, ____ no.
Patient is alert/oriented: ____ yes, ____ no. New confusion: ____ yes, ____ no.
Vital signs: temp ____, pulse _____, resp ______, b/p ______, 02 _____ %, ____ liters.
Glucose level: _____. Insulin: ___ yes, ___ no. Type: __________ # of units ____.

NURSING CARE FOR ______________________________

DATE ____________________, DAY NUMBER ____________________

INITIAL NIGHT SHIFT EXAM:

My nurse has ______ # of patients. CNA ___yes, ___no. Charge nurse ________________
Nurse ________________ RN/LPN came in at ____________ am/pm. Left at ___________ am/pm.
Did nurse wash hands and wear gloves before touching patient: _______ yes, ______ no.
Wash hands after touching patient and before leaving the room: _______ yes, ______ no.
Don't hesitate to request staff to wash their hands. This will help decrease the risk of spreading potentially lethal germs.
Did nurse wear protective gear (isolation precautions only): _______ yes, ______ no.
Did nurse provide oral care (to be done every two hours if unable to provide for self, also decreases risk of pneumonia, infections, and aspiration): _______ yes, ______ no.
If able to provide own oral care, then supplies at bedside: ________ yes, ______ no.
Was patient repositioned (every two hours if unable to turn self): _______ yes ______ no.
Head of bed at __________ degrees. This is important for patients on ventilators or on tube feedings. Anything less than thirty degrees places patients at risk for aspiration of stomach contents into the lungs causing aspiration pneumonia.
Checked for incontinence and skin breakdown: _____ yes, _____ no.
Patient's linens wet or soiled: _____yes, _____ no. Linens changed: ____ yes, ____ no.
Time linens changed: ________ am/pm. Any skin redness or breakdown: ____ yes, ____ no.
If yes, what stage is pressure ulcer: ______________. Acquired when: ________________.
List wounds not associated with pressure ulcers and how acquired: ________________
____.
Mattress type: ____.
Specialty mattresses are important to help prevent pressure ulcers)
If patient on ventilator or has tracheostomy, suction performed: ______ yes, ______ no.
Did nurse listen to lung sounds: _____ yes, _____ no.
Does patient have chest tubes: ____ yes, ____ no. Functioning _____ yes, _____ no.
Bowel sounds: _______ yes, _______ no. Bowel sounds active: _______ yes, ______ no.
Neurological exam: _______ yes, ______ no. Follow commands: _______ yes, ______ no.
Is patient alert and oriented to person, place, time, and events: _____ yes, _____ no.
If confused, patient is not oriented to: ___ person, ___ place, ___ time, ___ event.
Confusion began (time and date): ____.
Glasgow coma scale (checks conscious scale of patient): ___________________________.
Intracranial pressure monitoring: _____ yes, _____ no.
If yes, pressure is at ________ mm mercury. (Normal is one to fifteen).
Moves extremities: ___ yes, ___ no.
Paralysis: (inability to move extremities) _______ yes, _______ no.
If yes, extremities affected and when paralysis began: ____________________________.
Is patient in pain: ____ yes, ____ no. Describe pain and location ________________.
Patient able to eat: ____ yes, ____ no. What type of diet? ________________________.
If patient on tube feedings list type: ____________ at __________ cc/ml per hour.
Nausea ____, vomiting ____. If so, describe: ______________________________________.
Patient has: Nasal gastric tube ______, Dobhoff tube _____, Peg or gastric tube _____.
When was feeding tube placed and what site: ______________________________________.
Catheter for draining urine: ____ yes, ____ no. If so, when placed: _____________.
Find out policy for allowed time to remain in bladder. Too long may cause infections.)
IV site(s) where: ______________________ when placed: ____________________________.
IV fluids (types and rates): ______________, ______________, ______________________,
______________, ______________, ______________, ______________, ________________.
Is patient on oxygen: _____ yes, _____ no. If so, how much and route delivered (see oxygen routes): ____.
If patient on ventilator, list settings (see list on ventilator settings): _________
____.
Vital signs: temp ______, pulse ______, resp ______, b/p ______, o2 ______%,
current weight ______ pounds, ______ kg. Glucose level: ______
Insulin coverage: ____ yes, ____ no. Insulin type: _____________, # of units: ______.

NURSING CARE CONTINUED FOR ______________________
DATE ____________________, DAY NUMBER ____________________

FOLLOWING EXAMINATIONS FOR NIGHT SHIFT:

Nurse ______________, CNA ______________, in at _____ am/pm. Left at ______ am/pm.
Wash hands and wear gloves before touching patient: _______ yes, _______ no.
Wash hands before leaving room: ___ yes, ___ no. Wear protective gear: __ yes, __ no.
Clean stethoscope: __ yes, __ no. Oral care: __ yes, __ no. Suctioned: __ yes, __ no.
Repositioned: ___ yes, ___ no. Turned to: ___ left, ___ right, ___ backside ___.
Head of bed at: _______ degrees. Incontinence/skin breakdown: ____ yes, ____ no.
Linens wet or soiled: _____ yes, _____ no. Linens changed: _____ yes, ______ no.
Dressing changed: ____ yes, ____ no. Location: ____________________________.
IV site checked: _____ yes, _____ no. IV tubing labeled: _____ yes, _____no.
IV fluids at: ____.
Pain level (0-10 scale.0-no pain, 10 intolerable): ___________________________.
Location of pain: _______________. Medicated for pain: _____ yes, ____ no.
Patient is alert/oriented: ____ yes, ____ no. New confusion: ____ yes, ____ no.
Vital signs: temp ____, pulse _____, resp _____, b/p _____, 02 _____%, ____ liters.
Glucose level: _____. Insulin: ___ yes, ___ no. Type: _____________ # of units ____.

Nurse ______________, CNA ______________, in at _____ am/pm. Left at ______ am/pm.
Wash hands and wear gloves before touching patient: _______ yes, _______ no.
Wash hands before leaving room: ___ yes, ___ no. Wear protective gear: __ yes, __ no.
Clean stethoscope: __ yes, __ no. Oral care: __ yes, __ no. Suctioned: __ yes, __ no.
Repositioned: ___ yes, ___ no. Turned to: ___ left, ___ right, ___ backside ___.
Head of bed at: _______ degrees. Incontinence/skin breakdown: ____ yes, ____ no.
Linens wet or soiled: _____ yes, _____ no. Linens changed: _____ yes, ______ no.
Dressing changed: ____ yes, ____ no. Location: ____________________________.
IV site checked: _____ yes, _____ no. IV tubing labeled: _____ yes, _____no.
IV fluids at: ____.
Pain level (0-10 scale.0-no pain, 10 intolerable): ___________________________.
Location of pain: _______________. Medicated for pain: _____ yes, ____ no.
Patient is alert/oriented: ____ yes, ____ no. New confusion: ____ yes, ____ no.
Vital signs: temp ____, pulse _____, resp _____, b/p _____, 02 _____%, ____ liters.
Glucose level: _____. Insulin: ___ yes, ___ no. Type: _____________ # of units ____.

Nurse ______________, CNA ______________, in at _____ am/pm. Left at ______ am/pm.
Wash hands and wear gloves before touching patient: _______ yes, _______ no.
Wash hands before leaving room: ___ yes, ___ no. Wear protective gear: __ yes, __ no.
Clean stethoscope: __ yes, __ no. Oral care: __ yes, __ no. Suctioned: __ yes, __ no.
Repositioned: ___ yes, ___ no. Turned to: ___ left, ___ right, ___ backside ___.
Head of bed at: _______ degrees. Incontinence/skin breakdown: ____ yes, ____ no.
Linens wet or soiled: _____ yes, _____ no. Linens changed: _____ yes, ______ no.
Dressing changed: ____ yes, ____ no. Location: ____________________________.
IV site checked: _____ yes, _____ no. IV tubing labeled: _____ yes, _____no.
IV fluids at: ____.
Pain level (0-10 scale.0-no pain, 10 intolerable): ___________________________.
Location of pain: _______________. Medicated for pain: _____ yes, ____ no.
Patient is alert/oriented: ____ yes, ____ no. New confusion: ____ yes, ____ no.
Vital signs: temp ____, pulse _____, resp _____, b/p _____, 02 _____%, ____ liters.
Glucose level: _____. Insulin: ___ yes, ___ no. Type: _____________ # of units ____.

NURSING CARE CONTINUED FOR ______________________
DATE ____________________, DAY NUMBER ______________

FOLLOWING EXAMINATIONS FOR NIGHT SHIFT:

Nurse _______________, CNA _______________, in at _____ am/pm. Left at ______ am/pm.
Wash hands and wear gloves before touching patient: ________ yes, ________ no.
Wash hands before leaving room: ___ yes, ___ no. Wear protective gear: __ yes, __ no.
Clean stethoscope: __ yes, __ no. Oral care: __ yes, __ no. Suctioned: __ yes, __ no.
Repositioned: ___ yes, ___ no. Turned to: ___ left, ___ right, ___ backside ___.
Head of bed at: _______ degrees. Incontinence/skin breakdown: ____ yes, ____ no.
Linens wet or soiled: _____ yes, _____ no. Linens changed: _____ yes, _____ no.
Dressing changed: ____ yes, ____ no. Location: ______________________________.
IV site checked: _____ yes, _____ no. IV tubing labeled: _____ yes, _____ no.
IV fluids at: ____.
Pain level (0-10 scale.0-no pain, 10 intolerable): ___________________________.
Location of pain: ________________. Medicated for pain: _____ yes, _____ no.
Patient is alert/oriented: ____ yes, ____ no. New confusion: ____ yes, ____ no.
Vital signs: temp ____, pulse _____, resp ______, b/p ______, 02 _____ %, ____ liters.
Glucose level: _____. Insulin: ___ yes, ___ no. Type: ______________ # of units ____.

Nurse _______________, CNA _______________, in at _____ am/pm. Left at ______ am/pm.
Wash hands and wear gloves before touching patient: ________ yes, ________ no.
Wash hands before leaving room: ___ yes, ___ no. Wear protective gear: __ yes, __ no.
Clean stethoscope: __ yes, __ no. Oral care: __ yes, __ no. Suctioned: __ yes, __ no.
Repositioned: ___ yes, ___ no. Turned to: ___ left, ___ right, ___ backside ___.
Head of bed at: _______ degrees. Incontinence/skin breakdown: ____ yes, ____ no.
Linens wet or soiled: _____ yes, _____ no. Linens changed: _____ yes, _____ no.
Dressing changed: ____ yes, ____ no. Location: ______________________________.
IV site checked: _____ yes, _____ no. IV tubing labeled: _____ yes, _____ no.
IV fluids at: ____.
Pain level (0-10 scale.0-no pain, 10 intolerable): ___________________________.
Location of pain: ________________. Medicated for pain: _____ yes, _____ no.
Patient is alert/oriented: ____ yes, ____ no. New confusion: ____ yes, ____ no.
Vital signs: temp ____, pulse _____, resp ______, b/p ______, 02 _____ %, ____ liters.
Glucose level: _____. Insulin: ___ yes, ___ no. Type: ______________ # of units ____.

Nurse _______________, CNA _______________, in at _____ am/pm. Left at ______ am/pm.
Wash hands and wear gloves before touching patient: ________ yes, ________ no.
Wash hands before leaving room: ___ yes, ___ no. Wear protective gear: __ yes, __ no.
Clean stethoscope: __ yes, __ no. Oral care: __ yes, __ no. Suctioned: __ yes, __ no.
Repositioned: ___ yes, ___ no. Turned to: ___ left, ___ right, ___ backside ___.
Head of bed at: _______ degrees. Incontinence/skin breakdown: ____ yes, ____ no.
Linens wet or soiled: _____ yes, _____ no. Linens changed: _____ yes, _____ no.
Dressing changed: ____ yes, ____ no. Location: ______________________________.
IV site checked: _____ yes, _____ no. IV tubing labeled: _____ yes, _____ no.
IV fluids at: ____.
Pain level (0-10 scale.0-no pain, 10 intolerable): ___________________________.
Location of pain: ________________. Medicated for pain: _____ yes, _____ no.
Patient is alert/oriented: ____ yes, ____ no. New confusion: ____ yes, ____ no.
Vital signs: temp ____, pulse _____, resp ______, b/p ______, 02 _____ %, ____ liters.
Glucose level: _____. Insulin: ___ yes, ___ no. Type: ______________ # of units ____.

MEDICATION ADMINISTRATION LIST FOR ____________________
DATE ____________________ DAY NUMBER ____________________

List the medication for each day. Routes of administration: oral, thru feeding tube, intravenous (IV), intramuscular (IM), subcutaneous (SQ), epidural or a catheter in your spinal column, rectal, topical, eye drops, and ear drops.

Medication: ____________________ Route: ____________________ Time: ________________
Medication: ____________________ Route: ____________________ Time: ________________
Medication: ____________________ Route: ____________________ Time: ________________
Medication: ____________________ Route: ____________________ Time: ________________
Medication: ____________________ Route: ____________________ Time: ________________
Medication: ____________________ Route: ____________________ Time: ________________
Medication: ____________________ Route: ____________________ Time: ________________
Medication: ____________________ Route: ____________________ Time: ________________
Medication: ____________________ Route: ____________________ Time: ________________
Medication: ____________________ Route: ____________________ Time: ________________
Medication: ____________________ Route: ____________________ Time: ________________
Medication: ____________________ Route: ____________________ Time: ________________
Medication: ____________________ Route: ____________________ Time: ________________
Medication: ____________________ Route: ____________________ Time: ________________
Medication: ____________________ Route: ____________________ Time: ________________
Medication: ____________________ Route: ____________________ Time: ________________
Medication: ____________________ Route: ____________________ Time: ________________
Medication: ____________________ Route: ____________________ Time: ________________
Medication: ____________________ Route: ____________________ Time: ________________
Medication: ____________________ Route: ____________________ Time: ________________
Medication: ____________________ Route: ____________________ Time: ________________
Medication: ____________________ Route: ____________________ Time: ________________
Medication: ____________________ Route: ____________________ Time: ________________
Medication: ____________________ Route: ____________________ Time: ________________
Medication: ____________________ Route: ____________________ Time: ________________
Medication: ____________________ Route: ____________________ Time: ________________
Medication: ____________________ Route: ____________________ Time: ________________
Medication: ____________________ Route: ____________________ Time: ________________
Medication: ____________________ Route: ____________________ Time: ________________
Medication: ____________________ Route: ____________________ Time: ________________
Medication: ____________________ Route: ____________________ Time: ________________
Medication: ____________________ Route: ____________________ Time: ________________
Medication: ____________________ Route: ____________________ Time: ________________
Medication: ____________________ Route: ____________________ Time: ________________
Medication: ____________________ Route: ____________________ Time: ________________
Medication: ____________________ Route: ____________________ Time: ________________
Medication: ____________________ Route: ____________________ Time: ________________
Medication: ____________________ Route: ____________________ Time: ________________
Medication: ____________________ Route: ____________________ Time: ________________
Medication: ____________________ Route: ____________________ Time: ________________
Medication: ____________________ Route: ____________________ Time: ________________
Medication: ____________________ Route: ____________________ Time: ________________
Medication: ____________________ Route: ____________________ Time: ________________
Medication: ____________________ Route: ____________________ Time: ________________
Medication: ____________________ Route: ____________________ Time: ________________
Medication: ____________________ Route: ____________________ Time: ________________
Medication: ____________________ Route: ____________________ Time: ________________
Medication: ____________________ Route: ____________________ Time: ________________
Medication: ____________________ Route: ____________________ Time: ________________
Medication: ____________________ Route: ____________________ Time: ________________
Medication: ____________________ Route: ____________________ Time: ________________
Medication: ____________________ Route: ____________________ Time: ________________
Medication: ____________________ Route: ____________________ Time: ________________
Medication: ____________________ Route: ____________________ Time: ________________
Medication: ____________________ Route: ____________________ Time: ________________

NOTES FOR DAY NUMBER ______________________________

DATE ______________________________

MEDICAL JOURNAL FOR ______________________________

DATE ________________, DAY NUMBER ______________

VISITS FROM MY DOCTORS TODAY

Goals for today: ____

____

____.

Things to discuss with my doctor(s): ___________________________

____

____

Dr.____________ came in at ____ am/pm. Left at ____ am/pm.
We discussed ____.
Did doctor examine patient: ____ yes, ____ no.
Wash hands before touching patient: ____ yes, ____ no.
Wear gloves: ___ yes, ___ no. Clean stethoscope: ___ yes, ___ no.
Wear gown and mask (precautions only):___ yes, ____ no.
Wash hands before leaving the room: ____ yes, ____ no.

Dr.____________ came in at ____ am/pm. Left at ____ am/pm.
We discussed ____.
Did doctor examine patient: ____ yes, ____ no.
Wash hands before touching patient: ____ yes, ____ no.
Wear gloves: ___ yes, ___ no. Clean stethoscope: ___ yes, ___ no.
Wear gown and mask (precautions only):___ yes, ____ no.
Wash hands before leaving the room: ____ yes, ____ no.

Dr.____________ came in at ____ am/pm. Left at ____ am/pm.
We discussed ____.
Did doctor examine patient: ____ yes, ____ no.
Wash hands before touching patient: ____ yes, ____ no.
Wear gloves: ___ yes, ___ no. Clean stethoscope: ___ yes, ___ no.
Wear gown and mask (precautions only):___ yes, ____ no.
Wash hands before leaving the room: ____ yes, ____ no.

Dr.____________ came in at ____ am/pm. Left at ____ am/pm.
We discussed ____.
Did doctor examine patient: ____ yes, ____ no.
Wash hands before touching patient: ____ yes, ____ no.
Wear gloves: ___ yes, ___ no. Clean stethoscope: ___ yes, ___ no.
Wear gown and mask (precautions only):___ yes, ____ no.
Wash hands before leaving the room: ____ yes, ____ no.

Dr.____________ came in at ____ am/pm. Left at ____ am/pm.
We discussed ____.
Did doctor examine patient: ____ yes, ____ no.
Wash hands before touching patient: ____ yes, ____ no.
Wear gloves: ___ yes, ___ no. Clean stethoscope: ___ yes, ___ no.
Wear gown and mask (precautions only):___ yes, ____ no.
Wash hands before leaving the room: ____ yes, ____ no.

NURSING CARE FOR ____

DATE ______________________, DAY NUMBER ____________________

INITIAL DAY SHIFT EXAM:

My nurse has _____ # of patients. CNA ___yes, ___no. Charge nurse ____________
Nurse ____________ RN/LPN came in at ________ am/pm. Left at _________ am/pm.
Did nurse wash hands and wear gloves before touching patient: _____ yes, _____ no.
Wash hands after touching patient and before leaving the room: _____ yes, _____ no.
Don't hesitate to request staff to wash their hands. This will help decrease the risk of spreading potentially lethal germs.
Did nurse wear protective gear (isolation precautions only): ______ yes, _____ no.
Did nurse provide oral care (to be done every two hours if unable to provide for self, also decreases risk of pneumonia, infections, and aspiration): ______ yes, _____ no.
If able to provide own oral care, then supplies at bedside: ______ yes, ______ no.
Was patient repositioned (every two hours if unable to turn self): ____ yes ____ no.
Head of bed at ________ degrees. This is important for patients on ventilators or on tube feedings. Anything less than thirty degrees places patients at risk for aspiration of stomach contents into the lungs causing aspiration pneumonia.
Checked for incontinence and skin breakdown: ____ yes, ____ no.
Patient's linens wet or soiled: ____yes, ____ no. Linens changed: ____ yes, ____ no.
Time linens changed: ________ am/pm. Any skin redness or breakdown: ____ yes, ____ no.
If yes, what stage is pressure ulcer: ______. Acquired when: ____________________.
List wounds not associated with pressure ulcers and how acquired: _______________
____.
Mattress type: ____.
Specialty mattresses are important to help prevent pressure ulcers)
If patient on ventilator or has tracheostomy, suction performed: _____ yes, _____ no.
Did nurse listen to lung sounds: ____ yes, ____ no.
Does patient have chest tubes: ____yes, ____ no. Functioning _____ yes, _____ no.
Bowel sounds: _____ yes, ______ no. Bowel sounds active: ______ yes, ______ no.
Neurological exam: _____ yes, ______ no. Follow commands: ______ yes, ______ no.
Is patient alert and oriented to person, place, time, and events: _____ yes, ____ no.
If confused, patient is not oriented to: ___ person, ___ place, ___ time, ___ event.
Confusion began (time and date): ____.
Glasgow coma scale (checks conscious scale of patient): ___________________________.
Intracranial pressure monitoring: ______ yes, ______ no.
If yes, pressure is at ________ mm mercury. (Normal is one to fifteen).
Moves extremities: ___ yes, ___no.
Paralysis: (inability to move extremities) ______ yes, ______ no.
If yes, extremities affected and when paralysis began: ___________________________.
Is patient in pain: ____ yes, ____ no. Describe pain and location ______________.
Patient able to eat: ____ yes, ____ no. What type of diet? ______________________.
If patient on tube feedings list type: __________ at ________ cc/ml per hour.
Nausea ____, vomiting ____. If so, describe: ____________________________________.
Patient has: Nasal gastric tube _____, Dobhoff tube ____, Peg or gastric tube ____.
When was feeding tube placed and what site: _____________________________________.
Catheter for draining urine: ____ yes, ____ no. If so, when placed: ____________.
Find out policy for allowed time to remain in bladder. Too long may cause infections.)
IV site(s) where: ________________ when placed: _____________________________.
IV fluids (types and rates): ____,
______________________, ______________________, ______________________________.
Is patient on oxygen: ____ yes, ____ no. If so, how much and route delivered (see oxygen routes): ____.
If patient on ventilator, list settings (see list on ventilator settings): ________
____.
Vital signs: temp _____, pulse _____, resp _____, b/p _____, o2 _____%,
current weight _____ pounds, _____ kg. Glucose level: _____
Insulin coverage: ____ yes, ____ no. Insulin type: ___________, # of units: _____.

NURSING CARE CONTINUED FOR ______________________________
DATE ___________________, DAY NUMBER _________________

FOLLOWING EXAMINATIONS FOR DAY SHIFT:

Nurse _____________, CNA _____________, in at _____ am/pm. Left at ______ am/pm.
Wash hands and wear gloves before touching patient: _______ yes, ______ no.
Wash hands before leaving room: ___ yes, ___ no. Wear protective gear: __ yes, __ no.
Clean stethoscope: __ yes, __ no. Oral care: __ yes, __ no. Suctioned: __ yes, __ no.
Repositioned: ___ yes, ___ no. Turned to: ___ left, ___ right, ___ backside ___.
Head of bed at: _______ degrees. Incontinence/skin breakdown: ____ yes, ____ no.
Linens wet or soiled: ____ yes, _____ no. Linens changed: _____ yes, ______ no.
Dressing changed: ____ yes, ____ no. Location: ______________________________.
IV site checked: _____ yes, ____ no. IV tubing labeled: _____ yes, _____no.
IV fluids at: ____.
Pain level (0-10 scale.0-no pain, 10 intolerable): ___________________.
Location of pain: ___________________. Medicated for pain: ____ yes, ____ no.
Patient is alert/oriented: ____ yes, ____ no. New confusion: ____ yes, ____ no.
Vital signs: temp ____, pulse _____, resp _____, b/p _____, 02 _____ %, ____ liters.
Glucose level: _____. Insulin: ___ yes, ___ no. Type: ______________ # of units ____.

Nurse _____________, CNA _____________, in at _____ am/pm. Left at ______ am/pm.
Wash hands and wear gloves before touching patient: _______ yes, ______ no.
Wash hands before leaving room: ___ yes, ___ no. Wear protective gear: __ yes, __ no.
Clean stethoscope: __ yes, __ no. Oral care: __ yes, __ no. Suctioned: __ yes, __ no.
Repositioned: ___ yes, ___ no. Turned to: ___ left, ___ right, ___ backside ___.
Head of bed at: _______ degrees. Incontinence/skin breakdown: ____ yes, ____ no.
Linens wet or soiled: ____ yes, _____ no. Linens changed: _____ yes, ______ no.
Dressing changed: ____ yes, ____ no. Location: ______________________________.
IV site checked: _____ yes, ____ no. IV tubing labeled: _____ yes, _____no.
IV fluids at: ____.
Pain level (0-10 scale.0-no pain, 10 intolerable): ___________________.
Location of pain: ___________________. Medicated for pain: ____ yes, ____ no.
Patient is alert/oriented: ____ yes, ____ no. New confusion: ____ yes, ____ no.
Vital signs: temp ____, pulse _____, resp _____, b/p _____, 02 _____ %, ____ liters.
Glucose level: _____. Insulin: ___ yes, ___ no. Type: ______________ # of units ____.

Nurse _____________, CNA _____________, in at _____ am/pm. Left at ______ am/pm.
Wash hands and wear gloves before touching patient: _______ yes, ______ no.
Wash hands before leaving room: ___ yes, ___ no. Wear protective gear: __ yes, __ no.
Clean stethoscope: __ yes, __ no. Oral care: __ yes, __ no. Suctioned: __ yes, __ no.
Repositioned: ___ yes, ___ no. Turned to: ___ left, ___ right, ___ backside ___.
Head of bed at: _______ degrees. Incontinence/skin breakdown: ____ yes, ____ no.
Linens wet or soiled: ____ yes, _____ no. Linens changed: _____ yes, ______ no.
Dressing changed: ____ yes, ____ no. Location: ______________________________.
IV site checked: _____ yes, ____ no. IV tubing labeled: _____ yes, _____no.
IV fluids at: ____.
Pain level (0-10 scale.0-no pain, 10 intolerable): ___________________.
Location of pain: ___________________. Medicated for pain: ____ yes, ____ no.
Patient is alert/oriented: ____ yes, ____ no. New confusion: ____ yes, ____ no.
Vital signs: temp ____, pulse _____, resp _____, b/p _____, 02 _____ %, ____ liters.
Glucose level: _____. Insulin: ___ yes, ___ no. Type: ______________ # of units ____.

NURSING CARE CONTINUED FOR ______________________
DATE ____________________, DAY NUMBER ________________

FOLLOWING EXAMINATIONS FOR DAY SHIFT:

Nurse ____________, CNA ______________, in at ____ am/pm. Left at ______ am/pm.
Wash hands and wear gloves before touching patient: ____ yes, ___ no.
Wash hands before leaving room: ___ yes, ___ no. Wear protective gear: __ yes, __ no.
Clean stethoscope: __ yes, __ no. Oral care: __ yes, __ no. Suctioned: __ yes, __ no.
Repositioned: ___ yes, ___ no. Turned to: ___ left, ___ right, ____ backside ___.
Head of bed at: _______ degrees. Incontinence/skin breakdown: ____ yes, ____ no.
Linens wet or soiled: ____ yes, ____ no. Linens changed: ____ yes, ____ no.
Dressing changed: ____ yes, ____ no. Location: ______________________________.
IV site checked: _____ yes, _____ no. IV tubing labeled: ____ yes, ____no.
IV fluids at: ____.
Pain level (0-10 scale.0-no pain, 10 intolerable): ___________________________.
Location of pain: _______________. Medicated for pain: ____ yes, ____ no.
Patient is alert/oriented: ____ yes, ____ no. New confusion: ____ yes, ____ no.
Vital signs: temp ____, pulse ____, resp ____, b/p ______, 02 ____ %, ____ liters.
Glucose level: _____. Insulin: ____ yes, ___ no. Type: ________ # of units ____.

Nurse ____________, CNA ______________, in at ____ am/pm. Left at ______ am/pm.
Wash hands and wear gloves before touching patient: ____ yes, ___ no.
Wash hands before leaving room: ___ yes, ___ no. Wear protective gear: __ yes, __ no.
Clean stethoscope: __ yes, __ no. Oral care: __ yes, __ no. Suctioned: __ yes, __ no.
Repositioned: ___ yes, ___ no. Turned to: ___ left, ___ right, ____ backside ___.
Head of bed at: _______ degrees. Incontinence/skin breakdown: ____ yes, ____ no.
Linens wet or soiled: ____ yes, ____ no. Linens changed: ____ yes, ____ no.
Dressing changed: ____ yes, ____ no. Location: ______________________________.
IV site checked: _____ yes, _____ no. IV tubing labeled: ____ yes, ____no.
IV fluids at: ____.
Pain level (0-10 scale.0-no pain, 10 intolerable): ___________________________.
Location of pain: _______________. Medicated for pain: ____ yes, ____ no.
Patient is alert/oriented: ____ yes, ____ no. New confusion: ____ yes, ____ no.
Vital signs: temp ____, pulse ____, resp ____, b/p ______, 02 ____ %, ____ liters.
Glucose level: _____. Insulin: ____ yes, ___ no. Type: ________ # of units ____.

Nurse ____________, CNA ______________, in at ____ am/pm. Left at ______ am/pm.
Wash hands and wear gloves before touching patient: ____ yes, ___ no.
Wash hands before leaving room: ___ yes, ___ no. Wear protective gear: __ yes, __ no.
Clean stethoscope: __ yes, __ no. Oral care: __ yes, __ no. Suctioned: __ yes, __ no.
Repositioned: ___ yes, ___ no. Turned to: ___ left, ___ right, ____ backside ___.
Head of bed at: _______ degrees. Incontinence/skin breakdown: ____ yes, ____ no.
Linens wet or soiled: ____ yes, ____ no. Linens changed: ____ yes, ____ no.
Dressing changed: ____ yes, ____ no. Location: ______________________________.
IV site checked: _____ yes, _____ no. IV tubing labeled: ____ yes, ____no.
IV fluids at: ____.
Pain level (0-10 scale.0-no pain, 10 intolerable): ___________________________.
Location of pain: _______________. Medicated for pain: ____ yes, ____ no.
Patient is alert/oriented: ____ yes, ____ no. New confusion: ____ yes, ____ no.
Vital signs: temp ____, pulse ____, resp ____, b/p ______, 02 ____ %, ____ liters.
Glucose level: _____. Insulin: ____ yes, ___ no. Type: ________ # of units ____.

NURSING CARE FOR ______________________________

DATE ____________________, DAY NUMBER ____________________

INITIAL NIGHT SHIFT EXAM:

My nurse has ______ # of patients. CNA ___yes, ___no. Charge nurse ________________
Nurse ________________ RN/LPN came in at _________ am/pm. Left at __________ am/pm.
Did nurse wash hands and wear gloves before touching patient: ______ yes, ______ no.
Wash hands after touching patient and before leaving the room: ______ yes, ______ no.
Don't hesitate to request staff to wash their hands. This will help decrease the risk of spreading potentially lethal germs.
Did nurse wear protective gear (isolation precautions only): ______ yes, ______ no.
Did nurse provide oral care (to be done every two hours if unable to provide for self, also decreases risk of pneumonia, infections, and aspiration): _______ yes, ______ no.
If able to provide own oral care, then supplies at bedside: ______ yes, ______ no.
Was patient repositioned (every two hours if unable to turn self): _____ yes _____ no.
Head of bed at ________ degrees. This is important for patients on ventilators or on tube feedings. Anything less than thirty degrees places patients at risk for aspiration of stomach contents into the lungs causing aspiration pneumonia.
Checked for incontinence and skin breakdown: _____ yes, _____ no.
Patient's linens wet or soiled: ____ yes, ____ no. Linens changed: ____ yes, ____ no.
Time linens changed: _______ am/pm. Any skin redness or breakdown: ____ yes, ____ no.
If yes, what stage is pressure ulcer: ________. Acquired when: ________________.
List wounds not associated with pressure ulcers and how acquired: ______________
____.
Mattress type: ____.
Specialty mattresses are important to help prevent pressure ulcers)
If patient on ventilator or has tracheostomy, suction performed: _____ yes, _____ no.
Did nurse listen to lung sounds: _____ yes, _____ no.
Does patient have chest tubes: ____ yes, ____ no. Functioning _____ yes, _____ no.
Bowel sounds: ______ yes, ______ no. Bowel sounds active: ______ yes, ______ no.
Neurological exam: _____ yes, ______ no. Follow commands: ______ yes, ______ no.
Is patient alert and oriented to person, place, time, and events: _____ yes, _____ no.
If confused, patient is not oriented to: ____ person, ___ place, ___ time, ___ event.
Confusion began (time and date): ____.
Glasgow coma scale (checks conscious scale of patient): _________________________.
Intracranial pressure monitoring: _____ yes, _____ no.
If yes, pressure is at ________ mm mercury. (Normal is one to fifteen).
Moves extremities: ___ yes, ___ no.
Paralysis: (inability to move extremities) _______ yes, _______ no.
If yes, extremities affected and when paralysis began: ________________________.
Is patient in pain: ____ yes, ____ no. Describe pain and location ______________.
Patient able to eat: ____ yes, ____ no. What type of diet? _____________________.
If patient on tube feedings list type: ____________ at ___________ cc/ml per hour.
Nausea ____, vomiting ____. If so, describe: ___________________________________.
Patient has: Nasal gastric tube ______, Dobhoff tube _____, Peg or gastric tube _____.
When was feeding tube placed and what site: ____________________________________.
Catheter for draining urine: ____ yes, ____ no. If so, when placed: ____________
Find out policy for allowed time to remain in bladder. Too long may cause infections.)
IV site(s) where: ______________________ when placed: _________________________.
IV fluids (types and rates): _____________________, ____________________________,
__________________, ______________________, ____________________, ______________.
Is patient on oxygen: _____ yes, _____ no. If so, how much and route delivered
(see oxygen routes): ____.
If patient on ventilator, list settings (see list on ventilator settings): _________
____.
Vital signs: temp _____, pulse _____, resp ______, b/p _____, o2 _____%,
current weight _____ pounds, _____ kg. Glucose level: _____
Insulin coverage: ____ yes, ____ no. Insulin type: ___________, # of units: _____.

NURSING CARE CONTINUED FOR ____________________
DATE ____________________, DAY NUMBER ____________________

FOLLOWING EXAMINATIONS FOR NIGHT SHIFT:

Nurse __________, CNA __________, in at _____ am/pm. Left at _______ am/pm.
Wash hands and wear gloves before touching patient: _______yes, ___ no.
Wash hands before leaving room: ___ yes, ___ no. Wear protective gear: __ yes, __ no.
Clean stethoscope: __ yes, __ no. Oral care: __ yes, __ no. Suctioned: __ yes, __ no.
Repositioned: ___ yes, ___ no. Turned to: ___ left, ___ right, ___ backside ___.
Head of bed at: _______ degrees. Incontinence/skin breakdown: ____ yes, ___ no.
Linens wet or soiled: _____ yes, _____ no. Linens changed: _____ yes, ___ no.
Dressing changed: _____ yes, _____ no. Location: ____________________.
IV site checked: _____ yes, _____ no. IV tubing labeled: _____ yes, _____ no.
IV fluids at: ____.
Pain level (0-10 scale.0-no pain, 10 intolerable): ____________.
Location of pain: ____________. Medicated for pain: _____ yes, ___ no.
Patient is alert/oriented: ____ yes, ___ no. New confusion: ___ yes, ___ no.
Vital signs: temp ____, pulse ____, resp _____, b/p _____, 02 ___ %, ___ liters.
Glucose level: _____. Insulin: ___ yes, ___ no. Type: __________ # of units ___.

Nurse __________, CNA __________, in at _____ am/pm. Left at _______ am/pm.
Wash hands and wear gloves before touching patient: _______yes, ___ no.
Wash hands before leaving room: ___ yes, ___ no. Wear protective gear: __ yes, __ no.
Clean stethoscope: __ yes, __ no. Oral care: __ yes, __ no. Suctioned: __ yes, __ no.
Repositioned: ___ yes, ___ no. Turned to: ___ left, ___ right, ___ backside ___.
Head of bed at: _______ degrees. Incontinence/skin breakdown: ____ yes, ___ no.
Linens wet or soiled: _____ yes, _____ no. Linens changed: _____ yes, ___ no.
Dressing changed: _____ yes, _____ no. Location: ____________________.
IV site checked: _____ yes, _____ no. IV tubing labeled: _____ yes, _____ no.
IV fluids at: ____.
Pain level (0-10 scale.0-no pain, 10 intolerable): ____________.
Location of pain: ____________. Medicated for pain: _____ yes, ___ no.
Patient is alert/oriented: ____ yes, ___ no. New confusion: ___ yes, ___ no.
Vital signs: temp ____, pulse ____, resp _____, b/p _____, 02 ___ %, ___ liters.
Glucose level: _____. Insulin: ___ yes, ___ no. Type: __________ # of units ___.

Nurse __________, CNA __________, in at _____ am/pm. Left at _______ am/pm.
Wash hands and wear gloves before touching patient: _______yes, ___ no.
Wash hands before leaving room: ___ yes, ___ no. Wear protective gear: __ yes, __ no.
Clean stethoscope: __ yes, __ no. Oral care: __ yes, __ no. Suctioned: __ yes, __ no.
Repositioned: ___ yes, ___ no. Turned to: ___ left, ___ right, ___ backside ___.
Head of bed at: _______ degrees. Incontinence/skin breakdown: ____ yes, ___ no.
Linens wet or soiled: _____ yes, _____ no. Linens changed: _____ yes, ___ no.
Dressing changed: _____ yes, _____ no. Location: ____________________.
IV site checked: _____ yes, _____ no. IV tubing labeled: _____ yes, _____ no.
IV fluids at: ____.
Pain level (0-10 scale.0-no pain, 10 intolerable): ____________.
Location of pain: ____________. Medicated for pain: _____ yes, ___ no.
Patient is alert/oriented: ____ yes, ___ no. New confusion: ___ yes, ___ no.
Vital signs: temp ____, pulse ____, resp _____, b/p _____, 02 ___ %, ___ liters.
Glucose level: _____. Insulin: ___ yes, ___ no. Type: __________ # of units ___.

NURSING CARE CONTINUED FOR ______________________
DATE ____________________, DAY NUMBER ____________________

FOLLOWING EXAMINATIONS FOR NIGHT SHIFT:

Nurse ______________, CNA ______________, in at _____ am/pm. Left at ______ am/pm.
Wash hands and wear gloves before touching patient: ________ yes, ________ no.
Wash hands before leaving room: ___ yes, ___ no. Wear protective gear: __ yes, __ no.
Clean stethoscope: __ yes, __ no. Oral care: __ yes, __ no. Suctioned: __ yes, __ no.
Repositioned: ___ yes, ___ no. Turned to: ___ left, ___ right, ___ backside ___.
Head of bed at: _______ degrees. Incontinence/skin breakdown: ____ yes, ____ no.
Linens wet or soiled: _____ yes, _____ no. Linens changed: _____ yes, ______ no.
Dressing changed: ____ yes, ____ no. Location: ____________________________.
IV site checked: _____ yes, _____ no. IV tubing labeled: _____ yes, _____ no.
IV fluids at: ____.
Pain level (0-10 scale.0-no pain, 10 intolerable): ________________________.
Location of pain: ________________. Medicated for pain: _____ yes, ____ no.
Patient is alert/oriented: ____ yes, ____ no. New confusion: ____ yes, ____ no.
Vital signs: temp ____, pulse _____, resp _____, b/p ______, 02 _____ %, ____ liters.
Glucose level: _____. Insulin: ___ yes, ___ no. Type: _______________ # of units ____.

Nurse ______________, CNA ______________, in at _____ am/pm. Left at ______ am/pm.
Wash hands and wear gloves before touching patient: ________ yes, ________ no.
Wash hands before leaving room: ___ yes, ___ no. Wear protective gear: __ yes, __ no.
Clean stethoscope: __ yes, __ no. Oral care: __ yes, __ no. Suctioned: __ yes, __ no.
Repositioned: ___ yes, ___ no. Turned to: ___ left, ___ right, ___ backside ___.
Head of bed at: _______ degrees. Incontinence/skin breakdown: ____ yes, ____ no.
Linens wet or soiled: _____ yes, _____ no. Linens changed: _____ yes, ______ no.
Dressing changed: ____ yes, ____ no. Location: ____________________________.
IV site checked: _____ yes, _____ no. IV tubing labeled: _____ yes, _____ no.
IV fluids at: ____.
Pain level (0-10 scale.0-no pain, 10 intolerable): ________________________.
Location of pain: ________________. Medicated for pain: _____ yes, ____ no.
Patient is alert/oriented: ____ yes, ____ no. New confusion: ____ yes, ____ no.
Vital signs: temp ____, pulse _____, resp _____, b/p ______, 02 _____ %, ____ liters.
Glucose level: _____. Insulin: ___ yes, ___ no. Type: _______________ # of units ____.

Nurse ______________, CNA ______________, in at _____ am/pm. Left at ______ am/pm.
Wash hands and wear gloves before touching patient: ________ yes, ________ no.
Wash hands before leaving room: ___ yes, ___ no. Wear protective gear: __ yes, __ no.
Clean stethoscope: __ yes, __ no. Oral care: __ yes, __ no. Suctioned: __ yes, __ no.
Repositioned: ___ yes, ___ no. Turned to: ___ left, ___ right, ___ backside ___.
Head of bed at: _______ degrees. Incontinence/skin breakdown: ____ yes, ____ no.
Linens wet or soiled: _____ yes, _____ no. Linens changed: _____ yes, ______ no.
Dressing changed: ____ yes, ____ no. Location: ____________________________.
IV site checked: _____ yes, _____ no. IV tubing labeled: _____ yes, _____ no.
IV fluids at: ____.
Pain level (0-10 scale.0-no pain, 10 intolerable): ________________________.
Location of pain: ________________. Medicated for pain: _____ yes, ____ no.
Patient is alert/oriented: ____ yes, ____ no. New confusion: ____ yes, ____ no.
Vital signs: temp ____, pulse _____, resp _____, b/p ______, 02 _____ %, ____ liters.
Glucose level: _____. Insulin: ___ yes, ___ no. Type: _______________ # of units ____.

MEDICATION ADMINISTRATION LIST FOR ____________________
DATE ______________ DAY NUMBER ____________________

List the medication for each day. Routes of administration: oral, thru feeding tube, intravenous (IV), intramuscular (IM), subcutaneous (SQ), epidural or a catheter in your spinal column, rectal, topical, eye drops, and ear drops.

Medication: ______________ Route: ______________ Time: ______________
Medication: ______________ Route: ______________ Time: ______________
Medication: ______________ Route: ______________ Time: ______________
Medication: ______________ Route: ______________ Time: ______________
Medication: ______________ Route: ______________ Time: ______________
Medication: ______________ Route: ______________ Time: ______________
Medication: ______________ Route: ______________ Time: ______________
Medication: ______________ Route: ______________ Time: ______________
Medication: ______________ Route: ______________ Time: ______________
Medication: ______________ Route: ______________ Time: ______________
Medication: ______________ Route: ______________ Time: ______________
Medication: ______________ Route: ______________ Time: ______________
Medication: ______________ Route: ______________ Time: ______________
Medication: ______________ Route: ______________ Time: ______________
Medication: ______________ Route: ______________ Time: ______________
Medication: ______________ Route: ______________ Time: ______________
Medication: ______________ Route: ______________ Time: ______________
Medication: ______________ Route: ______________ Time: ______________
Medication: ______________ Route: ______________ Time: ______________
Medication: ______________ Route: ______________ Time: ______________
Medication: ______________ Route: ______________ Time: ______________
Medication: ______________ Route: ______________ Time: ______________
Medication: ______________ Route: ______________ Time: ______________
Medication: ______________ Route: ______________ Time: ______________
Medication: ______________ Route: ______________ Time: ______________
Medication: ______________ Route: ______________ Time: ______________
Medication: ______________ Route: ______________ Time: ______________
Medication: ______________ Route: ______________ Time: ______________
Medication: ______________ Route: ______________ Time: ______________
Medication: ______________ Route: ______________ Time: ______________
Medication: ______________ Route: ______________ Time: ______________
Medication: ______________ Route: ______________ Time: ______________
Medication: ______________ Route: ______________ Time: ______________
Medication: ______________ Route: ______________ Time: ______________
Medication: ______________ Route: ______________ Time: ______________
Medication: ______________ Route: ______________ Time: ______________
Medication: ______________ Route: ______________ Time: ______________
Medication: ______________ Route: ______________ Time: ______________
Medication: ______________ Route: ______________ Time: ______________
Medication: ______________ Route: ______________ Time: ______________
Medication: ______________ Route: ______________ Time: ______________
Medication: ______________ Route: ______________ Time: ______________
Medication: ______________ Route: ______________ Time: ______________
Medication: ______________ Route: ______________ Time: ______________
Medication: ______________ Route: ______________ Time: ______________
Medication: ______________ Route: ______________ Time: ______________
Medication: ______________ Route: ______________ Time: ______________
Medication: ______________ Route: ______________ Time: ______________
Medication: ______________ Route: ______________ Time: ______________
Medication: ______________ Route: ______________ Time: ______________
Medication: ______________ Route: ______________ Time: ______________
Medication: ______________ Route: ______________ Time: ______________
Medication: ______________ Route: ______________ Time: ______________
Medication: ______________ Route: ______________ Time: ______________

NOTES FOR DAY NUMBER ______________________________

DATE ______________________________

MEDICAL JOURNAL FOR ______________________________

DATE ____________________, DAY NUMBER ______________

VISITS FROM MY DOCTORS TODAY

Goals for today: ____
____
____.

Things to discuss with my doctor(s): ___________________________
____
____.

Dr.____________ came in at ____ am/pm. Left at ____ am/pm.
We discussed ____.
Did doctor examine patient: ____ yes, ____ no.
Wash hands before touching patient: ____ yes, ____ no.
Wear gloves: ____ yes, ___ no. Clean stethoscope: ____ yes, ____ no.
Wear gown and mask (precautions only):____ yes, ____ no.
Wash hands before leaving the room: ____ yes, ____ no.

Dr.____________ came in at ____ am/pm. Left at ____ am/pm.
We discussed ____.
Did doctor examine patient: ____ yes, ____ no.
Wash hands before touching patient: ____ yes, ____ no.
Wear gloves: ____ yes, ___ no. Clean stethoscope: ____ yes, ____ no.
Wear gown and mask (precautions only):____ yes, ____ no.
Wash hands before leaving the room: ____ yes, ____ no.

Dr.____________ came in at ____ am/pm. Left at ____ am/pm.
We discussed ____.
Did doctor examine patient: ____ yes, ____ no.
Wash hands before touching patient: ____ yes, ____ no.
Wear gloves: ____ yes, ___ no. Clean stethoscope: ____ yes, ____ no.
Wear gown and mask (precautions only):____ yes, ____ no.
Wash hands before leaving the room: ____ yes, ____ no.

Dr.____________ came in at ____ am/pm. Left at ____ am/pm.
We discussed ____.
Did doctor examine patient: ____ yes, ____ no.
Wash hands before touching patient: ____ yes, ____ no.
Wear gloves: ____ yes, ___ no. Clean stethoscope: ____ yes, ____ no.
Wear gown and mask (precautions only):____ yes, ____ no.
Wash hands before leaving the room: ____ yes, ____ no.

Dr.____________ came in at ____ am/pm. Left at ____ am/pm.
We discussed ____.
Did doctor examine patient: ____ yes, ____ no.
Wash hands before touching patient: ____ yes, ____ no.
Wear gloves: ____ yes, ___ no. Clean stethoscope: ____ yes, ____ no.
Wear gown and mask (precautions only):____ yes, ____ no.
Wash hands before leaving the room: ____ yes, ____ no.

NURSING CARE FOR ______________________________

DATE ________________, DAY NUMBER ________________

INITIAL DAY SHIFT EXAM:

My nurse has ______ # of patients. CNA ___yes, ___no. Charge nurse ______________
Nurse _______________ RN/LPN came in at _________ am/pm. Left at __________ am/pm.
Did nurse wash hands and wear gloves before touching patient: ______ yes, _______ no.
Wash hands after touching patient and before leaving the room: ______ yes, _______ no.
Don't hesitate to request staff to wash their hands. This will help decrease the risk of spreading potentially lethal germs.
Did nurse wear protective gear (isolation precautions only): _______ yes, _______ no.
Did nurse provide oral care (to be done every two hours if unable to provide for self, also decreases risk of pneumonia, infections, and aspiration): _______ yes, _______ no.
If able to provide own oral care, then supplies at bedside: ________ yes, ________ no.
Was patient repositioned (every two hours if unable to turn self): _____ yes _____ no.
Head of bed at _________ degrees. This is important for patients on ventilators or on tube feedings. Anything less than thirty degrees places patients at risk for aspiration of stomach contents into the lungs causing aspiration pneumonia.
Checked for incontinence and skin breakdown: _____ yes, _____ no.
Patient's linens wet or soiled: _____ yes, ____ no. Linens changed: ____ yes, ____ no.
Time linens changed: ________ am/pm. Any skin redness or breakdown: ____ yes, ____ no.
If yes, what stage is pressure ulcer: _________. Acquired when: ______________.
List wounds not associated with pressure ulcers and how acquired: ______________
____.
Mattress type: ____.
Specialty mattresses are important to help prevent pressure ulcers)
If patient on ventilator or has tracheostomy, suction performed: _____ yes, ______ no.
Did nurse listen to lung sounds: _____ yes, _____ no.
Does patient have chest tubes: ____ yes, ____ no. Functioning _____ yes, ______ no.
Bowel sounds: _______ yes, _______ no. Bowel sounds active: _______ yes, _______ no.
Neurological exam: ______ yes, ______ no. Follow commands: _______ yes, _______ no.
Is patient alert and oriented to person, place, time, and events: _____ yes, _____ no.
If confused, patient is not oriented to: ____ person, ___ place, ___ time, ___ event.
Confusion began (time and date): ____.
Glasgow coma scale (checks conscious scale of patient): ______________________.
Intracranial pressure monitoring: ______ yes, ______ no.
If yes, pressure is at ________ mm mercury. (Normal is one to fifteen).
Moves extremities: ___ yes, ___ no.
Paralysis: (inability to move extremities) ________ yes, ________ no.
If yes, extremities affected and when paralysis began: ________________________.
Is patient in pain: ____ yes, ____ no. Describe pain and location ______________.
Patient able to eat: ____ yes, ____ no. What type of diet? ____________________.
If patient on tube feedings list type: ______________ at ____________ cc/ml per hour.
Nausea ____, vomiting _____. If so, describe: ________________________________.
Patient has: Nasal gastric tube ______, Dobhoff tube _____, Peg or gastric tube ____.
When was feeding tube placed and what site: ___________________________________.
Catheter for draining urine: ____ yes, ____ no. If so, when placed: ___________.
Find out policy for allowed time to remain in bladder. Too long may cause infections.)
IV site(s) where: _________________________ when placed: ____________________.
IV fluids (types and rates): _______________________, _______________________,
_______________________, _______________________, _______________________,
Is patient on oxygen: _____ yes, _____ no. If so, how much and route delivered (see oxygen routes): ____.
If patient on ventilator, list settings (see list on ventilator settings): __________
____.
Vital signs: temp _____, pulse _____, resp _____, b/p _____, o2 ____%,
current weight ______ pounds, ______ kg. Glucose level: __________
Insulin coverage: ____ yes, ____ no. Insulin type: __________, # of units: _____.

NURSING CARE CONTINUED FOR ______________________
DATE ____________________, DAY NUMBER ______________

FOLLOWING EXAMINATIONS FOR DAY SHIFT:

Nurse __________, CNA __________, in at _____ am/pm. Left at _____ am/pm.
Wash hands and wear gloves before touching patient: _____ yes, _____ no.
Wash hands before leaving room: ___ yes, ___ no. Wear protective gear: __ yes, __ no.
Clean stethoscope: __ yes, __ no. Oral care: __ yes, __ no. Suctioned: __ yes, __ no.
Repositioned: ___ yes, ___ no. Turned to: ___ left, ___ right, ___ backside ___.
Head of bed at: _______ degrees. Incontinence/skin breakdown: ___ yes, ___ no.
Linens wet or soiled: ____ yes, ____ no. Linens changed: ____ yes, ____ no.
Dressing changed: ____ yes, ____ no. Location: ______________________.
IV site checked: ____ yes, ____ no. IV tubing labeled: ____ yes, ____ no.
IV fluids at: ____.
Pain level (0-10 scale.0-no pain, 10 intolerable): _______________.
Location of pain: __________. Medicated for pain: ____ yes, ____ no.
Patient is alert/oriented: ____ yes, ____ no. New confusion: ____ yes, ____ no.
Vital signs: temp ____, pulse ____, resp ____, b/p _____, 02 _____ %, ____ liters.
Glucose level: _____. Insulin: ___ yes, ___ no. Type: __________ # of units ____.

Nurse __________, CNA __________, in at _____ am/pm. Left at _____ am/pm.
Wash hands and wear gloves before touching patient: _____ yes, _____ no.
Wash hands before leaving room: ___ yes, ___ no. Wear protective gear: __ yes, __ no.
Clean stethoscope: __ yes, __ no. Oral care: __ yes, __ no. Suctioned: __ yes, __ no.
Repositioned: ___ yes, ___ no. Turned to: ___ left, ___ right, ___ backside ___.
Head of bed at: _______ degrees. Incontinence/skin breakdown: ___ yes, ___ no.
Linens wet or soiled: ____ yes, ____ no. Linens changed: ____ yes, ____ no.
Dressing changed: ____ yes, ____ no. Location: ______________________.
IV site checked: ____ yes, ____ no. IV tubing labeled: ____ yes, ____ no.
IV fluids at: ____.
Pain level (0-10 scale.0-no pain, 10 intolerable): _______________.
Location of pain: __________. Medicated for pain: ____ yes, ____ no.
Patient is alert/oriented: ____ yes, ____ no. New confusion: ____ yes, ____ no.
Vital signs: temp ____, pulse ____, resp ____, b/p _____, 02 _____ %, ____ liters.
Glucose level: _____. Insulin: ___ yes, ___ no. Type: __________ # of units ____.

Nurse __________, CNA __________, in at _____ am/pm. Left at _____ am/pm.
Wash hands and wear gloves before touching patient: _____ yes, _____ no.
Wash hands before leaving room: ___ yes, ___ no. Wear protective gear: __ yes, __ no.
Clean stethoscope: __ yes, __ no. Oral care: __ yes, __ no. Suctioned: __ yes, __ no.
Repositioned: ___ yes, ___ no. Turned to: ___ left, ___ right, ___ backside ___.
Head of bed at: _______ degrees. Incontinence/skin breakdown: ___ yes, ___ no.
Linens wet or soiled: ____ yes, ____ no. Linens changed: ____ yes, ____ no.
Dressing changed: ____ yes, ____ no. Location: ______________________.
IV site checked: ____ yes, ____ no. IV tubing labeled: ____ yes, ____ no.
IV fluids at: ____.
Pain level (0-10 scale.0-no pain, 10 intolerable): _______________.
Location of pain: __________. Medicated for pain: ____ yes, ____ no.
Patient is alert/oriented: ____ yes, ____ no. New confusion: ____ yes, ____ no.
Vital signs: temp ____, pulse ____, resp ____, b/p _____, 02 _____ %, ____ liters.
Glucose level: _____. Insulin: ___ yes, ___ no. Type: __________ # of units ____.

NURSING CARE CONTINUED FOR ______________________________
DATE ____________________, DAY NUMBER ______________________

FOLLOWING EXAMINATIONS FOR DAY SHIFT:

Nurse ____________, CNA ____________, in at _____ am/pm. Left at ______ am/pm.
Wash hands and wear gloves before touching patient: ________ yes, ________ no.
Wash hands before leaving room: ___ yes, ___ no. Wear protective gear: __ yes, __ no.
Clean stethoscope: __ yes, __ no. Oral care: __ yes, __ no. Suctioned: __ yes, __ no.
Repositioned: ___ yes, ___ no. Turned to: ___ left, ___ right, ___ backside ___.
Head of bed at: ______ degrees. Incontinence/skin breakdown: ____ yes, ____ no.
Linens wet or soiled: _____ yes, _____ no. Linens changed: _____ yes, ______ no.
Dressing changed: ____ yes, ____ no. Location: __________________________.
IV site checked: _____ yes, _____ no. IV tubing labeled: _____ yes, _____no.
IV fluids at: ____.
Pain level (0-10 scale.0-no pain, 10 intolerable): ________________________.
Location of pain: ________________. Medicated for pain: ____ yes, ____ no.
Patient is alert/oriented: ____ yes, ____ no. New confusion: ____ yes, ____ no.
Vital signs: temp ____, pulse _____, resp _____, b/p ______, 02 _____%, ____ liters.
Glucose level: _____. Insulin: ___ yes, ___ no. Type: _____________ # of units ____.

Nurse ____________, CNA ____________, in at _____ am/pm. Left at ______ am/pm.
Wash hands and wear gloves before touching patient: ________ yes, ________ no.
Wash hands before leaving room: ___ yes, ___ no. Wear protective gear: __ yes, __ no.
Clean stethoscope: __ yes, __ no. Oral care: __ yes, __ no. Suctioned: __ yes, __ no.
Repositioned: ___ yes, ___ no. Turned to: ___ left, ___ right, ___ backside ___.
Head of bed at: ______ degrees. Incontinence/skin breakdown: ____ yes, ____ no.
Linens wet or soiled: _____ yes, _____ no. Linens changed: _____ yes, ______ no.
Dressing changed: ____ yes, ____ no. Location: __________________________.
IV site checked: _____ yes, _____ no. IV tubing labeled: _____ yes, _____no.
IV fluids at: ____.
Pain level (0-10 scale.0-no pain, 10 intolerable): ________________________.
Location of pain: ________________. Medicated for pain: ____ yes, ____ no.
Patient is alert/oriented: ____ yes, ____ no. New confusion: ____ yes, ____ no.
Vital signs: temp ____, pulse _____, resp _____, b/p ______, 02 _____%, ____ liters.
Glucose level: _____. Insulin: ___ yes, ___ no. Type: _____________ # of units ____.

Nurse ____________, CNA ____________, in at _____ am/pm. Left at ______ am/pm.
Wash hands and wear gloves before touching patient: ________ yes, ________ no.
Wash hands before leaving room: ___ yes, ___ no. Wear protective gear: __ yes, __ no.
Clean stethoscope: __ yes, __ no. Oral care: __ yes, __ no. Suctioned: __ yes, __ no.
Repositioned: ___ yes, ___ no. Turned to: ___ left, ___ right, ___ backside ___.
Head of bed at: ______ degrees. Incontinence/skin breakdown: ____ yes, ____ no.
Linens wet or soiled: _____ yes, _____ no. Linens changed: _____ yes, ______ no.
Dressing changed: ____ yes, ____ no. Location: __________________________.
IV site checked: _____ yes, _____ no. IV tubing labeled: _____ yes, _____no.
IV fluids at: ____.
Pain level (0-10 scale.0-no pain, 10 intolerable): ________________________.
Location of pain: ________________. Medicated for pain: ____ yes, ____ no.
Patient is alert/oriented: ____ yes, ____ no. New confusion: ____ yes, ____ no.
Vital signs: temp ____, pulse _____, resp _____, b/p ______, 02 _____%, ____ liters.
Glucose level: _____. Insulin: ___ yes, ___ no. Type: _____________ # of units ____.

NURSING CARE FOR ______________________________

DATE ____________________, DAY NUMBER ____________________

INITIAL NIGHT SHIFT EXAM:

My nurse has ______ # of patients. CNA ___yes, ___no. Charge nurse ______________
Nurse ______________ RN/LPN came in at __________ am/pm. Left at __________ am/pm.
Did nurse wash hands and wear gloves before touching patient: _______ yes, _______ no.
Wash hands after touching patient and before leaving the room: _______ yes, _______ no.
Don't hesitate to request staff to wash their hands. This will help decrease the risk of spreading potentially lethal germs.
Did nurse wear protective gear (isolation precautions only): _______ yes, _______ no.
Did nurse provide oral care (to be done every two hours if unable to provide for self, also decreases risk of pneumonia, infections, and aspiration): _______ yes, _______ no.
If able to provide own oral care, then supplies at bedside: _______ yes, _______ no.
Was patient repositioned (every two hours if unable to turn self): ______ yes ______ no.
Head of bed at __________ degrees. This is important for patients on ventilators or on tube feedings. Anything less than thirty degrees places patients at risk for aspiration of stomach contents into the lungs causing aspiration pneumonia.
Checked for incontinence and skin breakdown: ____ yes, ____ no.
Patient's linens wet or soiled: ____ yes, ____ no. Linens changed: ____ yes, ____ no.
Time linens changed: ________ am/pm. Any skin redness or breakdown: ____ yes, ____ no.
If yes, what stage is pressure ulcer: ______. Acquired when: ______________.
List wounds not associated with pressure ulcers and how acquired: ______________
____.
Mattress type: ______________
Specialty mattresses are important to help prevent pressure ulcers)
If patient on ventilator or has tracheostomy, suction performed: ______ yes, ______ no.
Did nurse listen to lung sounds: ____ yes, ____ no.
Does patient have chest tubes: ____ yes, ____ no. Functioning ______ yes, ______ no.
Bowel sounds: _______ yes, _______ no. Bowel sounds active: ______ yes, ______ no.
Neurological exam: ______ yes, ______ no. Follow commands: ______ yes, ______ no.
Is patient alert and oriented to person, place, time, and events: ____ yes, ____ no.
If confused, patient is not oriented to: ___ person, ___ place, ___ time, ___ event.
Confusion began (time and date): ____.
Glasgow coma scale (checks conscious scale of patient): ________________________.
Intracranial pressure monitoring: ____ yes, ____ no.
If yes, pressure is at ________ mm mercury. (Normal is one to fifteen).
Moves extremities: ___ yes, ___ no.
Paralysis: (inability to move extremities) ______ yes, ______ no.
If yes, extremities affected and when paralysis began: __________________________.
Is patient in pain: ____ yes, ____ no. Describe pain and location ______________.
Patient able to eat: ____ yes, ____ no. What type of diet? ______________________.
If patient on tube feedings list type: __________ at ________ cc/ml per hour.
Nausea ____, vomiting ____. If so, describe: ____________________________________.
Patient has: Nasal gastric tube _____, Dobhoff tube _____, Peg or gastric tube _____.
When was feeding tube placed and what site: ______________________________________.
Catheter for draining urine: ____ yes, ____ no. If so, when placed: ____________.
Find out policy for allowed time to remain in bladder. Too long may cause infections.)
IV site(s) where: ______________ when placed: ______________.
IV fluids (types and rates): ____________, ____________, ____________,
____________, ____________, ____________, ____________.
Is patient on oxygen: _____ yes, _____ no. If so, how much and route delivered (see oxygen routes): ____.
If patient on ventilator, list settings (see list on ventilator settings): __________
____.
Vital signs: temp ______, pulse ______, resp ______, b/p ______, o2 ______%,
current weight ______ pounds, ______ kg. Glucose level: ______
Insulin coverage: ____ yes, ____ no. Insulin type: ____________, # of units: ______.

NURSING CARE CONTINUED FOR ____________________
DATE ____________________, DAY NUMBER ____________________

FOLLOWING EXAMINATIONS FOR NIGHT SHIFT:

Nurse ______________, CNA ______________, in at _____ am/pm. Left at _______ am/pm.
Wash hands and wear gloves before touching patient: ________ yes, ________ no.
Wash hands before leaving room: ___ yes, ___ no. Wear protective gear: __ yes, __ no.
Clean stethoscope: __ yes, __ no. Oral care: __ yes, __ no. Suctioned: __ yes, __ no.
Repositioned: ___ yes, ___ no. Turned to: ___ left, ___ right, ___ backside ___.
Head of bed at: _______ degrees. Incontinence/skin breakdown: ___ yes, ___ no.
Linens wet or soiled: _____ yes, _____ no. Linens changed: _____ yes, ______ no.
Dressing changed: ____ yes, ____ no. Location: ____________________.
IV site checked: _____ yes, _____ no. IV tubing labeled: _____ yes, _____no.
IV fluids at: ____.
Pain level (0-10 scale.0-no pain, 10 intolerable): ____________________.
Location of pain: ________________. Medicated for pain: _____ yes, _____ no.
Patient is alert/oriented: ____ yes, ____ no. New confusion: ____ yes, ____ no.
Vital signs: temp ____, pulse _____, resp ______, b/p ______, 02 _____ %, ____ liters.
Glucose level: _____. Insulin: ___ yes, ___ no. Type: ______________ # of units ____.

Nurse ______________, CNA ______________, in at _____ am/pm. Left at _______ am/pm.
Wash hands and wear gloves before touching patient: ________ yes, ________ no.
Wash hands before leaving room: ___ yes, ___ no. Wear protective gear: __ yes, __ no.
Clean stethoscope: __ yes, __ no. Oral care: __ yes, __ no. Suctioned: __ yes, __ no.
Repositioned: ___ yes, ___ no. Turned to: ___ left, ___ right, ___ backside ___.
Head of bed at: _______ degrees. Incontinence/skin breakdown: ___ yes, ___ no.
Linens wet or soiled: _____ yes, _____ no. Linens changed: _____ yes, ______ no.
Dressing changed: ____ yes, ____ no. Location: ____________________.
IV site checked: _____ yes, _____ no. IV tubing labeled: _____ yes, _____no.
IV fluids at: ____.
Pain level (0-10 scale.0-no pain, 10 intolerable): ____________________.
Location of pain: ________________. Medicated for pain: _____ yes, _____ no.
Patient is alert/oriented: ____ yes, ____ no. New confusion: ____ yes, ____ no.
Vital signs: temp ____, pulse _____, resp ______, b/p ______, 02 _____ %, ____ liters.
Glucose level: _____. Insulin: ___ yes, ___ no. Type: ______________ # of units ____.

Nurse ______________, CNA ______________, in at _____ am/pm. Left at _______ am/pm.
Wash hands and wear gloves before touching patient: ________ yes, ________ no.
Wash hands before leaving room: ___ yes, ___ no. Wear protective gear: __ yes, __ no.
Clean stethoscope: __ yes, __ no. Oral care: __ yes, __ no. Suctioned: __ yes, __ no.
Repositioned: ___ yes, ___ no. Turned to: ___ left, ___ right, ___ backside ___.
Head of bed at: _______ degrees. Incontinence/skin breakdown: ___ yes, ___ no.
Linens wet or soiled: _____ yes, _____ no. Linens changed: _____ yes, ______ no.
Dressing changed: ____ yes, ____ no. Location: ____________________.
IV site checked: _____ yes, _____ no. IV tubing labeled: _____ yes, _____no.
IV fluids at: ____.
Pain level (0-10 scale.0-no pain, 10 intolerable): ____________________.
Location of pain: ________________. Medicated for pain: _____ yes, _____ no.
Patient is alert/oriented: ____ yes, ____ no. New confusion: ____ yes, ____ no.
Vital signs: temp ____, pulse _____, resp ______, b/p ______, 02 _____ %, ____ liters.
Glucose level: _____. Insulin: ___ yes, ___ no. Type: ______________ # of units ____.

NURSING CARE CONTINUED FOR ____________________
DATE ____________________, DAY NUMBER ____________________

FOLLOWING EXAMINATIONS FOR NIGHT SHIFT:

Nurse ____________, CNA ____________, in at ______ am/pm. Left at ______ am/pm.
Wash hands and wear gloves before touching patient: ______ yes, ______ no.
Wash hands before leaving room: ___ yes, ___ no. Wear protective gear: __ yes, __ no.
Clean stethoscope: __ yes, __ no. Oral care: __ yes, __ no. Suctioned: __ yes, __ no.
Repositioned: ___ yes, ___ no. Turned to: ___ left, ___ right, ___ backside ___.
Head of bed at: ______ degrees. Incontinence/skin breakdown: ____ yes, ____ no.
Linens wet or soiled: _____ yes, _____ no. Linens changed: _____ yes, _____ no.
Dressing changed: ____ yes, ____ no. Location: ____________________.
IV site checked: ____ yes, ____ no. IV tubing labeled: _____ yes, _____no.
IV fluids at: ____________________.
Pain level (0-10 scale.0-no pain, 10 intolerable): ____________.
Location of pain: ____________. Medicated for pain: _____ yes, _____ no.
Patient is alert/oriented: ____ yes, ____ no. New confusion: ____ yes, ____ no.
Vital signs: temp ____, pulse ____, resp ____, b/p ______, 02 ____ %, ____ liters.
Glucose level: _____. Insulin: ___ yes, ___ no. Type: ____________ # of units ____.

Nurse ____________, CNA ____________, in at ______ am/pm. Left at ______ am/pm.
Wash hands and wear gloves before touching patient: ______ yes, ______ no.
Wash hands before leaving room: ___ yes, ___ no. Wear protective gear: __ yes, __ no.
Clean stethoscope: __ yes, __ no. Oral care: __ yes, __ no. Suctioned: __ yes, __ no.
Repositioned: ___ yes, ___ no. Turned to: ___ left, ___ right, ___ backside ___.
Head of bed at: ______ degrees. Incontinence/skin breakdown: ____ yes, ____ no.
Linens wet or soiled: _____ yes, _____ no. Linens changed: _____ yes, _____ no.
Dressing changed: ____ yes, ____ no. Location: ____________________.
IV site checked: ____ yes, ____ no. IV tubing labeled: _____ yes, _____no.
IV fluids at: ____________________.
Pain level (0-10 scale.0-no pain, 10 intolerable): ____________.
Location of pain: ____________. Medicated for pain: _____ yes, _____ no.
Patient is alert/oriented: ____ yes, ____ no. New confusion: ____ yes, ____ no.
Vital signs: temp ____, pulse ____, resp ____, b/p ______, 02 ____ %, ____ liters.
Glucose level: _____. Insulin: ___ yes, ___ no. Type: ____________ # of units ____.

Nurse ____________, CNA ____________, in at ______ am/pm. Left at ______ am/pm.
Wash hands and wear gloves before touching patient: ______ yes, ______ no.
Wash hands before leaving room: ___ yes, ___ no. Wear protective gear: __ yes, __ no.
Clean stethoscope: __ yes, __ no. Oral care: __ yes, __ no. Suctioned: __ yes, __ no.
Repositioned: ___ yes, ___ no. Turned to: ___ left, ___ right, ___ backside ___.
Head of bed at: ______ degrees. Incontinence/skin breakdown: ____ yes, ____ no.
Linens wet or soiled: _____ yes, _____ no. Linens changed: _____ yes, _____ no.
Dressing changed: ____ yes, ____ no. Location: ____________________.
IV site checked: ____ yes, ____ no. IV tubing labeled: _____ yes, _____no.
IV fluids at: ____________________.
Pain level (0-10 scale.0-no pain, 10 intolerable): ____________.
Location of pain: ____________. Medicated for pain: _____ yes, _____ no.
Patient is alert/oriented: ____ yes, ____ no. New confusion: ____ yes, ____ no.
Vital signs: temp ____, pulse ____, resp ____, b/p ______, 02 ____ %, ____ liters.
Glucose level: _____. Insulin: ___ yes, ___ no. Type: ____________ # of units ____.

MEDICATION ADMINISTRATION LIST FOR ____________________
DATE ________________ DAY NUMBER ____________________

List the medication for each day. Routes of administration: oral, thru feeding tube, intravenous (IV), intramuscular (IM), subcutaneous (SQ), epidural or a catheter in your spinal column, rectal, topical, eye drops, and ear drops.

Medication: ________________ Route: ________________ Time: ____________
Medication: ________________ Route: ________________ Time: ____________
Medication: ________________ Route: ________________ Time: ____________
Medication: ________________ Route: ________________ Time: ____________
Medication: ________________ Route: ________________ Time: ____________
Medication: ________________ Route: ________________ Time: ____________
Medication: ________________ Route: ________________ Time: ____________
Medication: ________________ Route: ________________ Time: ____________
Medication: ________________ Route: ________________ Time: ____________
Medication: ________________ Route: ________________ Time: ____________
Medication: ________________ Route: ________________ Time: ____________
Medication: ________________ Route: ________________ Time: ____________
Medication: ________________ Route: ________________ Time: ____________
Medication: ________________ Route: ________________ Time: ____________
Medication: ________________ Route: ________________ Time: ____________
Medication: ________________ Route: ________________ Time: ____________
Medication: ________________ Route: ________________ Time: ____________
Medication: ________________ Route: ________________ Time: ____________
Medication: ________________ Route: ________________ Time: ____________
Medication: ________________ Route: ________________ Time: ____________
Medication: ________________ Route: ________________ Time: ____________
Medication: ________________ Route: ________________ Time: ____________
Medication: ________________ Route: ________________ Time: ____________
Medication: ________________ Route: ________________ Time: ____________
Medication: ________________ Route: ________________ Time: ____________
Medication: ________________ Route: ________________ Time: ____________
Medication: ________________ Route: ________________ Time: ____________
Medication: ________________ Route: ________________ Time: ____________
Medication: ________________ Route: ________________ Time: ____________
Medication: ________________ Route: ________________ Time: ____________
Medication: ________________ Route: ________________ Time: ____________
Medication: ________________ Route: ________________ Time: ____________
Medication: ________________ Route: ________________ Time: ____________
Medication: ________________ Route: ________________ Time: ____________
Medication: ________________ Route: ________________ Time: ____________
Medication: ________________ Route: ________________ Time: ____________
Medication: ________________ Route: ________________ Time: ____________
Medication: ________________ Route: ________________ Time: ____________
Medication: ________________ Route: ________________ Time: ____________
Medication: ________________ Route: ________________ Time: ____________
Medication: ________________ Route: ________________ Time: ____________
Medication: ________________ Route: ________________ Time: ____________
Medication: ________________ Route: ________________ Time: ____________
Medication: ________________ Route: ________________ Time: ____________
Medication: ________________ Route: ________________ Time: ____________
Medication: ________________ Route: ________________ Time: ____________
Medication: ________________ Route: ________________ Time: ____________
Medication: ________________ Route: ________________ Time: ____________
Medication: ________________ Route: ________________ Time: ____________
Medication: ________________ Route: ________________ Time: ____________
Medication: ________________ Route: ________________ Time: ____________
Medication: ________________ Route: ________________ Time: ____________
Medication: ________________ Route: ________________ Time: ____________
Medication: ________________ Route: ________________ Time: ____________

NOTES FOR DAY NUMBER ______________________

DATE ______________________

MEDICAL JOURNAL FOR ______________________________

DATE ____________________, DAY NUMBER ________________

VISITS FROM MY DOCTORS TODAY

Goals for today: ____
____
____.

Things to discuss with my doctor(s): ______________________________
____
____

Dr.______________ came in at _____ am/pm. Left at _____ am/pm.
We discussed ____.
Did doctor examine patient: _____ yes, _____ no.
Wash hands before touching patient: _____ yes, _____ no.
Wear gloves: ____ yes, ___ no. Clean stethoscope: ____ yes, ____ no.
Wear gown and mask (precautions only):____ yes, _____ no.
Wash hands before leaving the room: _____ yes, _____ no.

Dr.______________ came in at _____ am/pm. Left at _____ am/pm.
We discussed ____.
Did doctor examine patient: _____ yes, _____ no.
Wash hands before touching patient: _____ yes, _____ no.
Wear gloves: ____ yes, ___ no. Clean stethoscope: ____ yes, ____ no.
Wear gown and mask (precautions only):____ yes, _____ no.
Wash hands before leaving the room: _____ yes, _____ no.

Dr.______________ came in at _____ am/pm. Left at _____ am/pm.
We discussed ____.
Did doctor examine patient: _____ yes, _____ no.
Wash hands before touching patient: _____ yes, _____ no.
Wear gloves: ____ yes, ___ no. Clean stethoscope: ____ yes, ____ no.
Wear gown and mask (precautions only):____ yes, _____ no.
Wash hands before leaving the room: _____ yes, _____ no.

Dr.______________ came in at _____ am/pm. Left at _____ am/pm.
We discussed ____.
Did doctor examine patient: _____ yes, _____ no.
Wash hands before touching patient: _____ yes, _____ no.
Wear gloves: ____ yes, ___ no. Clean stethoscope: ____ yes, ____ no.
Wear gown and mask (precautions only):____ yes, _____ no.
Wash hands before leaving the room: _____ yes, _____ no.

Dr.______________ came in at _____ am/pm. Left at _____ am/pm.
We discussed ____.
Did doctor examine patient: _____ yes, _____ no.
Wash hands before touching patient: _____ yes, _____ no.
Wear gloves: ____ yes, ___ no. Clean stethoscope: ____ yes, ____ no.
Wear gown and mask (precautions only):____ yes, _____ no.
Wash hands before leaving the room: _____ yes, _____ no.

NURSING CARE FOR ____________________

DATE ______________, DAY NUMBER ______________

INITIAL DAY SHIFT EXAM:

My nurse has _____ # of patients. CNA ___yes, ___no. Charge nurse ____________
Nurse ____________ RN/LPN came in at ________ am/pm. Left at _________ am/pm.
Did nurse wash hands and wear gloves before touching patient: _____ yes, _____ no.
Wash hands after touching patient and before leaving the room: _____ yes, _____ no.
Don't hesitate to request staff to wash their hands. This will help decrease the risk of spreading potentially lethal germs.
Did nurse wear protective gear (isolation precautions only): _____ yes, _____ no.
Did nurse provide oral care (to be done every two hours if unable to provide for self, also decreases risk of pneumonia, infections, and aspiration): _____ yes, _____ no.
If able to provide own oral care, then supplies at bedside: _____ yes, _____ no.
Was patient repositioned (every two hours if unable to turn self): _____ yes _____ no.
Head of bed at ________ degrees. This is important for patients on ventilators or on tube feedings. Anything less than thirty degrees places patients at risk for aspiration of stomach contents into the lungs causing aspiration pneumonia.
Checked for incontinence and skin breakdown: _____ yes, _____ no.
Patient's linens wet or soiled: ____ yes, ____ no. Linens changed: ____ yes, ____ no.
Time linens changed: ________ am/pm. Any skin redness or breakdown: ____ yes, ____ no.
If yes, what stage is pressure ulcer: ________. Acquired when: ____________.
List wounds not associated with pressure ulcers and how acquired: ____________
____
Mattress type: ____
Specialty mattresses are important to help prevent pressure ulcers)
If patient on ventilator or has tracheostomy, suction performed: _____ yes, _____ no.
Did nurse listen to lung sounds: _____ yes, _____ no.
Does patient have chest tubes: ____ yes, ____ no. Functioning _____ yes, _____ no.
Bowel sounds: _____ yes, _____ no. Bowel sounds active: _____ yes, _____ no.
Neurological exam: _____ yes, _____ no. Follow commands: _____ yes, _____ no.
Is patient alert and oriented to person, place, time, and events: _____ yes, _____ no.
If confused, patient is not oriented to: ___ person, ___ place, ___ time, ___ event.
Confusion began (time and date): ____
Glasgow coma scale (checks conscious scale of patient): ______________________
Intracranial pressure monitoring: _____ yes, _____ no.
If yes, pressure is at ________ mm mercury. (Normal is one to fifteen).
Moves extremities: ___ yes, ___ no.
Paralysis: (inability to move extremities) _______ yes, _______ no.
If yes, extremities affected and when paralysis began: ____________________.
Is patient in pain: ____ yes, ____ no. Describe pain and location ____________
Patient able to eat: ____ yes, ____ no. What type of diet? ____________________
If patient on tube feedings list type: ____________ at ______ cc/ml per hour.
Nausea ____, vomiting ____. If so, describe: ______________________________.
Patient has: Nasal gastric tube _____, Dobhoff tube _____, Peg or gastric tube _____.
When was feeding tube placed and what site: ______________________________.
Catheter for draining urine: ____ yes, ____ no. If so, when placed: __________.
Find out policy for allowed time to remain in bladder. Too long may cause infections.)
IV site(s) where: ________________ when placed: ____________________________.
IV fluids (types and rates): ____________________, ____________________________,
____________________, ____________________, ____________________________.
Is patient on oxygen: _____ yes, _____ no. If so, how much and route delivered
(see oxygen routes): ____.
If patient on ventilator, list settings (see list on ventilator settings): ________
____.
Vital signs: temp _____, pulse _____, resp _____, b/p _____, o2 _____%,
current weight _____ pounds, _____ kg. Glucose level: _____
Insulin coverage: ____ yes, ____ no. Insulin type: ____________, # of units: _____.

NURSING CARE CONTINUED FOR ________________________
DATE ____________________, DAY NUMBER ____________________

FOLLOWING EXAMINATIONS FOR DAY SHIFT:

Nurse ______________, CNA ______________, in at _____ am/pm. Left at ______ am/pm.
Wash hands and wear gloves before touching patient: ______ yes, ______ no.
Wash hands before leaving room: ___ yes, ___ no. Wear protective gear: __ yes, __ no.
Clean stethoscope: __ yes, __ no. Oral care: __ yes, __ no. Suctioned: __ yes, __ no.
Repositioned: ___ yes, ___ no. Turned to: ___ left, ___ right, ___ backside ___.
Head of bed at: _______ degrees. Incontinence/skin breakdown: ____ yes, ____ no.
Linens wet or soiled: ____ yes, ____ no. Linens changed: ____ yes, ______ no.
Dressing changed: ____ yes, ____ no. Location: ______________________________.
IV site checked: _____ yes, _____ no. IV tubing labeled: _____ yes, _____ no.
IV fluids at: ____.
Pain level (0-10 scale.0-no pain, 10 intolerable): ___________________________.
Location of pain: ________________. Medicated for pain: ____ yes, ____ no.
Patient is alert/oriented: ____ yes, ____ no. New confusion: ____ yes, ____ no.
Vital signs: temp ____, pulse _____, resp _____, b/p _____, 02 _____ %, ____ liters.
Glucose level: _____. Insulin: ___ yes, ___ no. Type: ______________ # of units ____.

Nurse ______________, CNA ______________, in at _____ am/pm. Left at ______ am/pm.
Wash hands and wear gloves before touching patient: ______ yes, ______ no.
Wash hands before leaving room: ___ yes, ___ no. Wear protective gear: __ yes, __ no.
Clean stethoscope: __ yes, __ no. Oral care: __ yes, __ no. Suctioned: __ yes, __ no.
Repositioned: ___ yes, ___ no. Turned to: ___ left, ___ right, ___ backside ___.
Head of bed at: _______ degrees. Incontinence/skin breakdown: ____ yes, ____ no.
Linens wet or soiled: ____ yes, ____ no. Linens changed: ____ yes, ______ no.
Dressing changed: ____ yes, ____ no. Location: ______________________________.
IV site checked: _____ yes, _____ no. IV tubing labeled: _____ yes, _____ no.
IV fluids at: ____.
Pain level (0-10 scale.0-no pain, 10 intolerable): ___________________________.
Location of pain: ________________. Medicated for pain: ____ yes, ____ no.
Patient is alert/oriented: ____ yes, ____ no. New confusion: ____ yes, ____ no.
Vital signs: temp ____, pulse _____, resp _____, b/p _____, 02 _____ %, ____ liters.
Glucose level: _____. Insulin: ___ yes, ___ no. Type: ______________ # of units ____.

Nurse ______________, CNA ______________, in at _____ am/pm. Left at ______ am/pm.
Wash hands and wear gloves before touching patient: ______ yes, ______ no.
Wash hands before leaving room: ___ yes, ___ no. Wear protective gear: __ yes, __ no.
Clean stethoscope: __ yes, __ no. Oral care: __ yes, __ no. Suctioned: __ yes, __ no.
Repositioned: ___ yes, ___ no. Turned to: ___ left, ___ right, ___ backside ___.
Head of bed at: _______ degrees. Incontinence/skin breakdown: ____ yes, ____ no.
Linens wet or soiled: ____ yes, ____ no. Linens changed: ____ yes, ______ no.
Dressing changed: ____ yes, ____ no. Location: ______________________________.
IV site checked: _____ yes, _____ no. IV tubing labeled: _____ yes, _____ no.
IV fluids at: ____.
Pain level (0-10 scale.0-no pain, 10 intolerable): ___________________________.
Location of pain: ________________. Medicated for pain: ____ yes, ____ no.
Patient is alert/oriented: ____ yes, ____ no. New confusion: ____ yes, ____ no.
Vital signs: temp ____, pulse _____, resp _____, b/p _____, 02 _____ %, ____ liters.
Glucose level: _____. Insulin: ___ yes, ___ no. Type: ______________ # of units ____.

NURSING CARE CONTINUED FOR ____________________
DATE ____________________, DAY NUMBER ____________

FOLLOWING EXAMINATIONS FOR DAY SHIFT:

Nurse ______________, CNA ______________, in at _____ am/pm. Left at _______ am/pm.
Wash hands and wear gloves before touching patient: _____ yes, _____ no.
Wash hands before leaving room: ___ yes, ___ no. Wear protective gear: __ yes, __ no.
Clean stethoscope: __ yes, __ no. Oral care: __ yes, __ no. Suctioned: __ yes, __ no.
Repositioned: ___ yes, ___ no. Turned to: ___ left, ___ right, ___ backside ___.
Head of bed at: _______ degrees. Incontinence/skin breakdown: ____ yes, ____ no.
Linens wet or soiled: ____ yes, ____ no. Linens changed: _____ yes, ____ no.
Dressing changed: ____ yes, ____ no. Location: _______________________.
IV site checked: _____ yes, _____ no. IV tubing labeled: _____ yes, ____ no.
IV fluids at: ____.
Pain level (0-10 scale.0-no pain, 10 intolerable): ______________.
Location of pain: ______________. Medicated for pain: ____ yes, ____ no.
Patient is alert/oriented: ____ yes, ____ no. New confusion: ____ yes, ____ no.
Vital signs: temp ____, pulse ____, resp _____, b/p _____, 02 _____ %, ____ liters.
Glucose level: _____. Insulin: ___ yes, ___ no. Type: _____________ # of units ___.

Nurse ______________, CNA ______________, in at _____ am/pm. Left at _______ am/pm.
Wash hands and wear gloves before touching patient: _____ yes, _____ no.
Wash hands before leaving room: ___ yes, ___ no. Wear protective gear: __ yes, __ no.
Clean stethoscope: __ yes, __ no. Oral care: __ yes, __ no. Suctioned: __ yes, __ no.
Repositioned: ___ yes, ___ no. Turned to: ___ left, ___ right, ___ backside ___.
Head of bed at: _______ degrees. Incontinence/skin breakdown: ____ yes, ____ no.
Linens wet or soiled: ____ yes, ____ no. Linens changed: _____ yes, ____ no.
Dressing changed: ____ yes, ____ no. Location: _______________________.
IV site checked: _____ yes, _____ no. IV tubing labeled: _____ yes, ____ no.
IV fluids at: ____.
Pain level (0-10 scale.0-no pain, 10 intolerable): ______________.
Location of pain: ______________. Medicated for pain: ____ yes, ____ no.
Patient is alert/oriented: ____ yes, ____ no. New confusion: ____ yes, ____ no.
Vital signs: temp ____, pulse ____, resp _____, b/p _____, 02 _____ %, ____ liters.
Glucose level: _____. Insulin: ___ yes, ___ no. Type: _____________ # of units ___.

Nurse ______________, CNA ______________, in at _____ am/pm. Left at _______ am/pm.
Wash hands and wear gloves before touching patient: _____ yes, _____ no.
Wash hands before leaving room: ___ yes, ___ no. Wear protective gear: __ yes, __ no.
Clean stethoscope: __ yes, __ no. Oral care: __ yes, __ no. Suctioned: __ yes, __ no.
Repositioned: ___ yes, ___ no. Turned to: ___ left, ___ right, ___ backside ___.
Head of bed at: _______ degrees. Incontinence/skin breakdown: ____ yes, ____ no.
Linens wet or soiled: ____ yes, ____ no. Linens changed: _____ yes, ____ no.
Dressing changed: ____ yes, ____ no. Location: _______________________.
IV site checked: _____ yes, _____ no. IV tubing labeled: _____ yes, ____ no.
IV fluids at: ____.
Pain level (0-10 scale.0-no pain, 10 intolerable): ______________.
Location of pain: ______________. Medicated for pain: ____ yes, ____ no.
Patient is alert/oriented: ____ yes, ____ no. New confusion: ____ yes, ____ no.
Vital signs: temp ____, pulse ____, resp _____, b/p _____, 02 _____ %, ____ liters.
Glucose level: _____. Insulin: ___ yes, ___ no. Type: _____________ # of units ___.

NURSING CARE FOR ______________________________

DATE ____________________, DAY NUMBER ____________________

INITIAL NIGHT SHIFT EXAM:

My nurse has ______ # of patients. CNA ___yes, ___no. Charge nurse ______________
Nurse ______________ RN/LPN came in at _________ am/pm. Left at __________ am/pm.
Did nurse wash hands and wear gloves before touching patient: ______ yes, ______ no.
Wash hands after touching patient and before leaving the room: ______ yes, ______ no.
Don't hesitate to request staff to wash their hands. This will help decrease the risk of spreading potentially lethal germs.
Did nurse wear protective gear (isolation precautions only): ______ yes, ______ no.
Did nurse provide oral care (to be done every two hours if unable to provide for self, also decreases risk of pneumonia, infections, and aspiration): ______ yes, ______ no.
If able to provide own oral care, then supplies at bedside: ______ yes, ______ no.
Was patient repositioned (every two hours if unable to turn self): _____ yes _____ no.
Head of bed at ________ degrees. This is important for patients on ventilators or on tube feedings. Anything less than thirty degrees places patients at risk for aspiration of stomach contents into the lungs causing aspiration pneumonia.
Checked for incontinence and skin breakdown: _____ yes, _____ no.
Patient's linens wet or soiled: _____ yes, ____ no. Linens changed: ____ yes, ____ no.
Time linens changed: ________ am/pm. Any skin redness or breakdown: ____ yes, ____ no.
If yes, what stage is pressure ulcer: _______. Acquired when: ____________________.
List wounds not associated with pressure ulcers and how acquired: ______________
____.
Mattress type: ____.
Specialty mattresses are important to help prevent pressure ulcers)
If patient on ventilator or has tracheostomy, suction performed: _____ yes, ______ no.
Did nurse listen to lung sounds: _____ yes, ______ no.
Does patient have chest tubes: ____ yes, ____ no. Functioning _____ yes, ______ no.
Bowel sounds: _______ yes, ______ no. Bowel sounds active: ______ yes, ______ no.
Neurological exam: ______ yes, ______ no. Follow commands: ______ yes, ______ no.
Is patient alert and oriented to person, place, time, and events: _____ yes, _____ no.
If confused, patient is not oriented to: ____ person, ___ place, ___ time, ___ event.
Confusion began (time and date): ____.
Glasgow coma scale (checks conscious scale of patient): ______________________.
Intracranial pressure monitoring: ______ yes, _____ no.
If yes, pressure is at ________ mm mercury. (Normal is one to fifteen).
Moves extremities: ___ yes, ___ no.
Paralysis: (inability to move extremities) _______ yes, _______ no.
If yes, extremities affected and when paralysis began: ______________________.
Is patient in pain: ____ yes, ____ no. Describe pain and location ______________.
Patient able to eat: ____ yes, ____ no. What type of diet? ___________________.
If patient on tube feedings list type: _____________ at __________ cc/ml per hour.
Nausea ____, vomiting _____. If so, describe: ________________________________.
Patient has: Nasal gastric tube ______, Dobhoff tube _____, Peg or gastric tube _____.
When was feeding tube placed and what site: ___________________________________.
Catheter for draining urine: ____ yes, ____ no. If so, when placed: ____________.
Find out policy for allowed time to remain in bladder. Too long may cause infections.)
IV site(s) where: ______________________________ when placed: ______________.
IV fluids (types and rates): ______________________, ______________________,
______________________, ______________________, ______________________.
Is patient on oxygen: _____ yes, _____ no. If so, how much and route delivered
(see oxygen routes): ____.
If patient on ventilator, list settings (see list on ventilator settings): __________
____.
Vital signs: temp ______, pulse ______, resp ______, b/p ______, o2 ______%,
current weight ______ pounds, ______ kg. Glucose level: ______
Insulin coverage: ____ yes, ____ no. Insulin type: ____________, # of units: ______.

NURSING CARE CONTINUED FOR ____________________
DATE ____________________, DAY NUMBER ____________________

FOLLOWING EXAMINATIONS FOR NIGHT SHIFT:

Nurse ____________, CNA ____________, in at _____ am/pm. Left at _______ am/pm.
Wash hands and wear gloves before touching patient: _____yes, ____ no.
Wash hands before leaving room: ___ yes, ___ no. Wear protective gear: __ yes, __ no.
Clean stethoscope: __ yes, __ no. Oral care: __ yes, __ no. Suctioned: __ yes, __ no.
Repositioned: ___ yes, ___ no. Turned to: ___ left, ___ right, ___ backside ___.
Head of bed at: ______ degrees. Incontinence/skin breakdown: ___ yes, ___ no.
Linens wet or soiled: _____ yes, _____ no. Linens changed: _____ yes, ____ no.
Dressing changed: _____ yes, _____ no. Location: ____________________
IV site checked: _____ yes, _____ no. IV tubing labeled: ____ yes, ____ no.
IV fluids at: ____.
Pain level (0-10 scale.0-no pain, 10 intolerable): ____________________.
Location of pain: ____________. Medicated for pain: ____ yes, ____ no.
Patient is alert/oriented: ___ yes, ___ no. New confusion: ___ yes, ___ no.
Vital signs: temp ____, pulse ____, resp _____, b/p _____, 02 ____ %, ___ liters.
Glucose level: _____. Insulin: ___ yes, ___ no. Type: __________ # of units ___.

Nurse ____________, CNA ____________, in at _____ am/pm. Left at _______ am/pm.
Wash hands and wear gloves before touching patient: _____yes, ____ no.
Wash hands before leaving room: ___ yes, ___ no. Wear protective gear: __ yes, __ no.
Clean stethoscope: __ yes, __ no. Oral care: __ yes, __ no. Suctioned: __ yes, __ no.
Repositioned: ___ yes, ___ no. Turned to: ___ left, ___ right, ___ backside ___.
Head of bed at: ______ degrees. Incontinence/skin breakdown: ___ yes, ___ no.
Linens wet or soiled: _____ yes, _____ no. Linens changed: _____ yes, ____ no.
Dressing changed: _____ yes, _____ no. Location: ____________________
IV site checked: _____ yes, _____ no. IV tubing labeled: ____ yes, ____ no.
IV fluids at: ____.
Pain level (0-10 scale.0-no pain, 10 intolerable): ____________________.
Location of pain: ____________. Medicated for pain: ____ yes, ____ no.
Patient is alert/oriented: ___ yes, ___ no. New confusion: ___ yes, ___ no.
Vital signs: temp ____, pulse ____, resp _____, b/p _____, 02 ____ %, ___ liters.
Glucose level: _____. Insulin: ___ yes, ___ no. Type: __________ # of units ___.

Nurse ____________, CNA ____________, in at _____ am/pm. Left at _______ am/pm.
Wash hands and wear gloves before touching patient: _____yes, ____ no.
Wash hands before leaving room: ___ yes, ___ no. Wear protective gear: __ yes, __ no.
Clean stethoscope: __ yes, __ no. Oral care: __ yes, __ no. Suctioned: __ yes, __ no.
Repositioned: ___ yes, ___ no. Turned to: ___ left, ___ right, ___ backside ___.
Head of bed at: ______ degrees. Incontinence/skin breakdown: ___ yes, ___ no.
Linens wet or soiled: _____ yes, _____ no. Linens changed: _____ yes, ____ no.
Dressing changed: _____ yes, _____ no. Location: ____________________
IV site checked: _____ yes, _____ no. IV tubing labeled: ____ yes, ____ no.
IV fluids at: ____.
Pain level (0-10 scale.0-no pain, 10 intolerable): ____________________.
Location of pain: ____________. Medicated for pain: ____ yes, ____ no.
Patient is alert/oriented: ___ yes, ___ no. New confusion: ___ yes, ___ no.
Vital signs: temp ____, pulse ____, resp _____, b/p _____, 02 ____ %, ___ liters.
Glucose level: _____. Insulin: ___ yes, ___ no. Type: __________ # of units ___.

NURSING CARE CONTINUED FOR ____________________
DATE ____________________, DAY NUMBER ____________________

FOLLOWING EXAMINATIONS FOR NIGHT SHIFT:

Nurse ____________, CNA ____________, in at _____ am/pm. Left at ______ am/pm.
Wash hands and wear gloves before touching patient: ______ yes, ______ no.
Wash hands before leaving room: ___ yes, ___ no. Wear protective gear: __ yes, __ no.
Clean stethoscope: __ yes, __ no. Oral care: __ yes, __ no. Suctioned: __ yes, __ no.
Repositioned: ___ yes, ___ no. Turned to: ___ left, ___ right, ___ backside ___.
Head of bed at: _______ degrees. Incontinence/skin breakdown: ____ yes, ____ no.
Linens wet or soiled: _____ yes, _____ no. Linens changed: _____ yes, ______ no.
Dressing changed: ____ yes, ____ no. Location: ____________________.
IV site checked: _____ yes, _____ no. IV tubing labeled: _____ yes, _____no.
IV fluids at: ____.
Pain level (0-10 scale.0-no pain, 10 intolerable): ____________________.
Location of pain: ________________. Medicated for pain: _____ yes, ____ no.
Patient is alert/oriented: ____ yes, ____ no. New confusion: ____ yes, ____ no.
Vital signs: temp ____, pulse _____, resp ______, b/p ______, 02 _____ %, ____ liters.
Glucose level: _____. Insulin: ___ yes, ___ no. Type: ______________ # of units ____.

Nurse ____________, CNA ____________, in at _____ am/pm. Left at ______ am/pm.
Wash hands and wear gloves before touching patient: ______ yes, ______ no.
Wash hands before leaving room: ___ yes, ___ no. Wear protective gear: __ yes, __ no.
Clean stethoscope: __ yes, __ no. Oral care: __ yes, __ no. Suctioned: __ yes, __ no.
Repositioned: ___ yes, ___ no. Turned to: ___ left, ___ right, ___ backside ___.
Head of bed at: _______ degrees. Incontinence/skin breakdown: ____ yes, ____ no.
Linens wet or soiled: _____ yes, _____ no. Linens changed: _____ yes, ______ no.
Dressing changed: ____ yes, ____ no. Location: ____________________.
IV site checked: _____ yes, _____ no. IV tubing labeled: _____ yes, _____no.
IV fluids at: ____.
Pain level (0-10 scale.0-no pain, 10 intolerable): ____________________.
Location of pain: ________________. Medicated for pain: _____ yes, ____ no.
Patient is alert/oriented: ____ yes, ____ no. New confusion: ____ yes, ____ no.
Vital signs: temp ____, pulse _____, resp ______, b/p ______, 02 _____ %, ____ liters.
Glucose level: _____. Insulin: ___ yes, ___ no. Type: ______________ # of units ____.

Nurse ____________, CNA ____________, in at _____ am/pm. Left at ______ am/pm.
Wash hands and wear gloves before touching patient: ______ yes, ______ no.
Wash hands before leaving room: ___ yes, ___ no. Wear protective gear: __ yes, __ no.
Clean stethoscope: __ yes, __ no. Oral care: __ yes, __ no. Suctioned: __ yes, __ no.
Repositioned: ___ yes, ___ no. Turned to: ___ left, ___ right, ___ backside ___.
Head of bed at: _______ degrees. Incontinence/skin breakdown: ____ yes, ____ no.
Linens wet or soiled: _____ yes, _____ no. Linens changed: _____ yes, ______ no.
Dressing changed: ____ yes, ____ no. Location: ____________________.
IV site checked: _____ yes, _____ no. IV tubing labeled: _____ yes, _____no.
IV fluids at: ____.
Pain level (0-10 scale.0-no pain, 10 intolerable): ____________________.
Location of pain: ________________. Medicated for pain: _____ yes, ____ no.
Patient is alert/oriented: ____ yes, ____ no. New confusion: ____ yes, ____ no.
Vital signs: temp ____, pulse _____, resp ______, b/p ______, 02 _____ %, ____ liters.
Glucose level: _____. Insulin: ___ yes, ___ no. Type: ______________ # of units ____.

MEDICATION ADMINISTRATION LIST FOR ______________________
DATE ________________ DAY NUMBER ______________________

List the medication for each day. Routes of administration: oral, thru feeding tube, intravenous (IV), intramuscular (IM), subcutaneous (SQ), epidural or a catheter in your spinal column, rectal, topical, eye drops, and ear drops.

Medication: ________________ Route: ______________ Time: ____________
Medication: ________________ Route: ______________ Time: ____________
Medication: ________________ Route: ______________ Time: ____________
Medication: ________________ Route: ______________ Time: ____________
Medication: ________________ Route: ______________ Time: ____________
Medication: ________________ Route: ______________ Time: ____________
Medication: ________________ Route: ______________ Time: ____________
Medication: ________________ Route: ______________ Time: ____________
Medication: ________________ Route: ______________ Time: ____________
Medication: ________________ Route: ______________ Time: ____________
Medication: ________________ Route: ______________ Time: ____________
Medication: ________________ Route: ______________ Time: ____________
Medication: ________________ Route: ______________ Time: ____________
Medication: ________________ Route: ______________ Time: ____________
Medication: ________________ Route: ______________ Time: ____________
Medication: ________________ Route: ______________ Time: ____________
Medication: ________________ Route: ______________ Time: ____________
Medication: ________________ Route: ______________ Time: ____________
Medication: ________________ Route: ______________ Time: ____________
Medication: ________________ Route: ______________ Time: ____________
Medication: ________________ Route: ______________ Time: ____________
Medication: ________________ Route: ______________ Time: ____________
Medication: ________________ Route: ______________ Time: ____________
Medication: ________________ Route: ______________ Time: ____________
Medication: ________________ Route: ______________ Time: ____________
Medication: ________________ Route: ______________ Time: ____________
Medication: ________________ Route: ______________ Time: ____________
Medication: ________________ Route: ______________ Time: ____________
Medication: ________________ Route: ______________ Time: ____________
Medication: ________________ Route: ______________ Time: ____________
Medication: ________________ Route: ______________ Time: ____________
Medication: ________________ Route: ______________ Time: ____________
Medication: ________________ Route: ______________ Time: ____________
Medication: ________________ Route: ______________ Time: ____________
Medication: ________________ Route: ______________ Time: ____________
Medication: ________________ Route: ______________ Time: ____________
Medication: ________________ Route: ______________ Time: ____________
Medication: ________________ Route: ______________ Time: ____________
Medication: ________________ Route: ______________ Time: ____________
Medication: ________________ Route: ______________ Time: ____________
Medication: ________________ Route: ______________ Time: ____________
Medication: ________________ Route: ______________ Time: ____________
Medication: ________________ Route: ______________ Time: ____________
Medication: ________________ Route: ______________ Time: ____________
Medication: ________________ Route: ______________ Time: ____________
Medication: ________________ Route: ______________ Time: ____________
Medication: ________________ Route: ______________ Time: ____________
Medication: ________________ Route: ______________ Time: ____________
Medication: ________________ Route: ______________ Time: ____________
Medication: ________________ Route: ______________ Time: ____________
Medication: ________________ Route: ______________ Time: ____________
Medication: ________________ Route: ______________ Time: ____________
Medication: ________________ Route: ______________ Time: ____________
Medication: ________________ Route: ______________ Time: ____________

NOTES FOR DAY NUMBER ______

DATE ______

MEDICAL JOURNAL FOR ______________________________

DATE ____________________, DAY NUMBER ____________

VISITS FROM MY DOCTORS TODAY

Goals for today: ____
____
____.

Things to discuss with my doctor(s): ________________________________
____
____.

Dr.____________ came in at _____ am/pm. Left at _____ am/pm.
We discussed ____.
Did doctor examine patient: _____ yes, _____ no.
Wash hands before touching patient: _____ yes, _____ no.
Wear gloves: ____ yes, ___ no. Clean stethoscope: ____ yes, ____ no.
Wear gown and mask (precautions only):____ yes, _____ no.
Wash hands before leaving the room: _____ yes, _____ no.

Dr.____________ came in at _____ am/pm. Left at _____ am/pm.
We discussed ____.
Did doctor examine patient: _____ yes, _____ no.
Wash hands before touching patient: _____ yes, _____ no.
Wear gloves: ____ yes, ___ no. Clean stethoscope: ____ yes, ____ no.
Wear gown and mask (precautions only):____ yes, _____ no.
Wash hands before leaving the room: _____ yes, _____ no.

Dr.____________ came in at _____ am/pm. Left at _____ am/pm.
We discussed ____.
Did doctor examine patient: _____ yes, _____ no.
Wash hands before touching patient: _____ yes, _____ no.
Wear gloves: ____ yes, ___ no. Clean stethoscope: ____ yes, ____ no.
Wear gown and mask (precautions only):____ yes, _____ no.
Wash hands before leaving the room: _____ yes, _____ no.

Dr.____________ came in at _____ am/pm. Left at _____ am/pm.
We discussed ____.
Did doctor examine patient: _____ yes, _____ no.
Wash hands before touching patient: _____ yes, _____ no.
Wear gloves: ____ yes, ___ no. Clean stethoscope: ____ yes, ____ no.
Wear gown and mask (precautions only):____ yes, _____ no.
Wash hands before leaving the room: _____ yes, _____ no.

Dr.____________ came in at _____ am/pm. Left at _____ am/pm.
We discussed ____.
Did doctor examine patient: _____ yes, _____ no.
Wash hands before touching patient: _____ yes, _____ no.
Wear gloves: ____ yes, ___ no. Clean stethoscope: ____ yes, ____ no.
Wear gown and mask (precautions only):____ yes, _____ no.
Wash hands before leaving the room: _____ yes, _____ no.

NURSING CARE FOR ______________________________

DATE ______________, DAY NUMBER ______________

INITIAL DAY SHIFT EXAM:

My nurse has ______ # of patients. CNA ___yes, ___no. Charge nurse ____________
Nurse ______________ RN/LPN came in at _________ am/pm. Left at __________ am/pm.
Did nurse wash hands and wear gloves before touching patient: ______ yes, ______ no.
Wash hands after touching patient and before leaving the room: ______ yes, ______ no.
Don't hesitate to request staff to wash their hands. This will help decrease the risk of spreading potentially lethal germs.
Did nurse wear protective gear (isolation precautions only): _______ yes, _______ no.
Did nurse provide oral care (to be done every two hours if unable to provide for self, also decreases risk of pneumonia, infections, and aspiration): _______ yes, ______ no.
If able to provide own oral care, then supplies at bedside: _______ yes, _______ no.
Was patient repositioned (every two hours if unable to turn self): ____ yes ____ no.
Head of bed at ________ degrees. This is important for patients on ventilators or on tube feedings. Anything less than thirty degrees places patients at risk for aspiration of stomach contents into the lungs causing aspiration pneumonia.
Checked for incontinence and skin breakdown: _____ yes, _____ no.
Patient's linens wet or soiled: _____ yes, ____ no. Linens changed: ____ yes, ____ no.
Time linens changed: _______ am/pm. Any skin redness or breakdown: ____ yes, ____ no.
If yes, what stage is pressure ulcer: _______. Acquired when: ______________.
List wounds not associated with pressure ulcers and how acquired: ____________
____.
Mattress type: ____.
Specialty mattresses are important to help prevent pressure ulcers)
If patient on ventilator or has tracheostomy, suction performed: _____ yes, ______ no.
Did nurse listen to lung sounds: _____ yes, _____ no.
Does patient have chest tubes: ____ yes, ____ no. Functioning _____ yes, ______ no.
Bowel sounds: _______ yes, _______ no. Bowel sounds active: ______ yes, ______ no.
Neurological exam: _____ yes, ______ no. Follow commands: ______ yes, ______ no.
Is patient alert and oriented to person, place, time, and events: ____ yes, ____ no.
If confused, patient is not oriented to: ____ person, ___ place, ___ time, ___ event.
Confusion began (time and date): ______________________________.
Glasgow coma scale (checks conscious scale of patient): ______________.
Intracranial pressure monitoring: _____ yes, _____ no.
If yes, pressure is at ________ mm mercury. (Normal is one to fifteen).
Moves extremities: ___ yes, ___ no.
Paralysis: (inability to move extremities) ______ yes, _______ no.
If yes, extremities affected and when paralysis began: ______________.
Is patient in pain: ____ yes, ____ no. Describe pain and location ____________.
Patient able to eat: ____ yes, ____ no. What type of diet? ____________.
If patient on tube feedings list type: ______________ at ____________ cc/ml per hour.
Nausea ____, vomiting ____. If so, describe: ______________________.
Patient has: Nasal gastric tube _____, Dobhoff tube _____, Peg or gastric tube _____.
When was feeding tube placed and what site: ______________________.
Catheter for draining urine: ____ yes, ____ no. If so, when placed: __________
Find out policy for allowed time to remain in bladder. Too long may cause infections.)
IV site(s) where: __________________________ when placed: __________.
IV fluids (types and rates): ______________, ______________, ______________,
______________, ______________, ______________,
Is patient on oxygen: _____ yes, _____ no. If so, how much and route delivered (see oxygen routes): ______________________________________.
If patient on ventilator, list settings (see list on ventilator settings): ________
____.
Vital signs: temp _____, pulse _____, resp _____, b/p _____, o2 _____%,
current weight _____ pounds, _____ kg. Glucose level: ________
Insulin coverage: ____ yes, ____ no. Insulin type: ____________, # of units: _____.

NURSING CARE CONTINUED FOR ____________________
DATE ____________________, DAY NUMBER ____________________

FOLLOWING EXAMINATIONS FOR DAY SHIFT:

Nurse ____________, CNA ____________, in at _____ am/pm. Left at ______ am/pm.
Wash hands and wear gloves before touching patient: ______ yes, ______ no.
Wash hands before leaving room: ___ yes, ___ no. Wear protective gear: __ yes, __ no.
Clean stethoscope: __ yes, __ no. Oral care: __ yes, __ no. Suctioned: __ yes, __ no.
Repositioned: ___ yes, ___ no. Turned to: ___ left, ___ right, ___ backside ___.
Head of bed at: ______ degrees. Incontinence/skin breakdown: ____ yes, ____ no.
Linens wet or soiled: _____ yes, _____ no. Linens changed: _____ yes, _____ no.
Dressing changed: ____ yes, ____ no. Location: ____________________.
IV site checked: _____ yes, _____ no. IV tubing labeled: _____ yes, _____ no.
IV fluids at: ____.
Pain level (0-10 scale.0-no pain, 10 intolerable): ____________________.
Location of pain: ____________. Medicated for pain: ____ yes, ____ no.
Patient is alert/oriented: ___ yes, ___ no. New confusion: ___ yes, ___ no.
Vital signs: temp ____, pulse ____, resp ______, b/p ______, 02 ____ %, ____ liters.
Glucose level: _____. Insulin: ___ yes, ___ no. Type: ____________ # of units ____.

Nurse ____________, CNA ____________, in at _____ am/pm. Left at ______ am/pm.
Wash hands and wear gloves before touching patient: ______ yes, ______ no.
Wash hands before leaving room: ___ yes, ___ no. Wear protective gear: __ yes, __ no.
Clean stethoscope: __ yes, __ no. Oral care: __ yes, __ no. Suctioned: __ yes, __ no.
Repositioned: ___ yes, ___ no. Turned to: ___ left, ___ right, ___ backside ___.
Head of bed at: ______ degrees. Incontinence/skin breakdown: ____ yes, ____ no.
Linens wet or soiled: _____ yes, _____ no. Linens changed: _____ yes, _____ no.
Dressing changed: ____ yes, ____ no. Location: ____________________.
IV site checked: _____ yes, _____ no. IV tubing labeled: _____ yes, _____ no.
IV fluids at: ____.
Pain level (0-10 scale.0-no pain, 10 intolerable): ____________________.
Location of pain: ____________. Medicated for pain: ____ yes, ____ no.
Patient is alert/oriented: ___ yes, ___ no. New confusion: ___ yes, ___ no.
Vital signs: temp ____, pulse ____, resp ______, b/p ______, 02 ____ %, ____ liters.
Glucose level: _____. Insulin: ___ yes, ___ no. Type: ____________ # of units ____.

Nurse ____________, CNA ____________, in at _____ am/pm. Left at ______ am/pm.
Wash hands and wear gloves before touching patient: ______ yes, ______ no.
Wash hands before leaving room: ___ yes, ___ no. Wear protective gear: __ yes, __ no.
Clean stethoscope: __ yes, __ no. Oral care: __ yes, __ no. Suctioned: __ yes, __ no.
Repositioned: ___ yes, ___ no. Turned to: ___ left, ___ right, ___ backside ___.
Head of bed at: ______ degrees. Incontinence/skin breakdown: ____ yes, ____ no.
Linens wet or soiled: _____ yes, _____ no. Linens changed: _____ yes, _____ no.
Dressing changed: ____ yes, ____ no. Location: ____________________.
IV site checked: _____ yes, _____ no. IV tubing labeled: _____ yes, _____ no.
IV fluids at: ____.
Pain level (0-10 scale.0-no pain, 10 intolerable): ____________________.
Location of pain: ____________. Medicated for pain: ____ yes, ____ no.
Patient is alert/oriented: ___ yes, ___ no. New confusion: ___ yes, ___ no.
Vital signs: temp ____, pulse ____, resp ______, b/p ______, 02 ____ %, ____ liters.
Glucose level: _____. Insulin: ___ yes, ___ no. Type: ____________ # of units ____.

NURSING CARE CONTINUED FOR ____________________
DATE ________________, DAY NUMBER ________________

FOLLOWING EXAMINATIONS FOR DAY SHIFT:

Nurse ____________, CNA ____________, in at _____ am/pm. Left at ______ am/pm.
Wash hands and wear gloves before touching patient: ______ yes, ______ no.
Wash hands before leaving room: __ yes, ___ no. Wear protective gear: __ yes, __ no.
Clean stethoscope: __ yes, __ no. Oral care: __ yes, __ no. Suctioned: __ yes, __ no.
Repositioned: ___ yes, ___ no. Turned to: ___ left, ___ right, ___ backside ___.
Head of bed at: _______ degrees. Incontinence/skin breakdown: ____ yes, ____ no.
Linens wet or soiled: _____ yes, _____ no. Linens changed: _____ yes, ______ no.
Dressing changed: ____ yes, ____ no. Location: ______________________________.
IV site checked: _____ yes, _____ no. IV tubing labeled: _____ yes, _____no.
IV fluids at: ____.
Pain level (0-10 scale.0-no pain, 10 intolerable): ___________________________.
Location of pain: ____________. Medicated for pain: _____ yes, _____ no.
Patient is alert/oriented: ____ yes, ____ no. New confusion: ____ yes, ____ no.
Vital signs: temp ____, pulse _____, resp _____, b/p ______, 02 _____ %, ____ liters.
Glucose level: _____. Insulin: ___ yes, ___ no. Type: ______________ # of units ____.

Nurse ____________, CNA ____________, in at _____ am/pm. Left at ______ am/pm.
Wash hands and wear gloves before touching patient: ______ yes, ______ no.
Wash hands before leaving room: __ yes, ___ no. Wear protective gear: __ yes, __ no.
Clean stethoscope: __ yes, __ no. Oral care: __ yes, __ no. Suctioned: __ yes, __ no.
Repositioned: ___ yes, ___ no. Turned to: ___ left, ___ right, ___ backside ___.
Head of bed at: _______ degrees. Incontinence/skin breakdown: ____ yes, ____ no.
Linens wet or soiled: _____ yes, _____ no. Linens changed: _____ yes, ______ no.
Dressing changed: ____ yes, ____ no. Location: ______________________________.
IV site checked: _____ yes, _____ no. IV tubing labeled: _____ yes, _____no.
IV fluids at: ____.
Pain level (0-10 scale.0-no pain, 10 intolerable): ___________________________.
Location of pain: ____________. Medicated for pain: _____ yes, _____ no.
Patient is alert/oriented: ____ yes, ____ no. New confusion: ____ yes, ____ no.
Vital signs: temp ____, pulse _____, resp _____, b/p ______, 02 _____ %, ____ liters.
Glucose level: _____. Insulin: ___ yes, ___ no. Type: ______________ # of units ____.

Nurse ____________, CNA ____________, in at _____ am/pm. Left at ______ am/pm.
Wash hands and wear gloves before touching patient: ______ yes, ______ no.
Wash hands before leaving room: __ yes, ___ no. Wear protective gear: __ yes, __ no.
Clean stethoscope: __ yes, __ no. Oral care: __ yes, __ no. Suctioned: __ yes, __ no.
Repositioned: ___ yes, ___ no. Turned to: ___ left, ___ right, ___ backside ___.
Head of bed at: _______ degrees. Incontinence/skin breakdown: ____ yes, ____ no.
Linens wet or soiled: _____ yes, _____ no. Linens changed: _____ yes, ______ no.
Dressing changed: ____ yes, ____ no. Location: ______________________________.
IV site checked: _____ yes, _____ no. IV tubing labeled: _____ yes, _____no.
IV fluids at: ____.
Pain level (0-10 scale.0-no pain, 10 intolerable): ___________________________.
Location of pain: ____________. Medicated for pain: _____ yes, _____ no.
Patient is alert/oriented: ____ yes, ____ no. New confusion: ____ yes, ____ no.
Vital signs: temp ____, pulse _____, resp _____, b/p ______, 02 _____ %, ____ liters.
Glucose level: _____. Insulin: ___ yes, ___ no. Type: ______________ # of units ____.

NURSING CARE FOR ____________________________

DATE ____________________, DAY NUMBER ______________

INITIAL NIGHT SHIFT EXAM:

My nurse has ______ # of patients. CNA ___yes, ___no. Charge nurse ______________
Nurse ____________ RN/LPN came in at __________ am/pm. Left at ___________ am/pm.
Did nurse wash hands and wear gloves before touching patient: ______ yes, ______ no.
Wash hands after touching patient and before leaving the room: ______ yes, ______ no.
Don't hesitate to request staff to wash their hands. This will help decrease the risk of spreading potentially lethal germs.
Did nurse wear protective gear (isolation precautions only): ______ yes, ______ no.
Did nurse provide oral care (to be done every two hours if unable to provide for self, also decreases risk of pneumonia, infections, and aspiration): ______ yes, ______ no.
If able to provide own oral care, then supplies at bedside: ______ yes, ______ no.
Was patient repositioned (every two hours if unable to turn self): ______ yes ______ no.
Head of bed at _________ degrees. This is important for patients on ventilators or on tube feedings. Anything less than thirty degrees places patients at risk for aspiration of stomach contents into the lungs causing aspiration pneumonia.
Checked for incontinence and skin breakdown: _____ yes, _____ no.
Patient's linens wet or soiled: _____ yes, _____ no. Linens changed: ____ yes, ____ no.
Time linens changed: _________ am/pm. Any skin redness or breakdown: ____ yes, ____ no.
If yes, what stage is pressure ulcer: ______. Acquired when: _________________.
List wounds not associated with pressure ulcers and how acquired: _______________
____
Mattress type: ____
Specialty mattresses are important to help prevent pressure ulcers)
If patient on ventilator or has tracheostomy, suction performed: _____ yes, _____ no.
Did nurse listen to lung sounds: _____ yes, _____ no.
Does patient have chest tubes: ____ yes, ____ no. Functioning _____ yes, _____ no.
Bowel sounds: ______ yes, ______ no. Bowel sounds active: ______ yes, ______ no.
Neurological exam: _____ yes, _____ no. Follow commands: ______ yes, ______ no.
Is patient alert and oriented to person, place, time, and events: _____ yes, _____ no.
If confused, patient is not oriented to: ___ person, ___ place, ___ time, ___ event.
Confusion began (time and date): ____
Glasgow coma scale (checks conscious scale of patient): _________________________
Intracranial pressure monitoring: _____ yes, _____ no.
If yes, pressure is at ________ mm mercury. (Normal is one to fifteen).
Moves extremities: ___ yes, ___ no.
Paralysis: (inability to move extremities) ________ yes, ________ no.
If yes, extremities affected and when paralysis began: __________________________
Is patient in pain: ____ yes, ____ no. Describe pain and location _______________.
Patient able to eat: ____ yes, ____ no. What type of diet? _____________________.
If patient on tube feedings list type: ____________ at __________ cc/ml per hour.
Nausea ____, vomiting _____. If so, describe: ______________________________.
Patient has: Nasal gastric tube ____, Dobhoff tube ____, Peg or gastric tube ____.
When was feeding tube placed and what site: ________________________________.
Catheter for draining urine: ____ yes, ____ no. If so, when placed: ____________.
Find out policy for allowed time to remain in bladder. Too long may cause infections.)
IV site(s) where: ___________________ when placed: ____________________________.
IV fluids (types and rates): _____________, _____________, _____________________,
_____________, _____________, _____________, _____________, _____________________.
Is patient on oxygen: _____ yes, _____ no. If so, how much and route delivered (see oxygen routes): ____.
If patient on ventilator, list settings (see list on ventilator settings): __________
____.
Vital signs: temp ______, pulse ______, resp ______, b/p ______, o2 ______%,
current weight ______ pounds, ______ kg. Glucose level: ______
Insulin coverage: ____ yes, ____ no. Insulin type: ____________, # of units: ______.

NURSING CARE CONTINUED FOR ______________________________
DATE ____________________, DAY NUMBER ____________________

FOLLOWING EXAMINATIONS FOR NIGHT SHIFT:

Nurse ____________, CNA ____________, in at _____ am/pm. Left at ______ am/pm.
Wash hands and wear gloves before touching patient: ______ yes, ______ no.
Wash hands before leaving room: ___ yes, ___ no. Wear protective gear: __ yes, __ no.
Clean stethoscope: __ yes, __ no. Oral care: __ yes, __ no. Suctioned: __ yes, __ no.
Repositioned: ___ yes, ___ no. Turned to: ___ left, ___ right, ___ backside ___.
Head of bed at: ______ degrees. Incontinence/skin breakdown: ____ yes, ____ no.
Linens wet or soiled: ____ yes, ____ no. Linens changed: ____ yes, _____ no.
Dressing changed: ____ yes, ____ no. Location: ____________________.
IV site checked: _____ yes, _____ no. IV tubing labeled: _____ yes, _____no.
IV fluids at: ____.
Pain level (0-10 scale.0-no pain, 10 intolerable): ____________________.
Location of pain: ______________. Medicated for pain: _____ yes, ____ no.
Patient is alert/oriented: ___ yes, ____ no. New confusion: ____ yes, ____ no.
Vital signs: temp ____, pulse _____, resp _____, b/p ______, 02 _____ %, ____ liters.
Glucose level: _____. Insulin: ___ yes, ___ no. Type: ____________ # of units ____.

Nurse ____________, CNA ____________, in at _____ am/pm. Left at ______ am/pm.
Wash hands and wear gloves before touching patient: ______ yes, ______ no.
Wash hands before leaving room: ___ yes, ___ no. Wear protective gear: __ yes, __ no.
Clean stethoscope: __ yes, __ no. Oral care: __ yes, __ no. Suctioned: __ yes, __ no.
Repositioned: ___ yes, ___ no. Turned to: ___ left, ___ right, ___ backside ___.
Head of bed at: ______ degrees. Incontinence/skin breakdown: ____ yes, ____ no.
Linens wet or soiled: ____ yes, ____ no. Linens changed: ____ yes, _____ no.
Dressing changed: ____ yes, ____ no. Location: ____________________.
IV site checked: _____ yes, _____ no. IV tubing labeled: _____ yes, _____no.
IV fluids at: ____.
Pain level (0-10 scale.0-no pain, 10 intolerable): ____________________.
Location of pain: ______________. Medicated for pain: _____ yes, ____ no.
Patient is alert/oriented: ____ yes, ____ no. New confusion: ____ yes, ____ no.
Vital signs: temp ____, pulse _____, resp _____, b/p ______, 02 _____ %, ____ liters.
Glucose level: _____. Insulin: ___ yes, ___ no. Type: ____________ # of units ____.

Nurse ____________, CNA ____________, in at _____ am/pm. Left at ______ am/pm.
Wash hands and wear gloves before touching patient: ______ yes, ______ no.
Wash hands before leaving room: ___ yes, ___ no. Wear protective gear: __ yes, __ no.
Clean stethoscope: __ yes, __ no. Oral care: __ yes, __ no. Suctioned: __ yes, __ no.
Repositioned: ___ yes, ___ no. Turned to: ___ left, ___ right, ___ backside ___.
Head of bed at: ______ degrees. Incontinence/skin breakdown: ____ yes, ____ no.
Linens wet or soiled: ____ yes, ____ no. Linens changed: ____ yes, _____ no.
Dressing changed: ____ yes, ____ no. Location: ____________________.
IV site checked: _____ yes, _____ no. IV tubing labeled: _____ yes, _____no.
IV fluids at: ____.
Pain level (0-10 scale.0-no pain, 10 intolerable): ____________________.
Location of pain: ______________. Medicated for pain: _____ yes, ____ no.
Patient is alert/oriented: ____ yes, ____ no. New confusion: ____ yes, ____ no.
Vital signs: temp ____, pulse _____, resp _____, b/p ______, 02 _____ %, ____ liters.
Glucose level: _____. Insulin: ___ yes, ___ no. Type: ____________ # of units ____.

NURSING CARE CONTINUED FOR ____________________
DATE ____________________, DAY NUMBER ____________________

FOLLOWING EXAMINATIONS FOR NIGHT SHIFT:

Nurse ______________, CNA ______________, in at _____ am/pm. Left at ______ am/pm.
Wash hands and wear gloves before touching patient: ________ yes, ________ no.
Wash hands before leaving room: ___ yes, ___ no. Wear protective gear: __ yes, __ no.
Clean stethoscope: __ yes, __ no. Oral care: __ yes, __ no. Suctioned: __ yes, __ no.
Repositioned: ___ yes, ___ no. Turned to: ___ left, ___ right, ___ backside ___.
Head of bed at: _______ degrees. Incontinence/skin breakdown: ____ yes, ____ no.
Linens wet or soiled: _____ yes, _____ no. Linens changed: _____ yes, _____ no.
Dressing changed: ____ yes, ____ no. Location: ____________________.
IV site checked: _____ yes, _____ no. IV tubing labeled: _____ yes, _____no.
IV fluids at: ____.
Pain level (0-10 scale.0-no pain, 10 intolerable): ____________________.
Location of pain: ______________. Medicated for pain: ____ yes, ____ no.
Patient is alert/oriented: ____ yes, ____ no. New confusion: ____ yes, ____ no.
Vital signs: temp ____, pulse ____, resp ____, b/p ______, 02 ____ %, ____ liters.
Glucose level: _____. Insulin: ___ yes, ___ no. Type: ____________ # of units ___.

Nurse ______________, CNA ______________, in at _____ am/pm. Left at ______ am/pm.
Wash hands and wear gloves before touching patient: ________ yes, ________ no.
Wash hands before leaving room: ___ yes, ___ no. Wear protective gear: __ yes, __ no.
Clean stethoscope: __ yes, __ no. Oral care: __ yes, __ no. Suctioned: __ yes, __ no.
Repositioned: ___ yes, ___ no. Turned to: ___ left, ___ right, ___ backside ___.
Head of bed at: _______ degrees. Incontinence/skin breakdown: ____ yes, ____ no.
Linens wet or soiled: _____ yes, _____ no. Linens changed: _____ yes, _____ no.
Dressing changed: ____ yes, ____ no. Location: ____________________.
IV site checked: _____ yes, _____ no. IV tubing labeled: _____ yes, _____no.
IV fluids at: ____.
Pain level (0-10 scale.0-no pain, 10 intolerable): ____________________.
Location of pain: ______________. Medicated for pain: ____ yes, ____ no.
Patient is alert/oriented: ____ yes, ____ no. New confusion: ____ yes, ____ no.
Vital signs: temp ____, pulse ____, resp ____, b/p ______, 02 ____ %, ____ liters.
Glucose level: _____. Insulin: ___ yes, ___ no. Type: ____________ # of units ___.

Nurse ______________, CNA ______________, in at _____ am/pm. Left at ______ am/pm.
Wash hands and wear gloves before touching patient: ________ yes, ________ no.
Wash hands before leaving room: ___ yes, ___ no. Wear protective gear: __ yes, __ no.
Clean stethoscope: __ yes, __ no. Oral care: __ yes, __ no. Suctioned: __ yes, __ no.
Repositioned: ___ yes, ___ no. Turned to: ___ left, ___ right, ___ backside ___.
Head of bed at: _______ degrees. Incontinence/skin breakdown: ____ yes, ____ no.
Linens wet or soiled: _____ yes, _____ no. Linens changed: _____ yes, _____ no.
Dressing changed: ____ yes, ____ no. Location: ____________________.
IV site checked: _____ yes, _____ no. IV tubing labeled: _____ yes, _____no.
IV fluids at: ____.
Pain level (0-10 scale.0-no pain, 10 intolerable): ____________________.
Location of pain: ______________. Medicated for pain: ____ yes, ____ no.
Patient is alert/oriented: ____ yes, ____ no. New confusion: ____ yes, ____ no.
Vital signs: temp ____, pulse ____, resp ____, b/p ______, 02 ____ %, ____ liters.
Glucose level: _____. Insulin: ___ yes, ___ no. Type: ____________ # of units ___

MEDICATION ADMINISTRATION LIST FOR ____________________
DATE ____________________ DAY NUMBER ____________________

List the medication for each day. Routes of administration: oral, thru feeding tube, intravenous (IV), intramuscular (IM), subcutaneous (SQ), epidural or a catheter in your spinal column, rectal, topical, eye drops, and ear drops.

Medication: ____________ Route: ____________ Time: ____________
Medication: ____________ Route: ____________ Time: ____________
Medication: ____________ Route: ____________ Time: ____________
Medication: ____________ Route: ____________ Time: ____________
Medication: ____________ Route: ____________ Time: ____________
Medication: ____________ Route: ____________ Time: ____________
Medication: ____________ Route: ____________ Time: ____________
Medication: ____________ Route: ____________ Time: ____________
Medication: ____________ Route: ____________ Time: ____________
Medication: ____________ Route: ____________ Time: ____________
Medication: ____________ Route: ____________ Time: ____________
Medication: ____________ Route: ____________ Time: ____________
Medication: ____________ Route: ____________ Time: ____________
Medication: ____________ Route: ____________ Time: ____________
Medication: ____________ Route: ____________ Time: ____________
Medication: ____________ Route: ____________ Time: ____________
Medication: ____________ Route: ____________ Time: ____________
Medication: ____________ Route: ____________ Time: ____________
Medication: ____________ Route: ____________ Time: ____________
Medication: ____________ Route: ____________ Time: ____________
Medication: ____________ Route: ____________ Time: ____________
Medication: ____________ Route: ____________ Time: ____________
Medication: ____________ Route: ____________ Time: ____________
Medication: ____________ Route: ____________ Time: ____________
Medication: ____________ Route: ____________ Time: ____________
Medication: ____________ Route: ____________ Time: ____________
Medication: ____________ Route: ____________ Time: ____________
Medication: ____________ Route: ____________ Time: ____________
Medication: ____________ Route: ____________ Time: ____________
Medication: ____________ Route: ____________ Time: ____________
Medication: ____________ Route: ____________ Time: ____________
Medication: ____________ Route: ____________ Time: ____________
Medication: ____________ Route: ____________ Time: ____________
Medication: ____________ Route: ____________ Time: ____________
Medication: ____________ Route: ____________ Time: ____________
Medication: ____________ Route: ____________ Time: ____________
Medication: ____________ Route: ____________ Time: ____________
Medication: ____________ Route: ____________ Time: ____________
Medication: ____________ Route: ____________ Time: ____________
Medication: ____________ Route: ____________ Time: ____________
Medication: ____________ Route: ____________ Time: ____________
Medication: ____________ Route: ____________ Time: ____________
Medication: ____________ Route: ____________ Time: ____________
Medication: ____________ Route: ____________ Time: ____________
Medication: ____________ Route: ____________ Time: ____________
Medication: ____________ Route: ____________ Time: ____________
Medication: ____________ Route: ____________ Time: ____________
Medication: ____________ Route: ____________ Time: ____________
Medication: ____________ Route: ____________ Time: ____________
Medication: ____________ Route: ____________ Time: ____________
Medication: ____________ Route: ____________ Time: ____________
Medication: ____________ Route: ____________ Time: ____________
Medication: ____________ Route: ____________ Time: ____________
Medication: ____________ Route: ____________ Time: ____________

NOTES FOR DAY NUMBER ______

DATE ______

MEDICAL JOURNAL FOR ______________________________

DATE ____________________, DAY NUMBER ______________

VISITS FROM MY DOCTORS TODAY

Goals for today: ____

____

____.

Things to discuss with my doctor(s): ________________________________

____

____

Dr.______________ came in at _____ am/pm. Left at _____ am/pm.
We discussed ____.
Did doctor examine patient: _____ yes, _____ no.
Wash hands before touching patient: _____ yes, _____ no.
Wear gloves: ____ yes, ___ no. Clean stethoscope: ____ yes, ____ no.
Wear gown and mask (precautions only):____ yes, _____ no.
Wash hands before leaving the room: _____ yes, _____ no.

Dr.______________ came in at _____ am/pm. Left at _____ am/pm.
We discussed ____.
Did doctor examine patient: _____ yes, _____ no.
Wash hands before touching patient: _____ yes, _____ no.
Wear gloves: ____ yes, ___ no. Clean stethoscope: ____ yes, ____ no.
Wear gown and mask (precautions only):____ yes, _____ no.
Wash hands before leaving the room: _____ yes, _____ no.

Dr.______________ came in at _____ am/pm. Left at _____ am/pm.
We discussed ____.
Did doctor examine patient: _____ yes, _____ no.
Wash hands before touching patient: _____ yes, _____ no.
Wear gloves: ____ yes, ___ no. Clean stethoscope: ____ yes, ____ no.
Wear gown and mask (precautions only):____ yes, _____ no.
Wash hands before leaving the room: _____ yes, _____ no.

Dr.______________ came in at _____ am/pm. Left at _____ am/pm.
We discussed ____.
Did doctor examine patient: _____ yes, _____ no.
Wash hands before touching patient: _____ yes, _____ no.
Wear gloves: ____ yes, ___ no. Clean stethoscope: ____ yes, ____ no.
Wear gown and mask (precautions only):____ yes, _____ no.
Wash hands before leaving the room: _____ yes, _____ no.

Dr.______________ came in at _____ am/pm. Left at _____ am/pm.
We discussed ____.
Did doctor examine patient: _____ yes, _____ no.
Wash hands before touching patient: _____ yes, _____ no.
Wear gloves: ____ yes, ___ no. Clean stethoscope: ____ yes, ____ no.
Wear gown and mask (precautions only):____ yes, _____ no.
Wash hands before leaving the room: _____ yes, _____ no.

NURSING CARE FOR ______________________________

DATE ____________________, DAY NUMBER __________________

INITIAL DAY SHIFT EXAM:

My nurse has _____ # of patients. CNA ___yes, ___no. Charge nurse ______________
Nurse ________________ RN/LPN came in at __________ am/pm. Left at _________ am/pm.
Did nurse wash hands and wear gloves before touching patient: ______ yes, ______ no.
Wash hands after touching patient and before leaving the room: ______ yes, ______ no.
Don't hesitate to request staff to wash their hands. This will help decrease the risk of spreading potentially lethal germs.
Did nurse wear protective gear (isolation precautions only): ______ yes, ______ no.
Did nurse provide oral care (to be done every two hours if unable to provide for self, also decreases risk of pneumonia, infections, and aspiration): ______ yes, ______ no.
If able to provide own oral care, then supplies at bedside: ______ yes, ______ no.
Was patient repositioned (every two hours if unable to turn self): ______ yes ______ no.
Head of bed at ________ degrees. This is important for patients on ventilators or on tube feedings. Anything less than thirty degrees places patients at risk for aspiration of stomach contents into the lungs causing aspiration pneumonia.
Checked for incontinence and skin breakdown: ____ yes, ____ no.
Patient's linens wet or soiled: ____ yes, ____ no. Linens changed: ____ yes, ____ no.
Time linens changed: ________ am/pm. Any skin redness or breakdown: ____ yes, ____ no.
If yes, what stage is pressure ulcer: ________. Acquired when: ______________.
List wounds not associated with pressure ulcers and how acquired: ______________
____
Mattress type: ____
Specialty mattresses are important to help prevent pressure ulcers)
If patient on ventilator or has tracheostomy, suction performed: ____ yes, ____ no.
Did nurse listen to lung sounds: ____ yes, ____ no.
Does patient have chest tubes: ____ yes, ____ no. Functioning ______ yes, ______ no.
Bowel sounds: ______ yes, ______ no. Bowel sounds active: ______ yes, ______ no.
Neurological exam: ______ yes, ______ no. Follow commands: ______ yes, ______ no.
Is patient alert and oriented to person, place, time, and events: ____ yes, ____ no.
If confused, patient is not oriented to: ____ person, ___ place, ___ time, ___ event.
Confusion began (time and date): ____
Glasgow coma scale (checks conscious scale of patient): __________________________
Intracranial pressure monitoring: ____ yes, ____ no.
If yes, pressure is at ________ mm mercury. (Normal is one to fifteen).
Moves extremities: ___ yes, ___ no.
Paralysis: (inability to move extremities) ______ yes, ______ no.
If yes, extremities affected and when paralysis began: __________________________
Is patient in pain: ____ yes, ____ no. Describe pain and location _______________
Patient able to eat: ____ yes, ____ no. What type of diet? _______________________
If patient on tube feedings list type: ______________ at ________ cc/ml per hour.
Nausea ____, vomiting ____. If so, describe: _____________________________________
Patient has: Nasal gastric tube ____, Dobhoff tube ____, Peg or gastric tube ____
When was feeding tube placed and what site: ______________________________________.
Catheter for draining urine: ____ yes, ____ no. If so, when placed: _____________.
Find out policy for allowed time to remain in bladder. Too long may cause infections.)
IV site(s) where: ______________________ when placed: ____________________________.
IV fluids (types and rates): ____________________, ____________________________,
____, ____________________________.
Is patient on oxygen: ____ yes, ____ no. If so, how much and route delivered (see oxygen routes): ____.
If patient on ventilator, list settings (see list on ventilator settings): ________
____.
Vital signs: temp _____, pulse _____, resp _____, b/p _____, o2 _____%,
current weight _____ pounds, _____ kg. Glucose level: _____
Insulin coverage: ____ yes, ____ no. Insulin type: ___________, # of units: _____.

NURSING CARE CONTINUED FOR ______________________
DATE __________________, DAY NUMBER __________________

FOLLOWING EXAMINATIONS FOR DAY SHIFT:

Nurse ____________, CNA ____________, in at _____ am/pm. Left at ______ am/pm.
Wash hands and wear gloves before touching patient: ______ yes, ______ no.
Wash hands before leaving room: ___ yes, ___ no. Wear protective gear: __ yes, __ no.
Clean stethoscope: __ yes, __ no. Oral care: __ yes, __ no. Suctioned: __ yes, __ no.
Repositioned: ___ yes, ___ no. Turned to: ___ left, ___ right, ___ backside ___.
Head of bed at: ______ degrees. Incontinence/skin breakdown: ____ yes, ____ no.
Linens wet or soiled: ____ yes, ____ no. Linens changed: _____ yes, _____ no.
Dressing changed: ____ yes, ____ no. Location: ____________________.
IV site checked: _____ yes, ____ no. IV tubing labeled: _____ yes, _____no.
IV fluids at: ____.
Pain level (0-10 scale.0-no pain, 10 intolerable): ________________.
Location of pain: __________. Medicated for pain: _____ yes, ____ no.
Patient is alert/oriented: ____ yes, ____ no. New confusion: ____ yes, ____ no.
Vital signs: temp ____, pulse _____, resp _____, b/p _____, 02 _____ %, ____ liters.
Glucose level: _____. Insulin: ___ yes, ___ no. Type: ____________ # of units ____.

Nurse ____________, CNA ____________, in at _____ am/pm. Left at ______ am/pm.
Wash hands and wear gloves before touching patient: ______ yes, ______ no.
Wash hands before leaving room: ___ yes, ___ no. Wear protective gear: __ yes, __ no.
Clean stethoscope: __ yes, __ no. Oral care: __ yes, __ no. Suctioned: __ yes, __ no.
Repositioned: ___ yes, ___ no. Turned to: ___ left, ___ right, ___ backside ___.
Head of bed at: ______ degrees. Incontinence/skin breakdown: ____ yes, ____ no.
Linens wet or soiled: ____ yes, ____ no. Linens changed: _____ yes, _____ no.
Dressing changed: ____ yes, ____ no. Location: ____________________.
IV site checked: _____ yes, ____ no. IV tubing labeled: _____ yes, _____no.
IV fluids at: ____.
Pain level (0-10 scale.0-no pain, 10 intolerable): ________________.
Location of pain: __________. Medicated for pain: _____ yes, ____ no.
Patient is alert/oriented: ____ yes, ____ no. New confusion: ____ yes, ____ no.
Vital signs: temp ____, pulse _____, resp _____, b/p _____, 02 _____ %, ____ liters.
Glucose level: _____. Insulin: ___ yes, ___ no. Type: ____________ # of units ____.

Nurse ____________, CNA ____________, in at _____ am/pm. Left at ______ am/pm.
Wash hands and wear gloves before touching patient: ______ yes, ______ no.
Wash hands before leaving room: ___ yes, ___ no. Wear protective gear: __ yes, __ no.
Clean stethoscope: __ yes, __ no. Oral care: __ yes, __ no. Suctioned: __ yes, __ no.
Repositioned: ___ yes, ___ no. Turned to: ___ left, ___ right, ___ backside ___.
Head of bed at: ______ degrees. Incontinence/skin breakdown: ____ yes, ____ no.
Linens wet or soiled: ____ yes, ____ no. Linens changed: _____ yes, _____ no.
Dressing changed: ____ yes, ____ no. Location: ____________________.
IV site checked: _____ yes, ____ no. IV tubing labeled: _____ yes, _____no.
IV fluids at: ____.
Pain level (0-10 scale.0-no pain, 10 intolerable): ________________.
Location of pain: __________. Medicated for pain: _____ yes, ____ no.
Patient is alert/oriented: ____ yes, ____ no. New confusion: ____ yes, ____ no.
Vital signs: temp ____, pulse _____, resp _____, b/p _____, 02 _____ %, ____ liters.
Glucose level: _____. Insulin: ___ yes, ___ no. Type: ____________ # of units ____.

NURSING CARE CONTINUED FOR ________________________
DATE ________________, DAY NUMBER ________________

FOLLOWING EXAMINATIONS FOR DAY SHIFT:

Nurse ____________, CNA ____________, in at ______ am/pm. Left at ______ am/pm.
Wash hands and wear gloves before touching patient: ____ yes, ____ no.
Wash hands before leaving room: __ yes, __ no. Wear protective gear: __ yes, __ no.
Clean stethoscope: __ yes, __ no. Oral care: __ yes, __ no. Suctioned: __ yes, __ no.
Repositioned: ___ yes, ___ no. Turned to: __ left, ___ right, ___ backside ___.
Head of bed at: ______ degrees. Incontinence/skin breakdown: ____ yes, ____ no.
Linens wet or soiled: ____ yes, ____ no. Linens changed: ____ yes, ____ no.
Dressing changed: ____ yes, ____ no. Location: ________________________.
IV site checked: _____ yes, _____ no. IV tubing labeled: ____ yes, ____no.
IV fluids at: ____.
Pain level (0-10 scale.0-no pain, 10 intolerable): ____________________.
Location of pain: ______________. Medicated for pain: ____ yes, ____ no.
Patient is alert/oriented: ____ yes, ____ no. New confusion: ____ yes, ____ no.
Vital signs: temp ____, pulse ____, resp _____, b/p _____, 02 ____ %, ____ liters.
Glucose level: _____. Insulin: ___ yes, ___ no. Type: __________ # of units ____.

Nurse ____________, CNA ____________, in at ______ am/pm. Left at ______ am/pm.
Wash hands and wear gloves before touching patient: ____ yes, ____ no.
Wash hands before leaving room: __ yes, __ no. Wear protective gear: __ yes, __ no.
Clean stethoscope: __ yes, __ no. Oral care: __ yes, __ no. Suctioned: __ yes, __ no.
Repositioned: ___ yes, ___ no. Turned to: __ left, ___ right, ___ backside ___.
Head of bed at: ______ degrees. Incontinence/skin breakdown: ____ yes, ____ no.
Linens wet or soiled: ____ yes, ____ no. Linens changed: ____ yes, ____ no.
Dressing changed: ____ yes, ____ no. Location: ________________________.
IV site checked: _____ yes, _____ no. IV tubing labeled: ____ yes, ____no.
IV fluids at: ____.
Pain level (0-10 scale.0-no pain, 10 intolerable): ____________________.
Location of pain: ______________. Medicated for pain: ____ yes, ____ no.
Patient is alert/oriented: ____ yes, ____ no. New confusion: ____ yes, ____ no.
Vital signs: temp ____, pulse ____, resp _____, b/p _____, 02 ____ %, ____ liters.
Glucose level: _____. Insulin: ___ yes, ___ no. Type: __________ # of units ____.

Nurse ____________, CNA ____________, in at ______ am/pm. Left at ______ am/pm.
Wash hands and wear gloves before touching patient: ____ yes, ____ no.
Wash hands before leaving room: __ yes, __ no. Wear protective gear: __ yes, __ no.
Clean stethoscope: __ yes, __ no. Oral care: __ yes, __ no. Suctioned: __ yes, __ no.
Repositioned: ___ yes, ___ no. Turned to: __ left, ___ right, ___ backside ___.
Head of bed at: ______ degrees. Incontinence/skin breakdown: ____ yes, ____ no.
Linens wet or soiled: ____ yes, ____ no. Linens changed: ____ yes, ____ no.
Dressing changed: ____ yes, ____ no. Location: ________________________.
IV site checked: _____ yes, _____ no. IV tubing labeled: ____ yes, ____no.
IV fluids at: ____.
Pain level (0-10 scale.0-no pain, 10 intolerable): ____________________.
Location of pain: ______________. Medicated for pain: ____ yes, ____ no.
Patient is alert/oriented: ____ yes, ____ no. New confusion: ____ yes, ____ no.
Vital signs: temp ____, pulse ____, resp _____, b/p _____, 02 ____ %, ____ liters.
Glucose level: _____. Insulin: ___ yes, ___ no. Type: __________ # of units ____.

NURSING CARE FOR ______________________________

DATE __________________, DAY NUMBER ____________________

INITIAL NIGHT SHIFT EXAM:

My nurse has ______ # of patients. CNA ___yes, ___no. Charge nurse ________________
Nurse ______________ RN/LPN came in at _________ am/pm. Left at __________ am/pm.
Did nurse wash hands and wear gloves before touching patient: _______ yes, _______ no.
Wash hands after touching patient and before leaving the room: _______ yes, _______ no.
Don't hesitate to request staff to wash their hands. This will help decrease the risk of spreading potentially lethal germs.
Did nurse wear protective gear (isolation precautions only): _______ yes, _______ no.
Did nurse provide oral care (to be done every two hours if unable to provide for self, also decreases risk of pneumonia, infections, and aspiration): _______ yes, ______ no.
If able to provide own oral care, then supplies at bedside: ________ yes, ________ no.
Was patient repositioned (every two hours if unable to turn self): _____ yes ______ no.
Head of bed at ________ degrees. This is important for patients on ventilators or on tube feedings. Anything less than thirty degrees places patients at risk for aspiration of stomach contents into the lungs causing aspiration pneumonia.
Checked for incontinence and skin breakdown: _____ yes, _____ no.
Patient's linens wet or soiled: _____ yes, _____ no. Linens changed: ____ yes, ____ no.
Time linens changed: _______ am/pm. Any skin redness or breakdown: ____ yes, ____ no.
If yes, what stage is pressure ulcer: ________. Acquired when: __________________.
List wounds not associated with pressure ulcers and how acquired: ________________
____.
Mattress type: ____.
Specialty mattresses are important to help prevent pressure ulcers)
If patient on ventilator or has tracheostomy, suction performed: _____ yes, ______ no.
Did nurse listen to lung sounds: _____ yes, _____ no.
Does patient have chest tubes: ____ yes, ____ no. Functioning _____ yes, ______ no.
Bowel sounds: _______ yes, ______ no. Bowel sounds active: _______ yes, _______ no.
Neurological exam: ______ yes, _______ no. Follow commands: _______ yes, _______ no.
Is patient alert and oriented to person, place, time, and events: _____ yes, _____ no.
If confused, patient is not oriented to: ____ person, ___ place, ___ time, ___ event.
Confusion began (time and date): ____.
Glasgow coma scale (checks conscious scale of patient): ________________________.
Intracranial pressure monitoring: ______ yes, ______ no.
If yes, pressure is at ________ mm mercury. (Normal is one to fifteen).
Moves extremities: ___ yes, ___ no.
Paralysis: (inability to move extremities) ________ yes, ________ no.
If yes, extremities affected and when paralysis began: __________________________.
Is patient in pain: ____ yes, ____ no. Describe pain and location ______________.
Patient able to eat: ____ yes, ____ no. What type of diet? _____________________.
If patient on tube feedings list type: ___________ at __________ cc/ml per hour.
Nausea ____, vomiting ____. If so, describe: ____________________________________.
Patient has: Nasal gastric tube ______, Dobhoff tube _____, Peg or gastric tube _____.
When was feeding tube placed and what site: ____________________________________.
Catheter for draining urine: ____ yes, ____ no. If so, when placed: ______________.
Find out policy for allowed time to remain in bladder. Too long may cause infections.)
IV site(s) where: ______________________________ when placed: __________________.
IV fluids (types and rates): _________________________, __________________________,
___________________________, ________________________, ___________________________,
Is patient on oxygen: _____ yes, _____ no. If so, how much and route delivered (see oxygen routes): ____.
If patient on ventilator, list settings (see list on ventilator settings): ___________
____.
Vital signs: temp ______, pulse ______, resp ______, b/p ______, o2 ______%,
current weight ______ pounds, ______ kg. Glucose level: ______
Insulin coverage: ____ yes, ____ no. Insulin type: ____________, # of units: ______.

NURSING CARE CONTINUED FOR ____________________
DATE ____________________, DAY NUMBER ____________________

FOLLOWING EXAMINATIONS FOR NIGHT SHIFT:

Nurse ____________, CNA ____________, in at ______ am/pm. Left at ______ am/pm.
Wash hands and wear gloves before touching patient: ______ yes, ______ no.
Wash hands before leaving room: ___ yes, ___ no. Wear protective gear: __ yes, __ no.
Clean stethoscope: __ yes, __ no. Oral care: __ yes, __ no. Suctioned: __ yes, __ no.
Repositioned: __ yes, ___ no. Turned to: ___ left, ___ right, ___ backside ___.
Head of bed at: ________ degrees. Incontinence/skin breakdown: ____ yes, ____ no.
Linens wet or soiled: ____ yes, ____ no. Linens changed: ____ yes, ____ no.
Dressing changed: ____ yes, ____ no. Location: ______________________________.
IV site checked: _____ yes, _____ no. IV tubing labeled: _____ yes, _____ no.
IV fluids at: ____.
Pain level (0-10 scale.0-no pain, 10 intolerable): ____________________________.
Location of pain: ______________. Medicated for pain: ____ yes, ____ no.
Patient is alert/oriented: ____ yes, ____ no. New confusion: ____ yes, ____ no.
Vital signs: temp ___, pulse ___, resp ___, b/p _____, 02 ____ %, ____ liters.
Glucose level: _____. Insulin: ___ yes, __ no. Type: __________ # of units ____.

Nurse ____________, CNA ____________, in at ______ am/pm. Left at ______ am/pm.
Wash hands and wear gloves before touching patient: ______ yes, ______ no.
Wash hands before leaving room: ___ yes, ___ no. Wear protective gear: __ yes, __ no.
Clean stethoscope: __ yes, __ no. Oral care: __ yes, __ no. Suctioned: __ yes, __ no.
Repositioned: __ yes, ___ no. Turned to: ___ left, ___ right, ___ backside ___.
Head of bed at: ________ degrees. Incontinence/skin breakdown: ____ yes, ____ no.
Linens wet or soiled: ____ yes, ____ no. Linens changed: ____ yes, ____ no.
Dressing changed: ____ yes, ____ no. Location: ______________________________.
IV site checked: _____ yes, _____ no. IV tubing labeled: _____ yes, _____ no.
IV fluids at: ____.
Pain level (0-10 scale.0-no pain, 10 intolerable): ____________________________.
Location of pain: ______________. Medicated for pain: ____ yes, ____ no.
Patient is alert/oriented: ____ yes, ____ no. New confusion: ____ yes, ____ no.
Vital signs: temp ___, pulse ___, resp ___, b/p _____, 02 ____ %, ____ liters.
Glucose level: _____. Insulin: ___ yes, __ no. Type: __________ # of units ____.

Nurse ____________, CNA ____________, in at ______ am/pm. Left at ______ am/pm.
Wash hands and wear gloves before touching patient: ______ yes, ______ no.
Wash hands before leaving room: ___ yes, ___ no. Wear protective gear: __ yes, __ no.
Clean stethoscope: __ yes, __ no. Oral care: __ yes, __ no. Suctioned: __ yes, __ no.
Repositioned: __ yes, ___ no. Turned to: ___ left, ___ right, ___ backside ___.
Head of bed at: ________ degrees. Incontinence/skin breakdown: ____ yes, ____ no.
Linens wet or soiled: ____ yes, ____ no. Linens changed: ____ yes, ____ no.
Dressing changed: ____ yes, ____ no. Location: ______________________________.
IV site checked: _____ yes, _____ no. IV tubing labeled: _____ yes, _____ no.
IV fluids at: ____.
Pain level (0-10 scale.0-no pain, 10 intolerable): ____________________________.
Location of pain: ______________. Medicated for pain: ____ yes, ____ no.
Patient is alert/oriented: ____ yes, ____ no. New confusion: ____ yes, ____ no.
Vital signs: temp ___, pulse ___, resp ___, b/p _____, 02 ____ %, ____ liters.
Glucose level: _____. Insulin: ___ yes, __ no. Type: __________ # of units ____.

NURSING CARE CONTINUED FOR ___________________________
DATE ____________________, DAY NUMBER ____________________

FOLLOWING EXAMINATIONS FOR NIGHT SHIFT:

Nurse ______________, CNA ____________, in at _____ am/pm. Left at ______ am/pm.
Wash hands and wear gloves before touching patient: _______ yes, _______ no.
Wash hands before leaving room: ___ yes, ___ no. Wear protective gear: __ yes, __ no.
Clean stethoscope: __ yes, __ no. Oral care: __ yes, __ no. Suctioned: __ yes, __ no.
Repositioned: ___ yes, ___ no. Turned to: ___ left, ___ right, ___ backside ___.
Head of bed at: _______ degrees. Incontinence/skin breakdown: ____ yes, ____ no.
Linens wet or soiled: _____ yes, _____ no. Linens changed: _____ yes, _____ no.
Dressing changed: ____ yes, ____ no. Location: ________________________.
IV site checked: _____ yes, _____ no. IV tubing labeled: _____ yes, _____no.
IV fluids at: ____.
Pain level (0-10 scale.0-no pain, 10 intolerable): ____________________.
Location of pain: ________________. Medicated for pain: _____ yes, _____ no.
Patient is alert/oriented: ____ yes, ____ no. New confusion: ____ yes, ____ no.
Vital signs: temp ____, pulse _____, resp _____, b/p _____, 02 _____ %, ____ liters.
Glucose level: _____. Insulin: ___ yes, ___ no. Type: _______________ # of units ____.

Nurse ______________, CNA ____________, in at _____ am/pm. Left at ______ am/pm.
Wash hands and wear gloves before touching patient: _______ yes, _______ no.
Wash hands before leaving room: ___ yes, ___ no. Wear protective gear: __ yes, __ no.
Clean stethoscope: __ yes, __ no. Oral care: __ yes, __ no. Suctioned: __ yes, __ no.
Repositioned: ___ yes, ___ no. Turned to: ___ left, ___ right, ___ backside ___.
Head of bed at: _______ degrees. Incontinence/skin breakdown: ____ yes, ____ no.
Linens wet or soiled: _____ yes, _____ no. Linens changed: _____ yes, _____ no.
Dressing changed: ____ yes, ____ no. Location: ________________________.
IV site checked: _____ yes, _____ no. IV tubing labeled: _____ yes, _____no.
IV fluids at: ____.
Pain level (0-10 scale.0-no pain, 10 intolerable): ____________________.
Location of pain: ________________. Medicated for pain: _____ yes, _____ no.
Patient is alert/oriented: ____ yes, ____ no. New confusion: ____ yes, ____ no.
Vital signs: temp ____, pulse _____, resp _____, b/p _____, 02 _____ %, ____ liters.
Glucose level: _____. Insulin: ___ yes, ___ no. Type: _______________ # of units ____.

Nurse ______________, CNA ____________, in at _____ am/pm. Left at ______ am/pm.
Wash hands and wear gloves before touching patient: _______ yes, _______ no.
Wash hands before leaving room: ___ yes, ___ no. Wear protective gear: __ yes, __ no.
Clean stethoscope: __ yes, __ no. Oral care: __ yes, __ no. Suctioned: __ yes, __ no.
Repositioned: ___ yes, ___ no. Turned to: ___ left, ___ right, ___ backside ___.
Head of bed at: _______ degrees. Incontinence/skin breakdown: ____ yes, ____ no.
Linens wet or soiled: _____ yes, _____ no. Linens changed: _____ yes, _____ no.
Dressing changed: ____ yes, ____ no. Location: ________________________.
IV site checked: _____ yes, _____ no. IV tubing labeled: _____ yes, _____no.
IV fluids at: ____.
Pain level (0-10 scale.0-no pain, 10 intolerable): ____________________.
Location of pain: ________________. Medicated for pain: _____ yes, _____ no.
Patient is alert/oriented: ____ yes, ____ no. New confusion: ____ yes, ____ no.
Vital signs: temp ____, pulse _____, resp _____, b/p _____, 02 _____ %, ____ liters.
Glucose level: _____. Insulin: ___ yes, ___ no. Type: _______________ # of units ____.

MEDICATION ADMINISTRATION LIST FOR ____________________
DATE ________________ DAY NUMBER ____________________

List the medication for each day. Routes of administration: oral, thru feeding tube, intravenous (IV), intramuscular (IM), subcutaneous (SQ), epidural or a catheter in your spinal column, rectal, topical, eye drops, and ear drops.

Medication: ____________ Route: ____________ Time: ____________
Medication: ____________ Route: ____________ Time: ____________
Medication: ____________ Route: ____________ Time: ____________
Medication: ____________ Route: ____________ Time: ____________
Medication: ____________ Route: ____________ Time: ____________
Medication: ____________ Route: ____________ Time: ____________
Medication: ____________ Route: ____________ Time: ____________
Medication: ____________ Route: ____________ Time: ____________
Medication: ____________ Route: ____________ Time: ____________
Medication: ____________ Route: ____________ Time: ____________
Medication: ____________ Route: ____________ Time: ____________
Medication: ____________ Route: ____________ Time: ____________
Medication: ____________ Route: ____________ Time: ____________
Medication: ____________ Route: ____________ Time: ____________
Medication: ____________ Route: ____________ Time: ____________
Medication: ____________ Route: ____________ Time: ____________
Medication: ____________ Route: ____________ Time: ____________
Medication: ____________ Route: ____________ Time: ____________
Medication: ____________ Route: ____________ Time: ____________
Medication: ____________ Route: ____________ Time: ____________
Medication: ____________ Route: ____________ Time: ____________
Medication: ____________ Route: ____________ Time: ____________
Medication: ____________ Route: ____________ Time: ____________
Medication: ____________ Route: ____________ Time: ____________
Medication: ____________ Route: ____________ Time: ____________
Medication: ____________ Route: ____________ Time: ____________
Medication: ____________ Route: ____________ Time: ____________
Medication: ____________ Route: ____________ Time: ____________
Medication: ____________ Route: ____________ Time: ____________
Medication: ____________ Route: ____________ Time: ____________
Medication: ____________ Route: ____________ Time: ____________
Medication: ____________ Route: ____________ Time: ____________
Medication: ____________ Route: ____________ Time: ____________
Medication: ____________ Route: ____________ Time: ____________
Medication: ____________ Route: ____________ Time: ____________
Medication: ____________ Route: ____________ Time: ____________
Medication: ____________ Route: ____________ Time: ____________
Medication: ____________ Route: ____________ Time: ____________
Medication: ____________ Route: ____________ Time: ____________
Medication: ____________ Route: ____________ Time: ____________
Medication: ____________ Route: ____________ Time: ____________
Medication: ____________ Route: ____________ Time: ____________
Medication: ____________ Route: ____________ Time: ____________
Medication: ____________ Route: ____________ Time: ____________
Medication: ____________ Route: ____________ Time: ____________
Medication: ____________ Route: ____________ Time: ____________
Medication: ____________ Route: ____________ Time: ____________
Medication: ____________ Route: ____________ Time: ____________
Medication: ____________ Route: ____________ Time: ____________
Medication: ____________ Route: ____________ Time: ____________
Medication: ____________ Route: ____________ Time: ____________
Medication: ____________ Route: ____________ Time: ____________
Medication: ____________ Route: ____________ Time: ____________
Medication: ____________ Route: ____________ Time: ____________

NOTES FOR DAY NUMBER ______________________________

DATE ______________________________

MEDICAL JOURNAL FOR ______________________________

DATE ____________________, DAY NUMBER ______________

VISITS FROM MY DOCTORS TODAY

Goals for today: ____
____
____.

Things to discuss with my doctor(s): ____________________________
____
____

Dr.____________ came in at _____ am/pm. Left at _____ am/pm.
We discussed ____.
Did doctor examine patient: _____ yes, _____ no.
Wash hands before touching patient: _____ yes, _____ no.
Wear gloves: ____ yes, ___ no. Clean stethoscope: ____ yes, ____ no.
Wear gown and mask (precautions only):____ yes, _____ no.
Wash hands before leaving the room: _____ yes, _____ no.

Dr.____________ came in at _____ am/pm. Left at _____ am/pm.
We discussed ____.
Did doctor examine patient: _____ yes, _____ no.
Wash hands before touching patient: _____ yes, _____ no.
Wear gloves: ____ yes, ___ no. Clean stethoscope: ____ yes, ____ no.
Wear gown and mask (precautions only):____ yes, _____ no.
Wash hands before leaving the room: _____ yes, _____ no.

Dr.____________ came in at _____ am/pm. Left at _____ am/pm.
We discussed ____.
Did doctor examine patient: _____ yes, _____ no.
Wash hands before touching patient: _____ yes, _____ no.
Wear gloves: ____ yes, ___ no. Clean stethoscope: ____ yes, ____ no.
Wear gown and mask (precautions only):____ yes, _____ no.
Wash hands before leaving the room: _____ yes, _____ no.

Dr.____________ came in at _____ am/pm. Left at _____ am/pm.
We discussed ____.
Did doctor examine patient: _____ yes, _____ no.
Wash hands before touching patient: _____ yes, _____ no.
Wear gloves: ____ yes, ___ no. Clean stethoscope: ____ yes, ____ no.
Wear gown and mask (precautions only):____ yes, _____ no.
Wash hands before leaving the room: _____ yes, _____ no.

Dr.____________ came in at _____ am/pm. Left at _____ am/pm.
We discussed ____.
Did doctor examine patient: _____ yes, _____ no.
Wash hands before touching patient: _____ yes, _____ no.
Wear gloves: ____ yes, ___ no. Clean stethoscope: ____ yes, ____ no.
Wear gown and mask (precautions only):____ yes, _____ no.
Wash hands before leaving the room: _____ yes, _____ no.

NURSING CARE FOR ______________________________

DATE ____________________, DAY NUMBER ____________________

INITIAL DAY SHIFT EXAM:

My nurse has ______ # of patients. CNA ___yes, ___no. Charge nurse ____________
Nurse ________________ RN/LPN came in at _________ am/pm. Left at __________ am/pm.
Did nurse wash hands and wear gloves before touching patient: ______ yes, ______ no.
Wash hands after touching patient and before leaving the room: ______ yes, ______ no.
Don't hesitate to request staff to wash their hands. This will help decrease the risk of spreading potentially lethal germs.
Did nurse wear protective gear (isolation precautions only): ______ yes, ______ no.
Did nurse provide oral care (to be done every two hours if unable to provide for self, also decreases risk of pneumonia, infections, and aspiration): ______ yes, ______ no.
If able to provide own oral care, then supplies at bedside: _______ yes, _______ no.
Was patient repositioned (every two hours if unable to turn self): _____ yes _____ no.
Head of bed at ________ degrees. This is important for patients on ventilators or on tube feedings. Anything less than thirty degrees places patients at risk for aspiration of stomach contents into the lungs causing aspiration pneumonia.
Checked for incontinence and skin breakdown: _____ yes, _____ no.
Patient's linens wet or soiled: _____ yes, _____ no. Linens changed: ____ yes, ____ no.
Time linens changed: _______ am/pm. Any skin redness or breakdown: ____ yes, ____ no.
If yes, what stage is pressure ulcer: _______. Acquired when: ____________________.
List wounds not associated with pressure ulcers and how acquired: ____________________
____.
Mattress type: ____.
Specialty mattresses are important to help prevent pressure ulcers)
If patient on ventilator or has tracheostomy, suction performed: _____ yes, _____ no.
Did nurse listen to lung sounds: _____ yes, _____ no.
Does patient have chest tubes: ____ yes, ____ no. Functioning _____ yes, _____ no.
Bowel sounds: _______ yes, _______ no. Bowel sounds active: _______ yes, _______ no.
Neurological exam: ______ yes, ______ no. Follow commands: _______ yes, _______ no.
Is patient alert and oriented to person, place, time, and events: _____ yes, _____ no.
If confused, patient is not oriented to: ___ person, ___ place, ___ time, ___ event.
Confusion began (time and date): ____.
Glasgow coma scale (checks conscious scale of patient): ___________________________.
Intracranial pressure monitoring: ______ yes, ______ no.
If yes, pressure is at ________ mm mercury. (Normal is one to fifteen).
Moves extremities: ___ yes, ___ no.
Paralysis: (inability to move extremities) _______ yes, _______ no.
If yes, extremities affected and when paralysis began: ___________________________.
Is patient in pain: ____ yes, ____ no. Describe pain and location ________________.
Patient able to eat: ____ yes, ____ no. What type of diet? _______________________.
If patient on tube feedings list type: _____________ at ___________ cc/ml per hour.
Nausea ____, vomiting _____. If so, describe: ____________________________________.
Patient has: Nasal gastric tube ______, Dobhoff tube _____, Peg or gastric tube _____.
When was feeding tube placed and what site: _______________________________________.
Catheter for draining urine: ____ yes, ____ no. If so, when placed: _______________.
Find out policy for allowed time to remain in bladder. Too long may cause infections.)
IV site(s) where: ____________________________ when placed: ________________________.
IV fluids (types and rates): ______________________, _____________________________,
______________________, ______________________, ____________________________________,
Is patient on oxygen: _____ yes, _____ no. If so, how much and route delivered
(see oxygen routes): ____.
If patient on ventilator, list settings (see list on ventilator settings): _________
____.
Vital signs: temp _____, pulse ______, resp ______, b/p ______, o2 _____%,
current weight ______ pounds, ______ kg. Glucose level: ______
Insulin coverage: ____ yes, ____ no. Insulin type: ____________, # of units: _____.

NURSING CARE CONTINUED FOR ____________________
DATE ____________________, DAY NUMBER ____________________

FOLLOWING EXAMINATIONS FOR DAY SHIFT:

Nurse ____________, CNA ____________, in at _____ am/pm. Left at _______ am/pm.
Wash hands and wear gloves before touching patient: _____ yes, _____ no.
Wash hands before leaving room: ___ yes, ___ no. Wear protective gear: __ yes, __ no.
Clean stethoscope: __ yes, __ no. Oral care: __ yes, __ no. Suctioned: __ yes, __ no.
Repositioned: ___ yes, ___ no. Turned to: ___ left, ___ right, ___ backside ___.
Head of bed at: _______ degrees. Incontinence/skin breakdown: ____ yes, ____ no.
Linens wet or soiled: _____ yes, _____ no. Linens changed: _____ yes, _____ no.
Dressing changed: _____ yes, _____ no. Location: ____________________.
IV site checked: _____ yes, _____ no. IV tubing labeled: _____ yes, _____ no.
IV fluids at: ____.
Pain level (0-10 scale.0-no pain, 10 intolerable): ____________.
Location of pain: ____________. Medicated for pain: _____ yes, _____ no.
Patient is alert/oriented: ___ yes, ___ no. New confusion: ___ yes, ___ no.
Vital signs: temp ____, pulse ____, resp ____, b/p _____, 02 _____ %, _____ liters.
Glucose level: _____. Insulin: ___ yes, ___ no. Type: __________ # of units ____.

Nurse ____________, CNA ____________, in at _____ am/pm. Left at _______ am/pm.
Wash hands and wear gloves before touching patient: _____ yes, _____ no.
Wash hands before leaving room: ___ yes, ___ no. Wear protective gear: __ yes, __ no.
Clean stethoscope: __ yes, __ no. Oral care: __ yes, __ no. Suctioned: __ yes, __ no.
Repositioned: ___ yes, ___ no. Turned to: ___ left, ___ right, ___ backside ___.
Head of bed at: _______ degrees. Incontinence/skin breakdown: ____ yes, ____ no.
Linens wet or soiled: _____ yes, _____ no. Linens changed: _____ yes, _____ no.
Dressing changed: _____ yes, _____ no. Location: ____________________.
IV site checked: _____ yes, _____ no. IV tubing labeled: _____ yes, _____ no.
IV fluids at: ____.
Pain level (0-10 scale.0-no pain, 10 intolerable): ____________.
Location of pain: ____________. Medicated for pain: _____ yes, _____ no.
Patient is alert/oriented: ___ yes, ___ no. New confusion: ___ yes, ___ no.
Vital signs: temp ____, pulse ____, resp ____, b/p _____, 02 _____ %, _____ liters.
Glucose level: _____. Insulin: ___ yes, ___ no. Type: __________ # of units ____.

Nurse ____________, CNA ____________, in at _____ am/pm. Left at _______ am/pm.
Wash hands and wear gloves before touching patient: _____ yes, _____ no.
Wash hands before leaving room: ___ yes, ___ no. Wear protective gear: __ yes, __ no.
Clean stethoscope: __ yes, __ no. Oral care: __ yes, __ no. Suctioned: __ yes, __ no.
Repositioned: ___ yes, ___ no. Turned to: ___ left, ___ right, ___ backside ___.
Head of bed at: _______ degrees. Incontinence/skin breakdown: ____ yes, ____ no.
Linens wet or soiled: _____ yes, _____ no. Linens changed: _____ yes, _____ no.
Dressing changed: _____ yes, _____ no. Location: ____________________.
IV site checked: _____ yes, _____ no. IV tubing labeled: _____ yes, _____ no.
IV fluids at: ____.
Pain level (0-10 scale.0-no pain, 10 intolerable): ____________.
Location of pain: ____________. Medicated for pain: _____ yes, _____ no.
Patient is alert/oriented: ___ yes, ___ no. New confusion: ___ yes, ___ no.
Vital signs: temp ____, pulse ____, resp ____, b/p _____, 02 _____ %, _____ liters.
Glucose level: _____. Insulin: ___ yes, ___ no. Type: __________ # of units ____.

NURSING CARE CONTINUED FOR ______________________________
DATE ____________________, DAY NUMBER ____________________

FOLLOWING EXAMINATIONS FOR DAY SHIFT:

Nurse __________, CNA __________, in at _____ am/pm. Left at _____ am/pm.
Wash hands and wear gloves before touching patient: _____ yes, _____ no.
Wash hands before leaving room: ___ yes, ___ no. Wear protective gear: __ yes, __ no.
Clean stethoscope: __ yes, __ no. Oral care: __ yes, __ no. Suctioned: __ yes, __ no.
Repositioned: ___ yes, ___ no. Turned to: ___ left, ___ right, ___ backside ___.
Head of bed at: _____ degrees. Incontinence/skin breakdown: ____ yes, ____ no.
Linens wet or soiled: _____ yes, _____ no. Linens changed: _____ yes, _____ no.
Dressing changed: ____ yes, ____ no. Location: ______________________.
IV site checked: ____ yes, ____ no. IV tubing labeled: _____ yes, _____no.
IV fluids at: ____.
Pain level (0-10 scale.0-no pain, 10 intolerable): ______________________.
Location of pain: ______________. Medicated for pain: _____ yes, ____ no.
Patient is alert/oriented: ____ yes, ____ no. New confusion: ____ yes, ____ no.
Vital signs: temp ____, pulse _____, resp _____, b/p _____, 02 _____ %, ____ liters.
Glucose level: _____. Insulin: ___ yes, ___ no. Type: ______________ # of units ____.

Nurse __________, CNA __________, in at _____ am/pm. Left at _____ am/pm.
Wash hands and wear gloves before touching patient: _____ yes, _____ no.
Wash hands before leaving room: ___ yes, ___ no. Wear protective gear: __ yes, __ no.
Clean stethoscope: __ yes, __ no. Oral care: __ yes, __ no. Suctioned: __ yes, __ no.
Repositioned: ___ yes, ___ no. Turned to: ___ left, ___ right, ___ backside ___.
Head of bed at: _____ degrees. Incontinence/skin breakdown: ____ yes, ____ no.
Linens wet or soiled: _____ yes, _____ no. Linens changed: _____ yes, _____ no.
Dressing changed: ____ yes, ____ no. Location: ______________________.
IV site checked: ____ yes, ____ no. IV tubing labeled: _____ yes, _____no.
IV fluids at: ____.
Pain level (0-10 scale.0-no pain, 10 intolerable): ______________________.
Location of pain: ______________. Medicated for pain: _____ yes, ____ no.
Patient is alert/oriented: ____ yes, ____ no. New confusion: ____ yes, ____ no.
Vital signs: temp ____, pulse _____, resp _____, b/p _____, 02 _____ %, ____ liters.
Glucose level: _____. Insulin: ___ yes, ___ no. Type: ______________ # of units ____.

Nurse __________, CNA __________, in at _____ am/pm. Left at _____ am/pm.
Wash hands and wear gloves before touching patient: _____ yes, _____ no.
Wash hands before leaving room: ___ yes, ___ no. Wear protective gear: __ yes, __ no.
Clean stethoscope: __ yes, __ no. Oral care: __ yes, __ no. Suctioned: __ yes, __ no.
Repositioned: ___ yes, ___ no. Turned to: ___ left, ___ right, ___ backside ___.
Head of bed at: _____ degrees. Incontinence/skin breakdown: ____ yes, ____ no.
Linens wet or soiled: _____ yes, _____ no. Linens changed: _____ yes, _____ no.
Dressing changed: ____ yes, ____ no. Location: ______________________.
IV site checked: ____ yes, ____ no. IV tubing labeled: _____ yes, _____no.
IV fluids at: ____.
Pain level (0-10 scale.0-no pain, 10 intolerable): ______________________.
Location of pain: ______________. Medicated for pain: _____ yes, ____ no.
Patient is alert/oriented: ____ yes, ____ no. New confusion: ____ yes, ____ no.
Vital signs: temp ____, pulse _____, resp _____, b/p _____, 02 _____ %, ____ liters.
Glucose level: _____. Insulin: ___ yes, ___ no. Type: ______________ # of units ____.

NURSING CARE FOR ____________________________

DATE __________________, DAY NUMBER __________________

INITIAL NIGHT SHIFT EXAM:

My nurse has _____ # of patients. CNA ___yes, ___no. Charge nurse ______________
Nurse ____________ RN/LPN came in at ________ am/pm. Left at __________ am/pm.
Did nurse wash hands and wear gloves before touching patient: _____ yes, _____ no.
Wash hands after touching patient and before leaving the room: _____ yes, _____ no.
Don't hesitate to request staff to wash their hands. This will help decrease the risk of spreading potentially lethal germs.
Did nurse wear protective gear (isolation precautions only): _____ yes, _____ no.
Did nurse provide oral care (to be done every two hours if unable to provide for self, also decreases risk of pneumonia, infections, and aspiration): _____ yes, _____ no.
If able to provide own oral care, then supplies at bedside: _____ yes, _____ no.
Was patient repositioned (every two hours if unable to turn self): ____ yes ____ no.
Head of bed at ________ degrees. This is important for patients on ventilators or on tube feedings. Anything less than thirty degrees places patients at risk for aspiration of stomach contents into the lungs causing aspiration pneumonia.
Checked for incontinence and skin breakdown: ____ yes, ____ no.
Patient's linens wet or soiled: ____ yes, ____ no. Linens changed: ____ yes, ____ no.
Time linens changed: _______ am/pm. Any skin redness or breakdown: ____ yes, ____ no.
If yes, what stage is pressure ulcer: _______. Acquired when: ______________.
List wounds not associated with pressure ulcers and how acquired: ______________
____.
Mattress type: ____.
Specialty mattresses are important to help prevent pressure ulcers)
If patient on ventilator or has tracheostomy, suction performed: _____ yes, _____ no.
Did nurse listen to lung sounds: ____ yes, ____ no.
Does patient have chest tubes: ____ yes, ____ no. Functioning _____ yes, _____ no.
Bowel sounds: _______ yes, _______ no. Bowel sounds active: ______ yes, ______ no.
Neurological exam: ______ yes, ______ no. Follow commands: _______ yes, ______ no.
Is patient alert and oriented to person, place, time, and events: ____ yes, ____ no.
If confused, patient is not oriented to: ____ person, ___ place, ___ time, ___ event.
Confusion began (time and date): ______________________________________.
Glasgow coma scale (checks conscious scale of patient): __________________.
Intracranial pressure monitoring: ____ yes, ____ no.
If yes, pressure is at ________ mm mercury. (Normal is one to fifteen).
Moves extremities: ___ yes, ___ no.
Paralysis: (inability to move extremities) _______ yes, _______ no.
If yes, extremities affected and when paralysis began: ____________________.
Is patient in pain: ___ yes, ____ no. Describe pain and location ______________.
Patient able to eat: ___ yes, ____ no. What type of diet? _____________________.
If patient on tube feedings list type: __________ at ________ cc/ml per hour.
Nausea ____, vomiting ____. If so, describe: ________________________________.
Patient has: Nasal gastric tube _____, Dobhoff tube _____, Peg or gastric tube _____.
When was feeding tube placed and what site: _______________________________.
Catheter for draining urine: ____ yes, ____ no. If so, when placed: __________.
Find out policy for allowed time to remain in bladder. Too long may cause infections.)
IV site(s) where: ____________________ when placed: ______________________.
IV fluids (types and rates): ____________________, ______________________,
____________________, ____________________, ______________________.
Is patient on oxygen: _____ yes, _____ no. If so, how much and route delivered (see oxygen routes): ____.
If patient on ventilator, list settings (see list on ventilator settings): ________
____.
Vital signs: temp _____, pulse _____, resp _____, b/p _____, o2 _____%,
current weight _____ pounds, _____ kg. Glucose level: _____
Insulin coverage: ____ yes, ____ no. Insulin type: ____________, # of units: _____.

NURSING CARE CONTINUED FOR ______________________________
DATE __________________, DAY NUMBER ____________________

FOLLOWING EXAMINATIONS FOR NIGHT SHIFT:

Nurse ______________, CNA ____________, in at _____ am/pm. Left at ______ am/pm.
Wash hands and wear gloves before touching patient: ________ yes, ________ no.
Wash hands before leaving room: ___ yes, ___ no. Wear protective gear: __ yes, __ no.
Clean stethoscope: __ yes, __ no. Oral care: __ yes, __ no. Suctioned: __ yes, __ no.
Repositioned: ___ yes, ___ no. Turned to: ___ left, ___ right, ___ backside ___.
Head of bed at: _______ degrees. Incontinence/skin breakdown: ____ yes, ____ no.
Linens wet or soiled: _____ yes, _____ no. Linens changed: _____ yes, ______ no.
Dressing changed: ____ yes, ____ no. Location: ____________________________.
IV site checked: _____ yes, _____ no. IV tubing labeled: _____ yes, _____no.
IV fluids at: ____.
Pain level (0-10 scale.0-no pain, 10 intolerable): ____________________________.
Location of pain: _____________. Medicated for pain: _____ yes, _____ no.
Patient is alert/oriented: ____ yes, ____ no. New confusion: ____ yes, ____ no.
Vital signs: temp ____, pulse _____, resp _____, b/p _____, 02 _____ %, ____ liters.
Glucose level: _____. Insulin: ___ yes, ___ no. Type: _____________ # of units ___.

Nurse ______________, CNA ____________, in at _____ am/pm. Left at ______ am/pm.
Wash hands and wear gloves before touching patient: ________ yes, ________ no.
Wash hands before leaving room: ___ yes, ___ no. Wear protective gear: __ yes, __ no.
Clean stethoscope: __ yes, __ no. Oral care: __ yes, __ no. Suctioned: __ yes, __ no.
Repositioned: ___ yes, ___ no. Turned to: ___ left, ___ right, ___ backside ___.
Head of bed at: _______ degrees. Incontinence/skin breakdown: ____ yes, ____ no.
Linens wet or soiled: _____ yes, _____ no. Linens changed: _____ yes, ______ no.
Dressing changed: ____ yes, ____ no. Location: ____________________________.
IV site checked: _____ yes, _____ no. IV tubing labeled: _____ yes, _____no.
IV fluids at: ____.
Pain level (0-10 scale.0-no pain, 10 intolerable): ____________________________.
Location of pain: _____________. Medicated for pain: _____ yes, _____ no.
Patient is alert/oriented: ____ yes, ____ no. New confusion: ____ yes, ____ no.
Vital signs: temp ____, pulse _____, resp _____, b/p _____, 02 _____ %, ____ liters.
Glucose level: _____. Insulin: ___ yes, ___ no. Type: _____________ # of units ___.

Nurse ______________, CNA ____________, in at _____ am/pm. Left at ______ am/pm.
Wash hands and wear gloves before touching patient: ________ yes, ________ no.
Wash hands before leaving room: ___ yes, ___ no. Wear protective gear: __ yes, __ no.
Clean stethoscope: __ yes, __ no. Oral care: __ yes, __ no. Suctioned: __ yes, __ no.
Repositioned: ___ yes, ___ no. Turned to: ___ left, ___ right, ___ backside ___.
Head of bed at: _______ degrees. Incontinence/skin breakdown: ____ yes, ____ no.
Linens wet or soiled: _____ yes, _____ no. Linens changed: _____ yes, ______ no.
Dressing changed: ____ yes, ____ no. Location: ____________________________.
IV site checked: _____ yes, _____ no. IV tubing labeled: _____ yes, _____no.
IV fluids at: ____.
Pain level (0-10 scale.0-no pain, 10 intolerable): ____________________________.
Location of pain: _____________. Medicated for pain: _____ yes, _____ no.
Patient is alert/oriented: ____ yes, ____ no. New confusion: ____ yes, ____ no.
Vital signs: temp ____, pulse _____, resp _____, b/p _____, 02 _____ %, ____ liters.
Glucose level: _____. Insulin: ___ yes, ___ no. Type: _____________ # of units ___.

NURSING CARE CONTINUED FOR ________________________
DATE ____________________, DAY NUMBER ____________________

FOLLOWING EXAMINATIONS FOR NIGHT SHIFT:

Nurse ______________, CNA ______________, in at _____ am/pm. Left at ______ am/pm.
Wash hands and wear gloves before touching patient: _______ yes, _______ no.
Wash hands before leaving room: ___ yes, ___ no. Wear protective gear: __ yes, __ no.
Clean stethoscope: __ yes, __ no. Oral care: __ yes, __ no. Suctioned: __ yes, __ no.
Repositioned: ___ yes, ___ no. Turned to: ___ left, ___ right, ___ backside ___.
Head of bed at: ______ degrees. Incontinence/skin breakdown: ____ yes, ____ no.
Linens wet or soiled: _____ yes, _____ no. Linens changed: _____ yes, _____ no.
Dressing changed: ____ yes, ____ no. Location: ______________________________.
IV site checked: _____ yes, _____ no. IV tubing labeled: _____ yes, _____no.
IV fluids at: ____.
Pain level (0-10 scale.0-no pain, 10 intolerable): ___________________________.
Location of pain: ________________. Medicated for pain: _____ yes, ____ no.
Patient is alert/oriented: ____ yes, ____ no. New confusion: ____ yes, ____ no.
Vital signs: temp ___, pulse ____, resp _____, b/p _____, 02 _____ %, ___ liters.
Glucose level: _____. Insulin: ___ yes, ___ no. Type: _______________ # of units ___.

Nurse ______________, CNA ______________, in at _____ am/pm. Left at ______ am/pm.
Wash hands and wear gloves before touching patient: _______ yes, _______ no.
Wash hands before leaving room: ___ yes, ___ no. Wear protective gear: __ yes, __ no.
Clean stethoscope: __ yes, __ no. Oral care: __ yes, __ no. Suctioned: __ yes, __ no.
Repositioned: ___ yes, ___ no. Turned to: ___ left, ___ right, ___ backside ___.
Head of bed at: ______ degrees. Incontinence/skin breakdown: ____ yes, ____ no.
Linens wet or soiled: _____ yes, _____ no. Linens changed: _____ yes, _____ no.
Dressing changed: ____ yes, ____ no. Location: ______________________________.
IV site checked: _____ yes, _____ no. IV tubing labeled: _____ yes, _____no.
IV fluids at: ____.
Pain level (0-10 scale.0-no pain, 10 intolerable): ___________________________.
Location of pain: ________________. Medicated for pain: _____ yes, ____ no.
Patient is alert/oriented: ____ yes, ____ no. New confusion: ____ yes, ____ no.
Vital signs: temp ___, pulse ____, resp _____, b/p _____, 02 _____ %, ___ liters.
Glucose level: _____. Insulin: ___ yes, ___ no. Type: _______________ # of units ___.

Nurse ______________, CNA ______________, in at _____ am/pm. Left at ______ am/pm.
Wash hands and wear gloves before touching patient: _______ yes, _______ no.
Wash hands before leaving room: ___ yes, ___ no. Wear protective gear: __ yes, __ no.
Clean stethoscope: __ yes, __ no. Oral care: __ yes, __ no. Suctioned: __ yes, __ no.
Repositioned: ___ yes, ___ no. Turned to: ___ left, ___ right, ___ backside ___.
Head of bed at: ______ degrees. Incontinence/skin breakdown: ____ yes, ____ no.
Linens wet or soiled: _____ yes, _____ no. Linens changed: _____ yes, _____ no.
Dressing changed: ____ yes, ____ no. Location: ______________________________.
IV site checked: _____ yes, _____ no. IV tubing labeled: _____ yes, _____no.
IV fluids at: ____.
Pain level (0-10 scale.0-no pain, 10 intolerable): ___________________________.
Location of pain: ________________. Medicated for pain: _____ yes, ____ no.
Patient is alert/oriented: ____ yes, ____ no. New confusion: ____ yes, ____ no.
Vital signs: temp ___, pulse ____, resp _____, b/p _____, 02 _____ %, ___ liters.
Glucose level: _____. Insulin: ___ yes, ___ no. Type: _______________ # of units ___

MEDICATION ADMINISTRATION LIST FOR ____________________
DATE ______________ DAY NUMBER ____________________

List the medication for each day. Routes of administration: oral, thru feeding tube, intravenous (IV), intramuscular (IM), subcutaneous (SQ), epidural or a catheter in your spinal column, rectal, topical, eye drops, and ear drops.

Medication: ______________ Route: ______________ Time: __________
Medication: ______________ Route: ______________ Time: __________
Medication: ______________ Route: ______________ Time: __________
Medication: ______________ Route: ______________ Time: __________
Medication: ______________ Route: ______________ Time: __________
Medication: ______________ Route: ______________ Time: __________
Medication: ______________ Route: ______________ Time: __________
Medication: ______________ Route: ______________ Time: __________
Medication: ______________ Route: ______________ Time: __________
Medication: ______________ Route: ______________ Time: __________
Medication: ______________ Route: ______________ Time: __________
Medication: ______________ Route: ______________ Time: __________
Medication: ______________ Route: ______________ Time: __________
Medication: ______________ Route: ______________ Time: __________
Medication: ______________ Route: ______________ Time: __________
Medication: ______________ Route: ______________ Time: __________
Medication: ______________ Route: ______________ Time: __________
Medication: ______________ Route: ______________ Time: __________
Medication: ______________ Route: ______________ Time: __________
Medication: ______________ Route: ______________ Time: __________
Medication: ______________ Route: ______________ Time: __________
Medication: ______________ Route: ______________ Time: __________
Medication: ______________ Route: ______________ Time: __________
Medication: ______________ Route: ______________ Time: __________
Medication: ______________ Route: ______________ Time: __________
Medication: ______________ Route: ______________ Time: __________
Medication: ______________ Route: ______________ Time: __________
Medication: ______________ Route: ______________ Time: __________
Medication: ______________ Route: ______________ Time: __________
Medication: ______________ Route: ______________ Time: __________
Medication: ______________ Route: ______________ Time: __________
Medication: ______________ Route: ______________ Time: __________
Medication: ______________ Route: ______________ Time: __________
Medication: ______________ Route: ______________ Time: __________
Medication: ______________ Route: ______________ Time: __________
Medication: ______________ Route: ______________ Time: __________
Medication: ______________ Route: ______________ Time: __________
Medication: ______________ Route: ______________ Time: __________
Medication: ______________ Route: ______________ Time: __________
Medication: ______________ Route: ______________ Time: __________
Medication: ______________ Route: ______________ Time: __________
Medication: ______________ Route: ______________ Time: __________
Medication: ______________ Route: ______________ Time: __________
Medication: ______________ Route: ______________ Time: __________
Medication: ______________ Route: ______________ Time: __________
Medication: ______________ Route: ______________ Time: __________
Medication: ______________ Route: ______________ Time: __________
Medication: ______________ Route: ______________ Time: __________
Medication: ______________ Route: ______________ Time: __________
Medication: ______________ Route: ______________ Time: __________
Medication: ______________ Route: ______________ Time: __________
Medication: ______________ Route: ______________ Time: __________
Medication: ______________ Route: ______________ Time: __________
Medication: ______________ Route: ______________ Time: __________

NOTES FOR DAY NUMBER ____________________

DATE ____________________

MEDICAL JOURNAL FOR ______________________________

DATE ____________________, DAY NUMBER ______________

VISITS FROM MY DOCTORS TODAY

Goals for today: ____

____

____.

Things to discuss with my doctor(s): ____________________________________

____

____

Dr.____________ came in at _____ am/pm. Left at _____ am/pm.
We discussed ____.
Did doctor examine patient: _____ yes, _____ no.
Wash hands before touching patient: _____ yes, _____ no.
Wear gloves: ____ yes, ___ no. Clean stethoscope: ____ yes, ____ no.
Wear gown and mask (precautions only):____ yes, _____ no.
Wash hands before leaving the room: _____ yes, _____ no.

Dr.____________ came in at _____ am/pm. Left at _____ am/pm.
We discussed ____.
Did doctor examine patient: _____ yes, _____ no.
Wash hands before touching patient: _____ yes, _____ no.
Wear gloves: ____ yes, ___ no. Clean stethoscope: ____ yes, ____ no.
Wear gown and mask (precautions only):____ yes, _____ no.
Wash hands before leaving the room: _____ yes, _____ no.

Dr.____________ came in at _____ am/pm. Left at _____ am/pm.
We discussed ____.
Did doctor examine patient: _____ yes, _____ no.
Wash hands before touching patient: _____ yes, _____ no.
Wear gloves: ____ yes, ___ no. Clean stethoscope: ____ yes, ____ no.
Wear gown and mask (precautions only):____ yes, _____ no.
Wash hands before leaving the room: _____ yes, _____ no.

Dr.____________ came in at _____ am/pm. Left at _____ am/pm.
We discussed ____.
Did doctor examine patient: _____ yes, _____ no.
Wash hands before touching patient: _____ yes, _____ no.
Wear gloves: ____ yes, ___ no. Clean stethoscope: ____ yes, ____ no.
Wear gown and mask (precautions only):____ yes, _____ no.
Wash hands before leaving the room: _____ yes, _____ no.

Dr.____________ came in at _____ am/pm. Left at _____ am/pm.
We discussed ____.
Did doctor examine patient: _____ yes, _____ no.
Wash hands before touching patient: _____ yes, _____ no.
Wear gloves: ____ yes, ___ no. Clean stethoscope: ____ yes, ____ no.
Wear gown and mask (precautions only):____ yes, _____ no.
Wash hands before leaving the room: _____ yes, _____ no.

NURSING CARE FOR ______________________________

DATE ____________________, DAY NUMBER ____________________

INITIAL DAY SHIFT EXAM:

My nurse has ______ # of patients. CNA ___yes, ___no. Charge nurse ______________
Nurse ____________ RN/LPN came in at ________ am/pm. Left at __________ am/pm.
Did nurse wash hands and wear gloves before touching patient: ______ yes, ______ no.
Wash hands after touching patient and before leaving the room: ______ yes, ______ no.
Don't hesitate to request staff to wash their hands. This will help decrease the risk of spreading potentially lethal germs.
Did nurse wear protective gear (isolation precautions only): ______ yes, ______ no.
Did nurse provide oral care (to be done every two hours if unable to provide for self, also decreases risk of pneumonia, infections, and aspiration): ______ yes, ______ no.
If able to provide own oral care, then supplies at bedside: ________ yes, ______ no.
Was patient repositioned (every two hours if unable to turn self): _____ yes ______ no.
Head of bed at ________ degrees. This is important for patients on ventilators or on tube feedings. Anything less than thirty degrees places patients at risk for aspiration of stomach contents into the lungs causing aspiration pneumonia.
Checked for incontinence and skin breakdown: ___ yes, ____ no.
Patient's linens wet or soiled: ____ yes, ___ no. Linens changed: ____ yes, ____ no.
Time linens changed: ________ am/pm. Any skin redness or breakdown: ___ yes, ____ no.
If yes, what stage is pressure ulcer: ______. Acquired when: ______________.
List wounds not associated with pressure ulcers and how acquired: ______________.
____
Mattress type: ____
Specialty mattresses are important to help prevent pressure ulcers)
If patient on ventilator or has tracheostomy, suction performed: ______ yes, ______ no.
Did nurse listen to lung sounds: _____ yes, ______ no.
Does patient have chest tubes: ____ yes, ____ no. Functioning _____ yes, _____ no.
Bowel sounds: _______ yes, ______ no. Bowel sounds active: ______ yes, ______ no.
Neurological exam: ______ yes, ______ no. Follow commands: ______ yes, ______ no.
Is patient alert and oriented to person, place, time, and events: _____yes, _____ no.
If confused, patient is not oriented to: ____ person, ___ place, ___ time, ___ event.
Confusion began (time and date): ____
Glasgow coma scale (checks conscious scale of patient): _______________________
Intracranial pressure monitoring: ____ yes, _____ no.
If yes, pressure is at ________ mm mercury. (Normal is one to fifteen).
Moves extremities: ___ yes, ___ no.
Paralysis: (inability to move extremities) ______ yes, ______ no.
If yes, extremities affected and when paralysis began: _________________________
Is patient in pain: ____ yes, _____ no. Describe pain and location ______________
Patient able to eat: ____ yes, ____ no. What type of diet? ______________________
If patient on tube feedings list type: ________ at ________ cc/ml per hour.
Nausea ____, vomiting _____. If so, describe: ________________________________.
Patient has: Nasal gastric tube ______, Dobhoff tube _____, Peg or gastric tube ____.
When was feeding tube placed and what site: ___________________________________.
Catheter for draining urine: ____ yes, ____ no. If so, when placed: ____________.
Find out policy for allowed time to remain in bladder. Too long may cause infections.)
IV site(s) where: ________________ when placed: ________________________________.
IV fluids (types and rates): ____,
____________________________, ____,
Is patient on oxygen: _____ yes, _____ no. If so, how much and route delivered (see oxygen routes): ____.
If patient on ventilator, list settings (see list on ventilator settings): ________
____.
Vital signs: temp ______, pulse ______, resp ______, b/p ______, o2 ______%,
current weight _____ pounds, _____ kg. Glucose level: ______
Insulin coverage: ____ yes, ____'no. Insulin type: ____________, # of units: _____.

NURSING CARE CONTINUED FOR ____________________________
DATE ____________________, DAY NUMBER ____________________

FOLLOWING EXAMINATIONS FOR DAY SHIFT:

Nurse ______________, CNA ______________, in at ______ am/pm. Left at _______ am/pm.
Wash hands and wear gloves before touching patient: _______ yes, _______ no.
Wash hands before leaving room: ___ yes, ___ no. Wear protective gear: __ yes, __ no.
Clean stethoscope: __ yes, __ no. Oral care: __ yes, __ no. Suctioned: __ yes, __ no.
Repositioned: ___ yes, ___ no. Turned to: ___ left, ___ right, ___ backside ___.
Head of bed at: ________ degrees. Incontinence/skin breakdown: ____ yes, ____ no.
Linens wet or soiled: _____ yes, _____ no. Linens changed: _____ yes, _____ no.
Dressing changed: ____ yes, ____ no. Location: ______________________________.
IV site checked: _____ yes, _____ no. IV tubing labeled: _____ yes, _____no.
IV fluids at: ____.
Pain level (0-10 scale.0-no pain, 10 intolerable): ____________________________.
Location of pain: ____________________. Medicated for pain: ____ yes, ____ no.
Patient is alert/oriented: ____ yes, ____ no. New confusion: ____ yes, ____ no.
Vital signs: temp ____, pulse _____, resp _____, b/p ______, 02 _____ %, ____ liters.
Glucose level: _____. Insulin: ___ yes, ___ no. Type: _______________ # of units ____.

Nurse ______________, CNA ______________, in at ______ am/pm. Left at _______ am/pm.
Wash hands and wear gloves before touching patient: _______ yes, _______ no.
Wash hands before leaving room: ___ yes, ___ no. Wear protective gear: __ yes, __ no.
Clean stethoscope: __ yes, __ no. Oral care: __ yes, __ no. Suctioned: __ yes, __ no.
Repositioned: ___ yes, ___ no. Turned to: ___ left, ___ right, ___ backside ___.
Head of bed at: ________ degrees. Incontinence/skin breakdown: ____ yes, ____ no.
Linens wet or soiled: _____ yes, _____ no. Linens changed: _____ yes, _____ no.
Dressing changed: ____ yes, ____ no. Location: ______________________________.
IV site checked: _____ yes, _____ no. IV tubing labeled: _____ yes, _____no.
IV fluids at: ____.
Pain level (0-10 scale.0-no pain, 10 intolerable): ____________________________.
Location of pain: ____________________. Medicated for pain: ____ yes, ____ no.
Patient is alert/oriented: ____ yes, ____ no. New confusion: ____ yes, ____ no.
Vital signs: temp ____, pulse _____, resp _____, b/p ______, 02 _____ %, ____ liters.
Glucose level: _____. Insulin: ___ yes, ___ no. Type: _______________ # of units ____.

Nurse ______________, CNA ______________, in at ______ am/pm. Left at _______ am/pm.
Wash hands and wear gloves before touching patient: _______ yes, _______ no.
Wash hands before leaving room: ___ yes, ___ no. Wear protective gear: __ yes, __ no.
Clean stethoscope: __ yes, __ no. Oral care: __ yes, __ no. Suctioned: __ yes, __ no.
Repositioned: ___ yes, ___ no. Turned to: ___ left, ___ right, ___ backside ___.
Head of bed at: ________ degrees. Incontinence/skin breakdown: ____ yes, ____ no.
Linens wet or soiled: _____ yes, _____ no. Linens changed: _____ yes, _____ no.
Dressing changed: ____ yes, ____ no. Location: ______________________________.
IV site checked: _____ yes, _____ no. IV tubing labeled: _____ yes, _____no.
IV fluids at: ____.
Pain level (0-10 scale.0-no pain, 10 intolerable): ____________________________.
Location of pain: ____________________. Medicated for pain: ____ yes, ____ no.
Patient is alert/oriented: ____ yes, ____ no. New confusion: ____ yes, ____ no.
Vital signs: temp ____, pulse _____, resp _____, b/p ______, 02 _____ %, ____ liters.
Glucose level: _____. Insulin: ___ yes, ___ no. Type: _______________ # of units ____.

NURSING CARE CONTINUED FOR ____________________
DATE ________________, DAY NUMBER ________________

FOLLOWING EXAMINATIONS FOR DAY SHIFT:

Nurse ____________, CNA ____________, in at ____ am/pm. Left at ____ am/pm.
Wash hands and wear gloves before touching patient: ____ yes, ____ no.
Wash hands before leaving room: ___ yes, ___ no. Wear protective gear: __ yes, __ no.
Clean stethoscope: __ yes, __ no. Oral care: __ yes, __ no. Suctioned: __ yes, __ no.
Repositioned: ___ yes, ___ no. Turned to: ___ left, ___ right, ___ backside ___.
Head of bed at: _______ degrees. Incontinence/skin breakdown: ___ yes, ___ no.
Linens wet or soiled: ____ yes, ____ no. Linens changed: ____ yes, ____ no.
Dressing changed: ____ yes, ____ no. Location: ____________________.
IV site checked: ____ yes, ____ no. IV tubing labeled: ____ yes, ____ no.
IV fluids at: ____.
Pain level (0-10 scale.0-no pain, 10 intolerable): ____________________.
Location of pain: ____________. Medicated for pain: ____ yes, ____ no.
Patient is alert/oriented: ____ yes, ____ no. New confusion: ____ yes, ____ no.
Vital signs: temp ____, pulse ____, resp ____, b/p ____, O2 ____%, ____ liters.
Glucose level: _____. Insulin: ___ yes, ___ no. Type: ________ # of units ____.

Nurse ____________, CNA ____________, in at ____ am/pm. Left at ____ am/pm.
Wash hands and wear gloves before touching patient: ____ yes, ____ no.
Wash hands before leaving room: ___ yes, ___ no. Wear protective gear: __ yes, __ no.
Clean stethoscope: __ yes, __ no. Oral care: __ yes, __ no. Suctioned: __ yes, __ no.
Repositioned: ___ yes, ___ no. Turned to: ___ left, ___ right, ___ backside ___.
Head of bed at: _______ degrees. Incontinence/skin breakdown: ___ yes, ___ no.
Linens wet or soiled: ____ yes, ____ no. Linens changed: ____ yes, ____ no.
Dressing changed: ____ yes, ____ no. Location: ____________________.
IV site checked: ____ yes, ____ no. IV tubing labeled: ____ yes, ____ no.
IV fluids at: ____.
Pain level (0-10 scale.0-no pain, 10 intolerable): ____________________.
Location of pain: ____________. Medicated for pain: ____ yes, ____ no.
Patient is alert/oriented: ____ yes, ____ no. New confusion: ____ yes, ____ no.
Vital signs: temp ____, pulse ____, resp ____, b/p ____, O2 ____%, ____ liters.
Glucose level: _____. Insulin: ___ yes, ___ no. Type: ________ # of units ____.

Nurse ____________, CNA ____________, in at ____ am/pm. Left at ____ am/pm.
Wash hands and wear gloves before touching patient: ____ yes, ____ no.
Wash hands before leaving room: ___ yes, ___ no. Wear protective gear: __ yes, __ no.
Clean stethoscope: __ yes, __ no. Oral care: __ yes, __ no. Suctioned: __ yes, __ no.
Repositioned: ___ yes, ___ no. Turned to: ___ left, ___ right, ___ backside ___.
Head of bed at: _______ degrees. Incontinence/skin breakdown: ___ yes, ___ no.
Linens wet or soiled: ____ yes, ____ no. Linens changed: ____ yes, ____ no.
Dressing changed: ____ yes, ____ no. Location: ____________________.
IV site checked: ____ yes, ____ no. IV tubing labeled: ____ yes, ____ no.
IV fluids at: ____.
Pain level (0-10 scale.0-no pain, 10 intolerable): ____________________.
Location of pain: ____________. Medicated for pain: ____ yes, ____ no.
Patient is alert/oriented: ____ yes, ____ no. New confusion: ____ yes, ____ no.
Vital signs: temp ____, pulse ____, resp ____, b/p ____, O2 ____%, ____ liters.
Glucose level: _____. Insulin: ___ yes, ___ no. Type: ________ # of units ____.

NURSING CARE FOR ______________________________

DATE ____________________, DAY NUMBER ______________________

INITIAL NIGHT SHIFT EXAM:

My nurse has _____ # of patients. CNA ___yes, ___no. Charge nurse ____________
Nurse ____________ RN/LPN came in at ________ am/pm. Left at _________ am/pm.
Did nurse wash hands and wear gloves before touching patient: ______ yes, ______ no.
Wash hands after touching patient and before leaving the room: ______ yes, ______ no.
Don't hesitate to request staff to wash their hands. This will help decrease the risk of spreading potentially lethal germs.
Did nurse wear protective gear (isolation precautions only): ______ yes, ______ no.
Did nurse provide oral care (to be done every two hours if unable to provide for self, also decreases risk of pneumonia, infections, and aspiration): ______ yes, ______ no.
If able to provide own oral care, then supplies at bedside: ______ yes, ______ no.
Was patient repositioned (every two hours if unable to turn self): _____ yes _____ no.
Head of bed at ________ degrees. This is important for patients on ventilators or on tube feedings. Anything less than thirty degrees places patients at risk for aspiration of stomach contents into the lungs causing aspiration pneumonia.
Checked for incontinence and skin breakdown: _____ yes, _____ no.
Patient's linens wet or soiled: _____ yes, ____ no. Linens changed: ____ yes, ____ no.
Time linens changed: _______ am/pm. Any skin redness or breakdown: ____ yes, ____ no.
If yes, what stage is pressure ulcer: ________. Acquired when: ______________.
List wounds not associated with pressure ulcers and how acquired: ____________
____.
Mattress type: ____.
Specialty mattresses are important to help prevent pressure ulcers)
If patient on ventilator or has tracheostomy, suction performed: _____ yes, _____ no.
Did nurse listen to lung sounds: _____ yes, _____ no.
Does patient have chest tubes: ____ yes, ____ no. Functioning _____ yes, _____ no.
Bowel sounds: ______ yes, ______ no. Bowel sounds active: ______ yes, ______ no.
Neurological exam: _____ yes, _____ no. Follow commands: ______ yes, ______ no.
Is patient alert and oriented to person, place, time, and events: _____ yes, _____ no.
If confused, patient is not oriented to: ___ person, ___ place, ___ time, ___ event.
Confusion began (time and date): ________________________________.
Glasgow coma scale (checks conscious scale of patient): ________________.
Intracranial pressure monitoring: _____ yes, _____ no.
If yes, pressure is at ________ mm mercury. (Normal is one to fifteen).
Moves extremities: ___ yes, ___ no.
Paralysis: (inability to move extremities) ______ yes, ______ no.
If yes, extremities affected and when paralysis began: ________________.
Is patient in pain: ____ yes, ____ no. Describe pain and location ____________.
Patient able to eat: ___ yes, ___ no. What type of diet? ____________________.
If patient on tube feedings list type: ____________ at __________ cc/ml per hour.
Nausea ____, vomiting ____. If so, describe: ______________________________.
Patient has: Nasal gastric tube _____, Dobhoff tube _____, Peg or gastric tube ____.
When was feeding tube placed and what site: ______________________________.
Catheter for draining urine: ___ yes, ___ no. If so, when placed: ____________.
Find out policy for allowed time to remain in bladder. Too long may cause infections.)
IV site(s) where: ______________________ when placed: ______________.
IV fluids (types and rates): ______________________, ______________________
______________________, ______________________, ______________________.
Is patient on oxygen: _____ yes, _____ no. If so, how much and route delivered
(see oxygen routes): ____.
If patient on ventilator, list settings (see list on ventilator settings): __________
____.
Vital signs: temp _____, pulse _____, resp _____, b/p _____, o2 _____%,
current weight _____ pounds, _____ kg. Glucose level: ______
Insulin coverage: ____ yes, ____ no. Insulin type: ____________, # of units: _____.

NURSING CARE CONTINUED FOR ____________________
DATE ____________________, DAY NUMBER ____________________

FOLLOWING EXAMINATIONS FOR NIGHT SHIFT:

Nurse ____________, CNA ____________, in at ______ am/pm. Left at _______ am/pm.
Wash hands and wear gloves before touching patient: _______ yes, _______ no.
Wash hands before leaving room: ___ yes, ___ no. Wear protective gear: __ yes, __ no.
Clean stethoscope: __ yes, __ no. Oral care: __ yes, __ no. Suctioned: __ yes, __ no.
Repositioned: ___ yes, ___ no. Turned to: ___ left, ___ right, ___ backside ___.
Head of bed at: _______ degrees. Incontinence/skin breakdown: ___ yes, ___ no.
Linens wet or soiled: _____ yes, _____ no. Linens changed: _____ yes, _____ no.
Dressing changed: ____ yes, ____ no. Location: ____________________.
IV site checked: _____ yes, _____ no. IV tubing labeled: _____ yes, _____ no.
IV fluids at: ____.
Pain level (0-10 scale.0-no pain, 10 intolerable): ____________________.
Location of pain: ____________. Medicated for pain: _____ yes, _____ no.
Patient is alert/oriented: ____ yes, ___ no. New confusion: ____ yes, ____ no.
Vital signs: temp ____, pulse _____, resp ______, b/p _______, 02 _____ %, _____ liters.
Glucose level: _____. Insulin: ___ yes, ___ no. Type: ____________ # of units ___.

Nurse ____________, CNA ____________, in at ______ am/pm. Left at _______ am/pm.
Wash hands and wear gloves before touching patient: _______ yes, _______ no.
Wash hands before leaving room: ___ yes, ___ no. Wear protective gear: __ yes, __ no.
Clean stethoscope: __ yes, __ no. Oral care: __ yes, __ no. Suctioned: __ yes, __ no.
Repositioned: ___ yes, ___ no. Turned to: ___ left, ___ right, ___ backside ___.
Head of bed at: _______ degrees. Incontinence/skin breakdown: ___ yes, ___ no.
Linens wet or soiled: _____ yes, _____ no. Linens changed: _____ yes, _____ no.
Dressing changed: ____ yes, ____ no. Location: ____________________.
IV site checked: _____ yes, _____ no. IV tubing labeled: _____ yes, _____ no.
IV fluids at: ____.
Pain level (0-10 scale.0-no pain, 10 intolerable): ____________________.
Location of pain: ____________. Medicated for pain: _____ yes, _____ no.
Patient is alert/oriented: ____ yes, ___ no. New confusion: ____ yes, ____ no.
Vital signs: temp ____, pulse _____, resp ______, b/p _______, 02 _____ %, _____ liters.
Glucose level: _____. Insulin: ___ yes, ___ no. Type: ____________ # of units ___.

Nurse ____________, CNA ____________, in at ______ am/pm. Left at _______ am/pm.
Wash hands and wear gloves before touching patient: _______ yes, _______ no.
Wash hands before leaving room: ___ yes, ___ no. Wear protective gear: __ yes, __ no.
Clean stethoscope: __ yes, __ no. Oral care: __ yes, __ no. Suctioned: __ yes, __ no.
Repositioned: ___ yes, ___ no. Turned to: ___ left, ___ right, ___ backside ___.
Head of bed at: _______ degrees. Incontinence/skin breakdown: ___ yes, ___ no.
Linens wet or soiled: _____ yes, _____ no. Linens changed: _____ yes, _____ no.
Dressing changed: ____ yes, ____ no. Location: ____________________.
IV site checked: _____ yes, _____ no. IV tubing labeled: _____ yes, _____ no.
IV fluids at: ____.
Pain level (0-10 scale.0-no pain, 10 intolerable): ____________________.
Location of pain: ____________. Medicated for pain: _____ yes, _____ no.
Patient is alert/oriented: ____ yes, ___ no. New confusion: ____ yes, ____ no.
Vital signs: temp ____, pulse _____, resp ______, b/p _______, 02 _____ %, _____ liters.
Glucose level: _____. Insulin: ___ yes, ___ no. Type: ____________ # of units ___.

NURSING CARE CONTINUED FOR ____________________
DATE ____________________, DAY NUMBER ____________________

FOLLOWING EXAMINATIONS FOR NIGHT SHIFT:

Nurse ____________, CNA ____________, in at _____ am/pm. Left at ______ am/pm.
Wash hands and wear gloves before touching patient: ______ yes, ______ no.
Wash hands before leaving room: ___ yes, ___ no. Wear protective gear: __ yes, __ no.
Clean stethoscope: __ yes, __ no. Oral care: __ yes, __ no. Suctioned: __ yes, __ no.
Repositioned: ___ yes, ___ no. Turned to: ___ left, ___ right, ___ backside ___.
Head of bed at: _______ degrees. Incontinence/skin breakdown: ____ yes, ____ no.
Linens wet or soiled: _____ yes, _____ no. Linens changed: _____ yes, _____ no.
Dressing changed: ____ yes, ____ no. Location: ____________________.
IV site checked: _____ yes, _____ no. IV tubing labeled: _____ yes, _____no.
IV fluids at: ____.
Pain level (0-10 scale.0-no pain, 10 intolerable): ____________________.
Location of pain: ______________. Medicated for pain: _____ yes, ___ no.
Patient is alert/oriented: ____ yes, ____ no. New confusion: ____ yes, ___ no.
Vital signs: temp ____, pulse _____, resp ______, b/p ______, 02 _____ %, ____ liters.
Glucose level: _____. Insulin: ___ yes, ___ no. Type: ____________ # of units ___.

Nurse ____________, CNA ____________, in at _____ am/pm. Left at ______ am/pm.
Wash hands and wear gloves before touching patient: ______ yes, ______ no.
Wash hands before leaving room: ___ yes, ___ no. Wear protective gear: __ yes, __ no.
Clean stethoscope: __ yes, __ no. Oral care: __ yes, __ no. Suctioned: __ yes, __ no.
Repositioned: ___ yes, ___ no. Turned to: ___ left, ___ right, ___ backside ___.
Head of bed at: _______ degrees. Incontinence/skin breakdown: ____ yes, ____ no.
Linens wet or soiled: _____ yes, _____ no. Linens changed: _____ yes, _____ no.
Dressing changed: ____ yes, ____ no. Location: ____________________.
IV site checked: _____ yes, _____ no. IV tubing labeled: _____ yes, _____no.
IV fluids at: ____.
Pain level (0-10 scale.0-no pain, 10 intolerable): ____________________.
Location of pain: ______________. Medicated for pain: _____ yes, ___ no.
Patient is alert/oriented: ____ yes, ____ no. New confusion: ____ yes, ___ no.
Vital signs: temp ____, pulse _____, resp ______, b/p ______, 02 _____ %, ____ liters.
Glucose level: _____. Insulin: ___ yes, ___ no. Type: ____________ # of units ___.

Nurse ____________, CNA ____________, in at _____ am/pm. Left at ______ am/pm.
Wash hands and wear gloves before touching patient: ______ yes, ______ no.
Wash hands before leaving room: ___ yes, ___ no. Wear protective gear: __ yes, __ no.
Clean stethoscope: __ yes, __ no. Oral care: __ yes, __ no. Suctioned: __ yes, __ no.
Repositioned: ___ yes, ___ no. Turned to: ___ left, ___ right, ___ backside ___.
Head of bed at: _______ degrees. Incontinence/skin breakdown: ____ yes, ____ no.
Linens wet or soiled: _____ yes, _____ no. Linens changed: _____ yes, _____ no.
Dressing changed: ____ yes, ____ no. Location: ____________________.
IV site checked: _____ yes, _____ no. IV tubing labeled: _____ yes, _____no.
IV fluids at: ____.
Pain level (0-10 scale.0-no pain, 10 intolerable): ____________________.
Location of pain: ______________. Medicated for pain: _____ yes, ___ no.
Patient is alert/oriented: ____ yes, ____ no. New confusion: ____ yes, ___ no.
Vital signs: temp ____, pulse _____, resp ______, b/p ______, 02 _____ %, ____ liters.
Glucose level: _____. Insulin: ___ yes, ___ no. Type: ____________ # of units ___.

MEDICATION ADMINISTRATION LIST FOR ____________________
DATE ________________ DAY NUMBER ____________________

List the medication for each day. Routes of administration: oral, thru feeding tube, intravenous (IV), intramuscular (IM), subcutaneous (SQ), epidural or a catheter in your spinal column, rectal, topical, eye drops, and ear drops.

Medication: ____________________ Route: ____________________ Time: ______________
Medication: ____________________ Route: ____________________ Time: ______________
Medication: ____________________ Route: ____________________ Time: ______________
Medication: ____________________ Route: ____________________ Time: ______________
Medication: ____________________ Route: ____________________ Time: ______________
Medication: ____________________ Route: ____________________ Time: ______________
Medication: ____________________ Route: ____________________ Time: ______________
Medication: ____________________ Route: ____________________ Time: ______________
Medication: ____________________ Route: ____________________ Time: ______________
Medication: ____________________ Route: ____________________ Time: ______________
Medication: ____________________ Route: ____________________ Time: ______________
Medication: ____________________ Route: ____________________ Time: ______________
Medication: ____________________ Route: ____________________ Time: ______________
Medication: ____________________ Route: ____________________ Time: ______________
Medication: ____________________ Route: ____________________ Time: ______________
Medication: ____________________ Route: ____________________ Time: ______________
Medication: ____________________ Route: ____________________ Time: ______________
Medication: ____________________ Route: ____________________ Time: ______________
Medication: ____________________ Route: ____________________ Time: ______________
Medication: ____________________ Route: ____________________ Time: ______________
Medication: ____________________ Route: ____________________ Time: ______________
Medication: ____________________ Route: ____________________ Time: ______________
Medication: ____________________ Route: ____________________ Time: ______________
Medication: ____________________ Route: ____________________ Time: ______________
Medication: ____________________ Route: ____________________ Time: ______________
Medication: ____________________ Route: ____________________ Time: ______________
Medication: ____________________ Route: ____________________ Time: ______________
Medication: ____________________ Route: ____________________ Time: ______________
Medication: ____________________ Route: ____________________ Time: ______________
Medication: ____________________ Route: ____________________ Time: ______________
Medication: ____________________ Route: ____________________ Time: ______________
Medication: ____________________ Route: ____________________ Time: ______________
Medication: ____________________ Route: ____________________ Time: ______________
Medication: ____________________ Route: ____________________ Time: ______________
Medication: ____________________ Route: ____________________ Time: ______________
Medication: ____________________ Route: ____________________ Time: ______________
Medication: ____________________ Route: ____________________ Time: ______________
Medication: ____________________ Route: ____________________ Time: ______________
Medication: ____________________ Route: ____________________ Time: ______________
Medication: ____________________ Route: ____________________ Time: ______________
Medication: ____________________ Route: ____________________ Time: ______________
Medication: ____________________ Route: ____________________ Time: ______________
Medication: ____________________ Route: ____________________ Time: ______________
Medication: ____________________ Route: ____________________ Time: ______________
Medication: ____________________ Route: ____________________ Time: ______________
Medication: ____________________ Route: ____________________ Time: ______________
Medication: ____________________ Route: ____________________ Time: ______________
Medication: ____________________ Route: ____________________ Time: ______________
Medication: ____________________ Route: ____________________ Time: ______________
Medication: ____________________ Route: ____________________ Time: ______________
Medication: ____________________ Route: ____________________ Time: ______________
Medication: ____________________ Route: ____________________ Time: ______________
Medication: ____________________ Route: ____________________ Time: ______________
Medication: ____________________ Route: ____________________ Time: ______________

NOTES FOR DAY NUMBER ______

DATE ______

MEDICAL JOURNAL FOR ______________________________

DATE ____________________, DAY NUMBER ______________

VISITS FROM MY DOCTORS TODAY

Goals for today: ____
____
____.

Things to discuss with my doctor(s): ____________________
____
____

Dr.____________ came in at ____ am/pm. Left at ____ am/pm.
We discussed ____.
Did doctor examine patient: _____ yes, _____ no.
Wash hands before touching patient: _____ yes, _____ no.
Wear gloves: ____ yes, ___ no. Clean stethoscope: ____ yes, ____ no.
Wear gown and mask (precautions only):____ yes, _____ no.
Wash hands before leaving the room: _____ yes, _____ no.

Dr.____________ came in at ____ am/pm. Left at ____ am/pm.
We discussed ____.
Did doctor examine patient: _____ yes, _____ no.
Wash hands before touching patient: _____ yes, _____ no.
Wear gloves: ____ yes, ___ no. Clean stethoscope: ____ yes, ____ no.
Wear gown and mask (precautions only):____ yes, _____ no.
Wash hands before leaving the room: _____ yes, _____ no.

Dr.____________ came in at ____ am/pm. Left at ____ am/pm.
We discussed ____.
Did doctor examine patient: _____ yes, _____ no.
Wash hands before touching patient: _____ yes, _____ no.
Wear gloves: ____ yes, ___ no. Clean stethoscope: ____ yes, ____ no.
Wear gown and mask (precautions only):____ yes, _____ no.
Wash hands before leaving the room: _____ yes, _____ no.

Dr.____________ came in at ____ am/pm. Left at ____ am/pm.
We discussed ____.
Did doctor examine patient: _____ yes, _____ no.
Wash hands before touching patient: _____ yes, _____ no.
Wear gloves: ____ yes, ___ no. Clean stethoscope: ____ yes, ____ no.
Wear gown and mask (precautions only):____ yes, _____ no.
Wash hands before leaving the room: _____ yes, _____ no.

Dr.____________ came in at ____ am/pm. Left at ____ am/pm.
We discussed ____.
Did doctor examine patient: _____ yes, _____ no.
Wash hands before touching patient: _____ yes, _____ no.
Wear gloves: ____ yes, ___ no. Clean stethoscope: ____ yes, ____ no.
Wear gown and mask (precautions only): ____ yes, _____ no.
Wash hands before leaving the room: _____ yes, _____ no.

NURSING CARE FOR ____________________

DATE ______________, DAY NUMBER ______________

INITIAL DAY SHIFT EXAM:

My nurse has _____ # of patients. CNA ___yes, ___no. Charge nurse _________
Nurse ____________ RN/LPN came in at ________ am/pm. Left at ________ am/pm.
Did nurse wash hands and wear gloves before touching patient: ______ yes, ______ no.
Wash hands after touching patient and before leaving the room: _____ yes, ______ no.
Don't hesitate to request staff to wash their hands. This will help decrease the risk of spreading potentially lethal germs.
Did nurse wear protective gear (isolation precautions only): ______ yes, ______ no.
Did nurse provide oral care (to be done every two hours if unable to provide for self, also decreases risk of pneumonia, infections, and aspiration): ______ yes, ______ no.
If able to provide own oral care, then supplies at bedside: ______ yes, ______ no.
Was patient repositioned (every two hours if unable to turn self): _____ yes _____ no.
Head of bed at ________ degrees. This is important for patients on ventilators or on tube feedings. Anything less than thirty degrees places patients at risk for aspiration of stomach contents into the lungs causing aspiration pneumonia.
Checked for incontinence and skin breakdown: _____ yes, _____ no.
Patient's linens wet or soiled: _____ yes, _____ no. Linens changed: ____ yes, ____ no.
Time linens changed: _______ am/pm. Any skin redness or breakdown: ____ yes, ____ no.
If yes, what stage is pressure ulcer: ________. Acquired when: __________.
List wounds not associated with pressure ulcers and how acquired: __________
____.
Mattress type: ______________________________________.
Specialty mattresses are important to help prevent pressure ulcers)
If patient on ventilator or has tracheostomy, suction performed: _____ yes, _____ no.
Did nurse listen to lung sounds: _____ yes, _____ no.
Does patient have chest tubes: ____ yes, ____ no. Functioning _____ yes, _____ no.
Bowel sounds: ______ yes, ______ no. Bowel sounds active: _____ yes, _____ no.
Neurological exam: _____ yes, _____ no. Follow commands: _____ yes, _____ no.
Is patient alert and oriented to person, place, time, and events: ____ yes, ____ no.
If confused, patient is not oriented to: ____ person, ___ place, ___ time, ___ event.
Confusion began (time and date): ______________________________.
Glasgow coma scale (checks conscious scale of patient): ____________________.
Intracranial pressure monitoring: _____ yes, _____ no.
If yes, pressure is at ________ mm mercury. (Normal is one to fifteen).
Moves extremities: ___ yes, ___ no.
Paralysis: (inability to move extremities) _______ yes, _______ no.
If yes, extremities affected and when paralysis began: ____________________.
Is patient in pain: ____ yes, ____ no. Describe pain and location ____________.
Patient able to eat: ____ yes, ____ no. What type of diet? ____________.
If patient on tube feedings list type: ____________ at __________ cc/ml per hour.
Nausea ____, vomiting _____. If so, describe: ____________________.
Patient has: Nasal gastric tube _____, Dobhoff tube _____, Peg or gastric tube _____.
When was feeding tube placed and what site: ____________________.
Catheter for draining urine: ____ yes, ____ no. If so, when placed: __________.
Find out policy for allowed time to remain in bladder. Too long may cause infections.)
IV site(s) where: ________________ when placed: ____________.
IV fluids (types and rates): ______________, ______________,
______________, ______________, ______________,
Is patient on oxygen: _____ yes, _____ no. If so, how much and route delivered (see oxygen routes): ______________________________.
If patient on ventilator, list settings (see list on ventilator settings): ______
____.
Vital signs: temp _____, pulse _____, resp _____, b/p _____, o2 _____%,
current weight _____ pounds, _____ kg. Glucose level: _____
Insulin coverage: ____ yes, ____ no. Insulin type: __________, # of units: _____.

NURSING CARE CONTINUED FOR ____________________
DATE ____________________, DAY NUMBER ____________________

FOLLOWING EXAMINATIONS FOR DAY SHIFT:

Nurse ____________, CNA ____________, in at _____ am/pm. Left at ______ am/pm.
Wash hands and wear gloves before touching patient: ______ yes, ____ no.
Wash hands before leaving room: ___ yes, ___ no. Wear protective gear: __ yes, __ no.
Clean stethoscope: __ yes, __ no. Oral care: __ yes, __ no. Suctioned: __ yes, __ no.
Repositioned: ___ yes, ___ no. Turned to: ___ left, ___ right, ___ backside ___.
Head of bed at: _____ degrees. Incontinence/skin breakdown: ____ yes, ____ no.
Linens wet or soiled: _____ yes, _____ no. Linens changed: _____ yes, _____ no.
Dressing changed: ____ yes, ____ no. Location: ____________________.
IV site checked: ____ yes, ____ no. IV tubing labeled: ____ yes, ____ no.
IV fluids at: ____.
Pain level (0-10 scale.0-no pain, 10 intolerable): ____________________.
Location of pain: ____________________. Medicated for pain: ____ yes, ____ no.
Patient is alert/oriented: ____ yes, ____ no. New confusion: ____ yes, ____ no.
Vital signs: temp ____, pulse ____, resp ____, b/p ____, 02 ____ %, ____ liters.
Glucose level: _____. Insulin: ___ yes, ___ no. Type: __________ # of units ____.

Nurse ____________, CNA ____________, in at _____ am/pm. Left at ______ am/pm.
Wash hands and wear gloves before touching patient: ______ yes, ____ no.
Wash hands before leaving room: ___ yes, ___ no. Wear protective gear: __ yes, __ no.
Clean stethoscope: __ yes, __ no. Oral care: __ yes, __ no. Suctioned: __ yes, __ no.
Repositioned: ___ yes, ___ no. Turned to: ___ left, ___ right, ___ backside ___.
Head of bed at: _____ degrees. Incontinence/skin breakdown: ____ yes, ____ no.
Linens wet or soiled: _____ yes, _____ no. Linens changed: _____ yes, _____ no.
Dressing changed: ____ yes, ____ no. Location: ____________________.
IV site checked: ____ yes, ____ no. IV tubing labeled: ____ yes, ____ no.
IV fluids at: ____.
Pain level (0-10 scale.0-no pain, 10 intolerable): ____________________.
Location of pain: ____________________. Medicated for pain: ____ yes, ____ no.
Patient is alert/oriented: ____ yes, ____ no. New confusion: ____ yes, ____ no.
Vital signs: temp ____, pulse ____, resp ____, b/p ____, 02 ____ %, ____ liters.
Glucose level: _____. Insulin: ___ yes, ___ no. Type: __________ # of units ____.

Nurse ____________, CNA ____________, in at _____ am/pm. Left at ______ am/pm.
Wash hands and wear gloves before touching patient: ______ yes, ____ no.
Wash hands before leaving room: ___ yes, ___ no. Wear protective gear: __ yes, __ no.
Clean stethoscope: __ yes, __ no. Oral care: __ yes, __ no. Suctioned: __ yes, __ no.
Repositioned: ___ yes, ___ no. Turned to: ___ left, ___ right, ___ backside ___.
Head of bed at: _____ degrees. Incontinence/skin breakdown: ____ yes, ____ no.
Linens wet or soiled: _____ yes, _____ no. Linens changed: _____ yes, _____ no.
Dressing changed: ____ yes, ____ no. Location: ____________________.
IV site checked: ____ yes, ____ no. IV tubing labeled: ____ yes, ____ no.
IV fluids at: ____.
Pain level (0-10 scale.0-no pain, 10 intolerable): ____________________.
Location of pain: ____________________. Medicated for pain: ____ yes, ____ no.
Patient is alert/oriented: ____ yes, ____ no. New confusion: ____ yes, ____ no.
Vital signs: temp ____, pulse ____, resp ____, b/p ____, 02 ____ %, ____ liters.
Glucose level: _____. Insulin: ___ yes, ___ no. Type: __________ # of units ____.

NURSING CARE CONTINUED FOR ____________________________
DATE ____________________, DAY NUMBER ______________________

FOLLOWING EXAMINATIONS FOR DAY SHIFT:

Nurse _____________, CNA _____________, in at _____ am/pm. Left at ______ am/pm.
Wash hands and wear gloves before touching patient: _______ yes, ______ no.
Wash hands before leaving room: ___ yes, ___ no. Wear protective gear: __ yes, __ no.
Clean stethoscope: __ yes, __ no. Oral care: __ yes, __ no. Suctioned: __ yes, __ no.
Repositioned: ___ yes, ___ no. Turned to: ___ left, ___ right, ___ backside ___.
Head of bed at: _______ degrees. Incontinence/skin breakdown: ____ yes, ____ no.
Linens wet or soiled: ____ yes, _____ no. Linens changed: _____ yes, ______ no.
Dressing changed: ____ yes, ____ no. Location: _________________________.
IV site checked: _____ yes, _____ no. IV tubing labeled: _____ yes, _____no.
IV fluids at: ____.
Pain level (0-10 scale.0-no pain, 10 intolerable): ________________.
Location of pain: ______________. Medicated for pain: ____ yes, ____ no.
Patient is alert/oriented: _____ yes, ____ no. New confusion: ____ yes, ____ no.
Vital signs: temp ____, pulse _____, resp ______, b/p ______, 02 _____ %, ____ liters.
Glucose level: _____. Insulin: ___ yes, ___ no. Type: ______________ # of units ____.

Nurse _____________, CNA _____________, in at _____ am/pm. Left at ______ am/pm.
Wash hands and wear gloves before touching patient: _______ yes, ______ no.
Wash hands before leaving room: ___ yes, ___ no. Wear protective gear: __ yes, __ no.
Clean stethoscope: __ yes, __ no. Oral care: __ yes, __ no. Suctioned: __ yes, __ no.
Repositioned: ___ yes, ___ no. Turned to: ___ left, ___ right, ___ backside ___.
Head of bed at: _______ degrees. Incontinence/skin breakdown: ____ yes, ____ no.
Linens wet or soiled: ____ yes, _____ no. Linens changed: _____ yes, ______ no.
Dressing changed: ____ yes, ____ no. Location: _________________________.
IV site checked: _____ yes, _____ no. IV tubing labeled: _____ yes, _____no.
IV fluids at: ____.
Pain level (0-10 scale.0-no pain, 10 intolerable): ________________.
Location of pain: ______________. Medicated for pain: ____ yes, ____ no.
Patient is alert/oriented: _____ yes, ____ no. New confusion: ____ yes, ____ no.
Vital signs: temp ____, pulse _____, resp ______, b/p ______, 02 _____ %, ____ liters.
Glucose level: _____. Insulin: ___ yes, ___ no. Type: ______________ # of units ____.

Nurse _____________, CNA _____________, in at _____ am/pm. Left at ______ am/pm.
Wash hands and wear gloves before touching patient: _______ yes, ______ no.
Wash hands before leaving room: ___ yes, ___ no. Wear protective gear: __ yes, __ no.
Clean stethoscope: __ yes, __ no. Oral care: __ yes, __ no. Suctioned: __ yes, __ no.
Repositioned: ___ yes, ___ no. Turned to: ___ left, ___ right, ___ backside ___.
Head of bed at: _______ degrees. Incontinence/skin breakdown: ____ yes, ____ no.
Linens wet or soiled: ____ yes, _____ no. Linens changed: _____ yes, ______ no.
Dressing changed: ____ yes, ____ no. Location: _________________________.
IV site checked: _____ yes, _____ no. IV tubing labeled: _____ yes, _____no.
IV fluids at: ____.
Pain level (0-10 scale.0-no pain, 10 intolerable): ________________.
Location of pain: ______________. Medicated for pain: ____ yes, ____ no.
Patient is alert/oriented: _____ yes, ____ no. New confusion: ____ yes, ____ no.
Vital signs: temp ____, pulse _____, resp ______, b/p ______, 02 _____ %, ____ liters.
Glucose level: _____. Insulin: ___ yes, ___ no. Type: ______________ # of units ____.

NURSING CARE FOR ______________________________

DATE ____________________, DAY NUMBER ____________________

INITIAL NIGHT SHIFT EXAM:

My nurse has ______ # of patients. CNA ___yes, ___no. Charge nurse _______________
Nurse ______________ RN/LPN came in at __________ am/pm. Left at __________ am/pm.
Did nurse wash hands and wear gloves before touching patient: ______ yes, ______ no.
Wash hands after touching patient and before leaving the room: ______ yes, ______ no.
Don't hesitate to request staff to wash their hands. This will help decrease the risk of spreading potentially lethal germs.
Did nurse wear protective gear (isolation precautions only): ________ yes, ______ no.
Did nurse provide oral care (to be done every two hours if unable to provide for self, also decreases risk of pneumonia, infections, and aspiration): ______ yes, ______ no.
If able to provide own oral care, then supplies at bedside: _______ yes, ______ no.
Was patient repositioned (every two hours if unable to turn self): _____ yes _____ no.
Head of bed at _________ degrees. This is important for patients on ventilators or on tube feedings. Anything less than thirty degrees places patients at risk for aspiration of stomach contents into the lungs causing aspiration pneumonia.
Checked for incontinence and skin breakdown: _____ yes, _____ no.
Patient's linens wet or soiled: _____yes, _____ no. Linens changed: ____ yes, ____ no.
Time linens changed: ________ am/pm. Any skin redness or breakdown: ____ yes, ____ no.
If yes, what stage is pressure ulcer: ______. Acquired when: ____________________.
List wounds not associated with pressure ulcers and how acquired: ______________
____.
Mattress type: ____.
Specialty mattresses are important to help prevent pressure ulcers)
If patient on ventilator or has tracheostomy, suction performed: _____ yes, _____ no.
Did nurse listen to lung sounds: _____ yes, _____ no.
Does patient have chest tubes: ____ yes, ____ no. Functioning _____ yes, _____ no.
Bowel sounds: ________ yes, ________ no. Bowel sounds active: ______ yes, ______ no.
Neurological exam: ______ yes, ______ no. Follow commands: _______ yes, ______ no.
Is patient alert and oriented to person, place, time, and events: _____yes, _____ no.
If confused, patient is not oriented to: ___ person, ___ place, ___ time, ___ event.
Confusion began (time and date): ____.
Glasgow coma scale (checks conscious scale of patient): __________________________.
Intracranial pressure monitoring: _____ yes, _____ no.
If yes, pressure is at ________ mm mercury. (Normal is one to fifteen).
Moves extremities: ___ yes, ___ no.
Paralysis: (inability to move extremities) ________ yes, ________ no.
If yes, extremities affected and when paralysis began: ___________________________.
Is patient in pain: ____ yes, ____ no. Describe pain and location _______________.
Patient able to eat: ____ yes, ____ no. What type of diet? ______________________.
If patient on tube feedings list type: _____________ at _____________ cc/ml per hour.
Nausea ____, vomiting ____ If so, describe: _____________________________________.
Patient has: Nasal gastric tube ______, Dobhoff tube _____, Peg or gastric tube _____.
When was feeding tube placed and what site: ____________________________________.
Catheter for draining urine: ____ yes, ____ no. If so, when placed: ______________.
Find out policy for allowed time to remain in bladder. Too long may cause infections.)
IV site(s) where: ____________________________ when placed: ____________________.
IV fluids (types and rates): _______________, _______________, _________________,
____________________, ____________________, ______________________________,
Is patient on oxygen: _____ yes, _____ no. If so, how much and route delivered (see oxygen routes): ____.
If patient on ventilator, list settings (see list on ventilator settings): __________
____.
Vital signs: temp ______, pulse ______, resp ______, b/p ______, o2 ______%,
current weight ______ pounds, ______ kg. Glucose level: ______
Insulin coverage: ____ yes, ____ no. Insulin type: _____________, # of units: ______.

NURSING CARE CONTINUED FOR ____________________________
DATE ____________________, DAY NUMBER ______________________

FOLLOWING EXAMINATIONS FOR NIGHT SHIFT:

Nurse ______________, CNA ______________, in at ______ am/pm. Left at _______ am/pm.
Wash hands and wear gloves before touching patient: ________ yes, ________ no.
Wash hands before leaving room: ___ yes, ___ no. Wear protective gear: __ yes, __ no.
Clean stethoscope: __ yes, __ no. Oral care: __ yes, __ no. Suctioned: __ yes, __ no.
Repositioned: ___ yes, ___ no. Turned to: ___ left, ___ right, ___ backside ___.
Head of bed at: ________ degrees. Incontinence/skin breakdown: ____ yes, ____ no.
Linens wet or soiled: _____ yes, _____ no. Linens changed: _____ yes, ______ no.
Dressing changed: ____ yes, ____ no. Location: ______________________________.
IV site checked: _____ yes, _____ no. IV tubing labeled: _____ yes, _____no.
IV fluids at: ____.
Pain level (0-10 scale.0-no pain, 10 intolerable): ________________________.
Location of pain: ______________. Medicated for pain: _____ yes, ____ no.
Patient is alert/oriented: ____ yes, ____ no. New confusion: ____ yes, ____ no.
Vital signs: temp ____, pulse _____, resp ______, b/p ______, 02 _____ %, ____ liters.
Glucose level: _____. Insulin: ___ yes, ___ no. Type: ______________ # of units ____.

Nurse ______________, CNA ______________, in at ______ am/pm. Left at _______ am/pm.
Wash hands and wear gloves before touching patient: ________ yes, ________ no.
Wash hands before leaving room: ___ yes, ___ no. Wear protective gear: __ yes, __ no.
Clean stethoscope: __ yes, __ no. Oral care: __ yes, __ no. Suctioned: __ yes, __ no.
Repositioned: ___ yes, ___ no. Turned to: ___ left, ___ right, ___ backside ___.
Head of bed at: ________ degrees. Incontinence/skin breakdown: ____ yes, ____ no.
Linens wet or soiled: _____ yes, _____ no. Linens changed: _____ yes, ______ no.
Dressing changed: ____ yes, ____ no. Location: ______________________________.
IV site checked: _____ yes, _____ no. IV tubing labeled: _____ yes, _____no.
IV fluids at: ____.
Pain level (0-10 scale.0-no pain, 10 intolerable): ________________________.
Location of pain: ______________. Medicated for pain: _____ yes, ____ no.
Patient is alert/oriented: ____ yes, ____ no. New confusion: ____ yes, ____ no.
Vital signs: temp ____, pulse _____, resp ______, b/p ______, 02 _____ %, ____ liters.
Glucose level: _____. Insulin: ___ yes, ___ no. Type: ______________ # of units ____.

Nurse ______________, CNA ______________, in at ______ am/pm. Left at _______ am/pm.
Wash hands and wear gloves before touching patient: ________ yes, ________ no.
Wash hands before leaving room: ___ yes, ___ no. Wear protective gear: __ yes, __ no.
Clean stethoscope: __ yes, __ no. Oral care: __ yes, __ no. Suctioned: __ yes, __ no.
Repositioned: ___ yes, ___ no. Turned to: ___ left, ___ right, ___ backside ___.
Head of bed at: ________ degrees. Incontinence/skin breakdown: ____ yes, ____ no.
Linens wet or soiled: _____ yes, _____ no. Linens changed: _____ yes, ______ no.
Dressing changed: ____ yes, ____ no. Location: ______________________________.
IV site checked: _____ yes, _____ no. IV tubing labeled: _____ yes, _____no.
IV fluids at: ____.
Pain level (0-10 scale.0-no pain, 10 intolerable): ________________________.
Location of pain: ______________. Medicated for pain: _____ yes, ____ no.
Patient is alert/oriented: ____ yes, ____ no. New confusion: ____ yes, ____ no.
Vital signs: temp ____, pulse _____, resp ______, b/p ______, 02 _____ %, ____ liters.
Glucose level: _____. Insulin: ___ yes, ___ no. Type: ______________ # of units ____.

NURSING CARE CONTINUED FOR ____________________
DATE ____________________, DAY NUMBER ____________________

FOLLOWING EXAMINATIONS FOR NIGHT SHIFT:

Nurse ____________, CNA ____________, in at _____ am/pm. Left at ______ am/pm.
Wash hands and wear gloves before touching patient: ______ yes, ______ no.
Wash hands before leaving room: ___ yes, ___ no. Wear protective gear: __ yes, __ no.
Clean stethoscope: __ yes, __ no. Oral care: __ yes, __ no. Suctioned: __ yes, __ no.
Repositioned: ___ yes, ___ no. Turned to: ___ left, ___ right, ___ backside ___.
Head of bed at: ________ degrees. Incontinence/skin breakdown: ____ yes, ____ no.
Linens wet or soiled: _____ yes, _____ no. Linens changed: _____ yes, _____ no.
Dressing changed: ____ yes, ____ no. Location: ____________________.
IV site checked: _____ yes, _____ no. IV tubing labeled: _____ yes, _____no.
IV fluids at: ____________________.
Pain level (0-10 scale.0-no pain, 10 intolerable): ____________.
Location of pain: ____________. Medicated for pain: ____ yes, ____ no.
Patient is alert/oriented: ____ yes, ____ no. New confusion: ____ yes, ____ no.
Vital signs: temp ____, pulse _____, resp _____, b/p ______, 02 _____ %, ____ liters.
Glucose level: _____. Insulin: ___ yes, ___ no. Type: ____________ # of units ____.

Nurse ____________, CNA ____________, in at _____ am/pm. Left at ______ am/pm.
Wash hands and wear gloves before touching patient: ______ yes, ______ no.
Wash hands before leaving room: ___ yes, ___ no. Wear protective gear: __ yes, __ no.
Clean stethoscope: __ yes, __ no. Oral care: __ yes, __ no. Suctioned: __ yes, __ no.
Repositioned: ___ yes, ___ no. Turned to: ___ left, ___ right, ___ backside ___.
Head of bed at: ________ degrees. Incontinence/skin breakdown: ____ yes, ____ no.
Linens wet or soiled: _____ yes, _____ no. Linens changed: _____ yes, _____ no.
Dressing changed: ____ yes, ____ no. Location: ____________________.
IV site checked: _____ yes, _____ no. IV tubing labeled: _____ yes, _____no.
IV fluids at: ____________________.
Pain level (0-10 scale.0-no pain, 10 intolerable): ____________.
Location of pain: ____________. Medicated for pain: ____ yes, ____ no.
Patient is alert/oriented: ____ yes, ____ no. New confusion: ____ yes, ____ no.
Vital signs: temp ____, pulse _____, resp _____, b/p ______, 02 _____ %, ____ liters.
Glucose level: _____. Insulin: ___ yes, ___ no. Type: ____________ # of units ____.

Nurse ____________, CNA ____________, in at _____ am/pm. Left at ______ am/pm.
Wash hands and wear gloves before touching patient: ______ yes, ______ no.
Wash hands before leaving room: ___ yes, ___ no. Wear protective gear: __ yes, __ no.
Clean stethoscope: __ yes, __ no. Oral care: __ yes, __ no. Suctioned: __ yes, __ no.
Repositioned: ___ yes, ___ no. Turned to: ___ left, ___ right, ___ backside ___.
Head of bed at: ________ degrees. Incontinence/skin breakdown: ____ yes, ____ no.
Linens wet or soiled: _____ yes, _____ no. Linens changed: _____ yes, _____ no.
Dressing changed: ____ yes, ____ no. Location: ____________________.
IV site checked: _____ yes, _____ no. IV tubing labeled: _____ yes, _____no.
IV fluids at: ____________________.
Pain level (0-10 scale.0-no pain, 10 intolerable): ____________.
Location of pain: ____________. Medicated for pain: ____ yes, ____ no.
Patient is alert/oriented: ____ yes, ____ no. New confusion: ____ yes, ____ no.
Vital signs: temp ____, pulse _____, resp _____, b/p ______, 02 _____ %, ____ liters.
Glucose level: _____. Insulin: ___ yes, ___ no. Type: ____________ # of units ____.

MEDICATION ADMINISTRATION LIST FOR ____________________
DATE ______________ DAY NUMBER ______________________

List the medication for each day. Routes of administration: oral, thru feeding tube, intravenous (IV), intramuscular (IM), subcutaneous (SQ), epidural or a catheter in your spinal column, rectal, topical, eye drops, and ear drops.

Medication: ______________ Route: ______________ Time: __________
Medication: ______________ Route: ______________ Time: __________
Medication: ______________ Route: ______________ Time: __________
Medication: ______________ Route: ______________ Time: __________
Medication: ______________ Route: ______________ Time: __________
Medication: ______________ Route: ______________ Time: __________
Medication: ______________ Route: ______________ Time: __________
Medication: ______________ Route: ______________ Time: __________
Medication: ______________ Route: ______________ Time: __________
Medication: ______________ Route: ______________ Time: __________
Medication: ______________ Route: ______________ Time: __________
Medication: ______________ Route: ______________ Time: __________
Medication: ______________ Route: ______________ Time: __________
Medication: ______________ Route: ______________ Time: __________
Medication: ______________ Route: ______________ Time: __________
Medication: ______________ Route: ______________ Time: __________
Medication: ______________ Route: ______________ Time: __________
Medication: ______________ Route: ______________ Time: __________
Medication: ______________ Route: ______________ Time: __________
Medication: ______________ Route: ______________ Time: __________
Medication: ______________ Route: ______________ Time: __________
Medication: ______________ Route: ______________ Time: __________
Medication: ______________ Route: ______________ Time: __________
Medication: ______________ Route: ______________ Time: __________
Medication: ______________ Route: ______________ Time: __________
Medication: ______________ Route: ______________ Time: __________
Medication: ______________ Route: ______________ Time: __________
Medication: ______________ Route: ______________ Time: __________
Medication: ______________ Route: ______________ Time: __________
Medication: ______________ Route: ______________ Time: __________
Medication: ______________ Route: ______________ Time: __________
Medication: ______________ Route: ______________ Time: __________
Medication: ______________ Route: ______________ Time: __________
Medication: ______________ Route: ______________ Time: __________
Medication: ______________ Route: ______________ Time: __________
Medication: ______________ Route: ______________ Time: __________
Medication: ______________ Route: ______________ Time: __________
Medication: ______________ Route: ______________ Time: __________
Medication: ______________ Route: ______________ Time: __________
Medication: ______________ Route: ______________ Time: __________
Medication: ______________ Route: ______________ Time: __________
Medication: ______________ Route: ______________ Time: __________
Medication: ______________ Route: ______________ Time: __________
Medication: ______________ Route: ______________ Time: __________
Medication: ______________ Route: ______________ Time: __________
Medication: ______________ Route: ______________ Time: __________
Medication: ______________ Route: ______________ Time: __________
Medication: ______________ Route: ______________ Time: __________
Medication: ______________ Route: ______________ Time: __________
Medication: ______________ Route: ______________ Time: __________
Medication: ______________ Route: ______________ Time: __________
Medication: ______________ Route: ______________ Time: __________
Medication: ______________ Route: ______________ Time: __________
Medication: ______________ Route: ______________ Time: __________

NOTES FOR DAY NUMBER ______________________

DATE ______________________

MEDICAL JOURNAL FOR ______________________________

DATE ____________________, DAY NUMBER _______________

VISITS FROM MY DOCTORS TODAY

Goals for today: ____

____

____.

Things to discuss with my doctor(s): ______________________________

____

____

Dr.____________ came in at ____ am/pm. Left at ____ am/pm.
We discussed ____.
Did doctor examine patient: ____ yes, ____ no.
Wash hands before touching patient: ____ yes, ____ no.
Wear gloves: ____ yes, ___ no. Clean stethoscope: ____ yes, ____ no.
Wear gown and mask (precautions only):____ yes, ____ no.
Wash hands before leaving the room: ____ yes, ____ no.

Dr.____________ came in at ____ am/pm. Left at ____ am/pm.
We discussed ____.
Did doctor examine patient: ____ yes, ____ no.
Wash hands before touching patient: ____ yes, ____ no.
Wear gloves: ____ yes, ___ no. Clean stethoscope: ____ yes, ____ no.
Wear gown and mask (precautions only):____ yes, ____ no.
Wash hands before leaving the room: ____ yes, ____ no.

Dr.____________ came in at ____ am/pm. Left at ____ am/pm.
We discussed ____.
Did doctor examine patient: ____ yes, ____ no.
Wash hands before touching patient: ____ yes, ____ no.
Wear gloves: ____ yes, ___ no. Clean stethoscope: ____ yes, ____ no.
Wear gown and mask (precautions only):____ yes, ____ no.
Wash hands before leaving the room: ____ yes, ____ no.

Dr.____________ came in at ____ am/pm. Left at ____ am/pm.
We discussed ____.
Did doctor examine patient: ____ yes, ____ no.
Wash hands before touching patient: ____ yes, ____ no.
Wear gloves: ____ yes, ___ no. Clean stethoscope: ____ yes, ____ no.
Wear gown and mask (precautions only):____ yes, ____ no.
Wash hands before leaving the room: ____ yes, ____ no.

Dr.____________ came in at ____ am/pm. Left at ____ am/pm.
We discussed ____.
Did doctor examine patient: ____ yes, ____ no.
Wash hands before touching patient: ____ yes, ____ no.
Wear gloves: ____ yes, ___ no. Clean stethoscope: ____ yes, ____ no.
Wear gown and mask (precautions only):____ yes, ____ no.
Wash hands before leaving the room: ____ yes, ____ no.

NURSING CARE FOR ______________________________

DATE ____________________, DAY NUMBER ________________

INITIAL DAY SHIFT EXAM:

My nurse has ______ # of patients. CNA ___yes, ___no. Charge nurse ________________
Nurse ______________ RN/LPN came in at __________ am/pm. Left at __________ am/pm.
Did nurse wash hands and wear gloves before touching patient: ______ yes, ______ no.
Wash hands after touching patient and before leaving the room: ______ yes, ______ no.
Don't hesitate to request staff to wash their hands. This will help decrease the risk of spreading potentially lethal germs.
Did nurse wear protective gear (isolation precautions only): ______ yes, ______ no.
Did nurse provide oral care (to be done every two hours if unable to provide for self, also decreases risk of pneumonia, infections, and aspiration): ______ yes, ______ no.
If able to provide own oral care, then supplies at bedside: ______ yes, ______ no.
Was patient repositioned (every two hours if unable to turn self): ______ yes ______ no.
Head of bed at ________ degrees. This is important for patients on ventilators or on tube feedings. Anything less than thirty degrees places patients at risk for aspiration of stomach contents into the lungs causing aspiration pneumonia.
Checked for incontinence and skin breakdown: ______ yes, ______ no.
Patient's linens wet or soiled: ______ yes, ______ no. Linens changed: ______ yes, ______ no.
Time linens changed: ________ am/pm. Any skin redness or breakdown: ______ yes, ______ no.
If yes, what stage is pressure ulcer: ______. Acquired when: ______________________.
List wounds not associated with pressure ulcers and how acquired: ____.
Mattress type: ____
Specialty mattresses are important to help prevent pressure ulcers)
If patient on ventilator or has tracheostomy, suction performed: ______ yes, ______ no.
Did nurse listen to lung sounds: ______ yes, ______ no.
Does patient have chest tubes: ______ yes, ______ no. Functioning ______ yes, ______ no.
Bowel sounds: ______ yes, ______ no. Bowel sounds active: ______ yes, ______ no.
Neurological exam: ______ yes, ______ no. Follow commands: ______ yes, ______ no.
Is patient alert and oriented to person, place, time, and events: ______ yes, ______ no.
If confused, patient is not oriented to: ___ person, ___ place, ___ time, ___ event.
Confusion began (time and date): ____.
Glasgow coma scale (checks conscious scale of patient): _________________________.
Intracranial pressure monitoring: ______ yes, ______ no.
If yes, pressure is at ________ mm mercury. (Normal is one to fifteen).
Moves extremities: ___ yes, ___ no.
Paralysis: (inability to move extremities) ______ yes, ______ no.
If yes, extremities affected and when paralysis began: ___________________________.
Is patient in pain: ____ yes, ____ no. Describe pain and location ______________________.
Patient able to eat: ____ yes, ____ no. What type of diet? ____________________________.
If patient on tube feedings list type: ______________ at ____________ cc/ml per hour.
Nausea ____, vomiting ____ If so, describe: ______________________________________.
Patient has: Nasal gastric tube ______, Dobhoff tube ______, Peg or gastric tube ______.
When was feeding tube placed and what site: ____________________________________.
Catheter for draining urine: ____ yes, ____ no. If so, when placed: ______________.
Find out policy for allowed time to remain in bladder. Too long may cause infections.)
IV site(s) where: __________________________ when placed: _____________________.
IV fluids (types and rates): ______________________, ______________________, ______________________, ______________________, ______________________.
Is patient on oxygen: ______ yes, ______ no. If so, how much and route delivered (see oxygen routes): ____.
If patient on ventilator, list settings (see list on ventilator settings): __________ ____.
Vital signs: temp ______, pulse ______, resp ______, b/p ______, o2 ______%,
current weight ______ pounds, ______ kg. Glucose level: ______
Insulin coverage: ____ yes, ____ no. Insulin type: ____________, # of units: ______.

NURSING CARE CONTINUED FOR ______________________
DATE ______________, DAY NUMBER ______________

FOLLOWING EXAMINATIONS FOR DAY SHIFT:

Nurse ____________, CNA ____________, in at _____ am/pm. Left at ______ am/pm.
Wash hands and wear gloves before touching patient: ______ yes, ______ no.
Wash hands before leaving room: ___ yes, ___ no. Wear protective gear: __ yes, __ no.
Clean stethoscope: __ yes, __ no. Oral care: __ yes, __ no. Suctioned: __ yes, __ no.
Repositioned: ___ yes, ___ no. Turned to: ___ left, ___ right, ___ backside ___.
Head of bed at: _______ degrees. Incontinence/skin breakdown: ____ yes, ___ no.
Linens wet or soiled: _____ yes, _____ no. Linens changed: _____ yes, ______ no.
Dressing changed: ____ yes, ____ no. Location: ______________________.
IV site checked: _____ yes, _____ no. IV tubing labeled: _____ yes, _____no.
IV fluids at: ____.
Pain level (0-10 scale.0-no pain, 10 intolerable): ______________________.
Location of pain: ______________. Medicated for pain: _____ yes, ___ no.
Patient is alert/oriented: ____ yes, ____ no. New confusion: ____ yes, ___ no.
Vital signs: temp ____, pulse _____, resp _____, b/p _____, 02 ____ %, ____ liters.
Glucose level: _____. Insulin: ___ yes, ___ no. Type: ___________ # of units ___.

Nurse ____________, CNA ____________, in at _____ am/pm. Left at ______ am/pm.
Wash hands and wear gloves before touching patient: ______ yes, ______ no.
Wash hands before leaving room: ___ yes, ___ no. Wear protective gear: __ yes, __ no.
Clean stethoscope: __ yes, __ no. Oral care: __ yes, __ no. Suctioned: __ yes, __ no.
Repositioned: ___ yes, ___ no. Turned to: ___ left, ___ right, ___ backside ___.
Head of bed at: _______ degrees. Incontinence/skin breakdown: ____ yes, ___ no.
Linens wet or soiled: _____ yes, _____ no. Linens changed: _____ yes, ______ no.
Dressing changed: ____ yes, ____ no. Location: ______________________.
IV site checked: _____ yes, _____ no. IV tubing labeled: _____ yes, _____no.
IV fluids at: ____.
Pain level (0-10 scale.0-no pain, 10 intolerable): ______________________.
Location of pain: ______________. Medicated for pain: _____ yes, ___ no.
Patient is alert/oriented: ____ yes, ____ no. New confusion: ____ yes, ___ no.
Vital signs: temp ____, pulse _____, resp _____, b/p _____, 02 ____ %, ____ liters.
Glucose level: _____. Insulin: ___ yes, ___ no. Type: ___________ # of units ___.

Nurse ____________, CNA ____________, in at _____ am/pm. Left at ______ am/pm.
Wash hands and wear gloves before touching patient: ______ yes, ______ no.
Wash hands before leaving room: ___ yes, ___ no. Wear protective gear: __ yes, __ no.
Clean stethoscope: __ yes, __ no. Oral care: __ yes, __ no. Suctioned: __ yes, __ no.
Repositioned: ___ yes, ___ no. Turned to: ___ left, ___ right, ___ backside ___.
Head of bed at: _______ degrees. Incontinence/skin breakdown: ____ yes, ___ no.
Linens wet or soiled: _____ yes, _____ no. Linens changed: _____ yes, ______ no.
Dressing changed: ____ yes, ____ no. Location: ______________________.
IV site checked: _____ yes, _____ no. IV tubing labeled: _____ yes, _____no.
IV fluids at: ____.
Pain level (0-10 scale.0-no pain, 10 intolerable): ______________________.
Location of pain: ______________. Medicated for pain: _____ yes, ___ no.
Patient is alert/oriented: ____ yes, ____ no. New confusion: ____ yes, ___ no.
Vital signs: temp ____, pulse _____, resp _____, b/p _____, 02 ____ %, ____ liters.
Glucose level: _____. Insulin: ___ yes, ___ no. Type: ___________ # of units ___.

NURSING CARE CONTINUED FOR ______________________________
DATE __________________, DAY NUMBER ________________

FOLLOWING EXAMINATIONS FOR DAY SHIFT:

Nurse ___________, CNA ____________, in at ______ am/pm. Left at _______ am/pm.
Wash hands and wear gloves before touching patient: ______ yes, ______ no.
Wash hands before leaving room: ___ yes, ___ no. Wear protective gear: __ yes, __ no.
Clean stethoscope: __ yes, __ no. Oral care: __ yes, __ no. Suctioned: __ yes, __ no.
Repositioned: ___ yes, ___ no. Turned to: ___ left, ___ right, ___ backside ___.
Head of bed at: ________ degrees. Incontinence/skin breakdown: ______ yes, ____ no.
Linens wet or soiled: _____ yes, ____ no. Linens changed: _____ yes, ____ no.
Dressing changed: ____ yes, _____ no. Location: ______________________________.
IV site checked: _____ yes, _____ no. IV tubing labeled: _____ yes, _____ no.
IV fluids at: ____.
Pain level (0-10 scale.0-no pain, 10 intolerable): ___________________________.
Location of pain: ____________. Medicated for pain: _______ yes, ____ no.
Patient is alert/oriented: ____ yes, ____ no. New confusion: ____ yes, ____ no.
Vital signs: temp ____, pulse _____, resp _____, b/p _____, 02 _____ %, _____ liters.
Glucose level: _____. Insulin: ___ yes, ___ no. Type: ___________ # of units _____.

Nurse ______________, CNA ____________, in at ______ am/pm. Left at _______ am/pm.
Wash hands and wear gloves before touching patient: ______ yes, ______ no.
Wash hands before leaving room: ___ yes, ___ no. Wear protective gear: __ yes, __ no.
Clean stethoscope: __ yes, __ no. Oral care: __ yes, __ no. Suctioned: __ yes, __ no.
Repositioned: ___ yes, ___ no. Turned to: ___ left, ___ right, ___ backside ___.
Head of bed at: ______ degrees. Incontinence/skin breakdown: ______ yes, ____ no.
Linens wet or soiled: _____ yes, ____ no. Linens changed: _____ yes, ____ no.
Dressing changed: ____ yes, _____ no. Location: ______________________________.
IV site checked: _____ yes, _____ no. IV tubing labeled: _____ yes, _____ no.
IV fluids at: ____.
Pain level (0-10 scale.0-no pain, 10 intolerable): ___________________________.
Location of pain: ____________. Medicated for pain: _______ yes, ____ no.
Patient is alert/oriented: ____ yes, ____ no. New confusion: ____ yes, ____ no.
Vital signs: temp ____, pulse _____, resp _____, b/p _____, 02 _____ %, _____ liters.
Glucose level: _____. Insulin: ___ yes, ___ no. Type: ___________ # of units _____.

Nurse ______________, CNA ______________, in at _____ am/pm. Left at _____ am/pm.
Wash hands and wear gloves before touching patient: ______ yes, ______ no.
Wash hands before leaving room: ___ yes, ___ no. Wear protective gear: __ yes, __ no.
Clean stethoscope: __ yes, __ no. Oral care: __ yes, __ no. Suctioned: __ yes, __ no.
Repositioned: ___ yes, ___ no. Turned to: ___ left, ___ right, ___ backside ___.
Head of bed at: ______ degrees. Incontinence/skin breakdown: ______ yes, ____ no.
Linens wet or soiled: _____ yes, ____ no. Linens changed: _____ yes, ____ no.
Dressing changed: ____ yes, _____ no. Location: ______________________________.
IV site checked: _____ yes, _____ no. IV tubing labeled: _____ yes, _____ no.
IV fluids at: ____.
Pain level (0-10 scale.0-no pain, 10 intolerable): ___________________________.
Location of pain: ____________. Medicated for pain: _____ yes, ____ no.
Patient is alert/oriented: ____ yes, ____ no. New confusion: ____ yes, ____ no.
Vital signs: temp ____, pulse _____, resp _____, b/p ______, 02 _____ %, _____ liters.
Glucose level: _____. Insulin: ___ yes, ___ no. Type: ______________ # of units _____.

NURSING CARE FOR ______________________________

DATE ____________________, DAY NUMBER ____________________

INITIAL NIGHT SHIFT EXAM:

My nurse has ______ # of patients. CNA ___yes, ___no. Charge nurse ________________
Nurse ________________ RN/LPN came in at __________ am/pm. Left at __________ am/pm.
Did nurse wash hands and wear gloves before touching patient: _______ yes, _______ no.
Wash hands after touching patient and before leaving the room: _______ yes, _______ no.
Don't hesitate to request staff to wash their hands. This will help decrease the risk of spreading potentially lethal germs.
Did nurse wear protective gear (isolation precautions only): _______ yes, _______ no.
Did nurse provide oral care (to be done every two hours if unable to provide for self, also decreases risk of pneumonia, infections, and aspiration): _______ yes, _______ no.
If able to provide own oral care, then supplies at bedside: ________ yes, ________ no.
Was patient repositioned (every two hours if unable to turn self): _____ yes _____ no.
Head of bed at ________ degrees. This is important for patients on ventilators or on tube feedings. Anything less than thirty degrees places patients at risk for aspiration of stomach contents into the lungs causing aspiration pneumonia.
Checked for incontinence and skin breakdown: _____ yes, _____ no.
Patient's linens wet or soiled: _____ yes, _____ no. Linens changed: ____ yes, ____ no.
Time linens changed: _______ am/pm. Any skin redness or breakdown: ____ yes, ____ no.
If yes, what stage is pressure ulcer: _______. Acquired when: ________________.
List wounds not associated with pressure ulcers and how acquired: ____________
____.
Mattress type: ____.
Specialty mattresses are important to help prevent pressure ulcers)
If patient on ventilator or has tracheostomy, suction performed: _____ yes, _____ no.
Did nurse listen to lung sounds: _____ yes, _____ no.
Does patient have chest tubes: ____ yes, ____ no. Functioning _____ yes, _____ no.
Bowel sounds: _______ yes, _______ no. Bowel sounds active: ______ yes, _______ no.
Neurological exam: ______ yes, ______ no. Follow commands: _______ yes, _______ no.
Is patient alert and oriented to person, place, time, and events: _____ yes, _____ no.
If confused, patient is not oriented to: ____ person, ___ place, ___ time, ___ event.
Confusion began (time and date): ______________________________________.
Glasgow coma scale (checks conscious scale of patient): ____________________.
Intracranial pressure monitoring: ______ yes, ______ no.
If yes, pressure is at ________ mm mercury. (Normal is one to fifteen).
Moves extremities: ___ yes, ___ no.
Paralysis: (inability to move extremities) _______ yes, _______ no.
If yes, extremities affected and when paralysis began: ____________________.
Is patient in pain: ____ yes, ____ no. Describe pain and location _____________.
Patient able to eat: ____ yes, ____ no. What type of diet? ____________________.
If patient on tube feedings list type: ____________ at ____________ cc/ml per hour.
Nausea ____, vomiting ____. If so, describe: ______________________________.
Patient has: Nasal gastric tube ______, Dobhoff tube _____, Peg or gastric tube _____.
When was feeding tube placed and what site: ______________________________.
Catheter for draining urine: ____ yes, ____ no. If so, when placed: ____________.
Find out policy for allowed time to remain in bladder. Too long may cause infections.)
IV site(s) where: ______________________ when placed: ____________________.
IV fluids (types and rates): ____________________, ____________________,
____________________, ____________________, ____________________,
Is patient on oxygen: _____ yes, _____ no. If so, how much and route delivered (see oxygen routes): ____.
If patient on ventilator, list settings (see list on ventilator settings): __________
____.
Vital signs: temp ______, pulse ______, resp ______, b/p ______, o2 ______%,
current weight ______ pounds, ______ kg. Glucose level: ______
Insulin coverage: ____ yes, ____ no. Insulin type: ____________, # of units: ______.

NURSING CARE CONTINUED FOR ____________________
DATE ____________________, DAY NUMBER ____________________

FOLLOWING EXAMINATIONS FOR NIGHT SHIFT:

Nurse ____________, CNA ____________, in at ______ am/pm. Left at ______ am/pm.
Wash hands and wear gloves before touching patient: ______ yes, ______ no.
Wash hands before leaving room: ___ yes, ___ no. Wear protective gear: __ yes, __ no.
Clean stethoscope: __ yes, __ no. Oral care: __ yes, __ no. Suctioned: __ yes, __ no.
Repositioned: ___ yes, ___ no. Turned to: ___ left, ___ right, ___ backside ___.
Head of bed at: ________ degrees. Incontinence/skin breakdown: ____ yes, ____ no.
Linens wet or soiled: ____ yes, ____ no. Linens changed: ____ yes, ____ no.
Dressing changed: ____ yes, ____ no. Location: ____________________.
IV site checked: _____ yes, _____ no. IV tubing labeled: _____ yes, _____no.
IV fluids at: ____.
Pain level (0-10 scale.0-no pain, 10 intolerable): ____________________.
Location of pain: ____________. Medicated for pain: ____ yes, ____ no.
Patient is alert/oriented: ____ yes, ____ no. New confusion: ____yes, ____ no.
Vital signs: temp ____, pulse ____, resp ______, b/p ______, 02 ____ %, ___ liters.
Glucose level: _____. Insulin: ___ yes, ___ no. Type: ____________ # of units ___.

Nurse ____________, CNA ____________, in at ______ am/pm. Left at ______ am/pm.
Wash hands and wear gloves before touching patient: ______ yes, ______ no.
Wash hands before leaving room: ___ yes, ___ no. Wear protective gear: __ yes, __ no.
Clean stethoscope: __ yes, __ no. Oral care: __ yes, __ no. Suctioned: __ yes, __ no.
Repositioned: ___ yes, ___ no. Turned to: ___ left, ___ right, ___ backside ___.
Head of bed at: ________ degrees. Incontinence/skin breakdown: ____ yes, ____ no.
Linens wet or soiled: ____ yes, ____ no. Linens changed: ____ yes, ____ no.
Dressing changed: ____ yes, ____ no. Location: ____________________.
IV site checked: _____ yes, _____ no. IV tubing labeled: _____ yes, _____no.
IV fluids at: ____.
Pain level (0-10 scale.0-no pain, 10 intolerable): ____________________.
Location of pain: ____________. Medicated for pain: ____ yes, ____ no.
Patient is alert/oriented: ____ yes, ____ no. New confusion: ____yes, ____ no.
Vital signs: temp ____, pulse ____, resp ______, b/p ______, 02 ____ %, ___ liters.
Glucose level: _____. Insulin: ___ yes, ___ no. Type: ____________ # of units ___.

Nurse ____________, CNA ____________, in at ______ am/pm. Left at ______ am/pm.
Wash hands and wear gloves before touching patient: ______ yes, ______ no.
Wash hands before leaving room: ___ yes, ___ no. Wear protective gear: __ yes, __ no.
Clean stethoscope: __ yes, __ no. Oral care: __ yes, __ no. Suctioned: __ yes, __ no.
Repositioned: ___ yes, ___ no. Turned to: ___ left, ___ right, ___ backside ___.
Head of bed at: ________ degrees. Incontinence/skin breakdown: ____ yes, ____ no.
Linens wet or soiled: ____ yes, ____ no. Linens changed: ____ yes, ____ no.
Dressing changed: ____ yes, ____ no. Location: ____________________.
IV site checked: _____ yes, _____ no. IV tubing labeled: _____ yes, _____no.
IV fluids at: ____.
Pain level (0-10 scale.0-no pain, 10 intolerable): ____________________.
Location of pain: ____________. Medicated for pain: ____ yes, ____ no.
Patient is alert/oriented: ____ yes, ____ no. New confusion: ____yes, ____ no.
Vital signs: temp ____, pulse ____, resp ______, b/p ______, 02 ____ %, ___ liters.
Glucose level: _____. Insulin: ___ yes, ___ no. Type: ____________ # of units ___.

NURSING CARE CONTINUED FOR ____________________________
DATE __________________, DAY NUMBER ___________________

FOLLOWING EXAMINATIONS FOR NIGHT SHIFT:

Nurse ____________, CNA ____________, in at _____ am/pm. Left at ______ am/pm.
Wash hands and wear gloves before touching patient: _______ yes, _______ no.
Wash hands before leaving room: ___ yes, ___ no. Wear protective gear: __ yes, __ no.
Clean stethoscope: __ yes, __ no. Oral care: __ yes, __ no. Suctioned: __ yes, __ no.
Repositioned: ___ yes, ___ no. Turned to: ___ left, ___ right, ___ backside ___.
Head of bed at: ______ degrees. Incontinence/skin breakdown: ____ yes, ____ no.
Linens wet or soiled: ____ yes, _____ no. Linens changed: _____ yes, _____ no.
Dressing changed: ____ yes, ____ no. Location: ____________________________.
IV site checked: _____ yes, _____ no. IV tubing labeled: _____ yes, _____no.
IV fluids at: ____.
Pain level (0-10 scale.0-no pain, 10 intolerable): _________________________.
Location of pain: ________________. Medicated for pain: _____ yes, ____ no.
Patient is alert/oriented: ____ yes, ____ no. New confusion: ____ yes, ____ no.
Vital signs: temp ____, pulse ____, resp _____, b/p _____, 02 _____ %, ____ liters.
Glucose level: _____. Insulin: ___ yes, ___ no. Type: ___________ # of units ____.

Nurse ____________, CNA ____________, in at _____ am/pm. Left at ______ am/pm.
Wash hands and wear gloves before touching patient: _______ yes, _______ no.
Wash hands before leaving room: ___ yes, ___ no. Wear protective gear: __ yes, __ no.
Clean stethoscope: __ yes, __ no. Oral care: __ yes, __ no. Suctioned: __ yes, __ no.
Repositioned: ___ yes, ___ no. Turned to: ___ left, ___ right, ___ backside ___.
Head of bed at: ______ degrees. Incontinence/skin breakdown: ____ yes, ____ no.
Linens wet or soiled: ____ yes, _____ no. Linens changed: _____ yes, _____ no.
Dressing changed: ____ yes, ____ no. Location: ____________________________.
IV site checked: _____ yes, _____ no. IV tubing labeled: _____ yes, _____no.
IV fluids at: ____.
Pain level (0-10 scale.0-no pain, 10 intolerable): _________________________.
Location of pain: ________________. Medicated for pain: _____ yes, ____ no.
Patient is alert/oriented: ____ yes, ____ no. New confusion: ____ yes, ____ no.
Vital signs: temp ____, pulse ____, resp _____, b/p _____, 02 _____ %, ____ liters.
Glucose level: _____. Insulin: ___ yes, ___ no. Type: ___________ # of units ____.

Nurse ____________, CNA ____________, in at _____ am/pm. Left at ______ am/pm.
Wash hands and wear gloves before touching patient: _______ yes, _______ no.
Wash hands before leaving room: ___ yes, ___ no. Wear protective gear: __ yes, __ no.
Clean stethoscope: __ yes, __ no. Oral care: __ yes, __ no. Suctioned: __ yes, __ no.
Repositioned: ___ yes, ___ no. Turned to: ___ left, ___ right, ___ backside ___.
Head of bed at: ______ degrees. Incontinence/skin breakdown: ____ yes, ____ no.
Linens wet or soiled: ____ yes, _____ no. Linens changed: _____ yes, _____ no.
Dressing changed: ____ yes, ____ no. Location: ____________________________.
IV site checked: _____ yes, _____ no. IV tubing labeled: _____ yes, _____no.
IV fluids at: ____.
Pain level (0-10 scale.0-no pain, 10 intolerable): _________________________.
Location of pain: ________________. Medicated for pain: _____ yes, ____ no.
Patient is alert/oriented: ____ yes, ____ no. New confusion: ____ yes, ____ no.
Vital signs: temp ____, pulse ____, resp _____, b/p _____, 02 _____ %, ____ liters.
Glucose level: _____. Insulin: ___ yes, ___ no. Type: ___________ # of units ____.

MEDICATION ADMINISTRATION LIST FOR ____________________
DATE ______________ DAY NUMBER ____________________

List the medication for each day. Routes of administration: oral, thru feeding tube, intravenous (IV), intramuscular (IM), subcutaneous (SQ), epidural or a catheter in your spinal column, rectal, topical, eye drops, and ear drops.

Medication: ______________ Route: ______________ Time: ______________
Medication: ______________ Route: ______________ Time: ______________
Medication: ______________ Route: ______________ Time: ______________
Medication: ______________ Route: ______________ Time: ______________
Medication: ______________ Route: ______________ Time: ______________
Medication: ______________ Route: ______________ Time: ______________
Medication: ______________ Route: ______________ Time: ______________
Medication: ______________ Route: ______________ Time: ______________
Medication: ______________ Route: ______________ Time: ______________
Medication: ______________ Route: ______________ Time: ______________
Medication: ______________ Route: ______________ Time: ______________
Medication: ______________ Route: ______________ Time: ______________
Medication: ______________ Route: ______________ Time: ______________
Medication: ______________ Route: ______________ Time: ______________
Medication: ______________ Route: ______________ Time: ______________
Medication: ______________ Route: ______________ Time: ______________
Medication: ______________ Route: ______________ Time: ______________
Medication: ______________ Route: ______________ Time: ______________
Medication: ______________ Route: ______________ Time: ______________
Medication: ______________ Route: ______________ Time: ______________
Medication: ______________ Route: ______________ Time: ______________
Medication: ______________ Route: ______________ Time: ______________
Medication: ______________ Route: ______________ Time: ______________
Medication: ______________ Route: ______________ Time: ______________
Medication: ______________ Route: ______________ Time: ______________
Medication: ______________ Route: ______________ Time: ______________
Medication: ______________ Route: ______________ Time: ______________
Medication: ______________ Route: ______________ Time: ______________
Medication: ______________ Route: ______________ Time: ______________
Medication: ______________ Route: ______________ Time: ______________
Medication: ______________ Route: ______________ Time: ______________
Medication: ______________ Route: ______________ Time: ______________
Medication: ______________ Route: ______________ Time: ______________
Medication: ______________ Route: ______________ Time: ______________
Medication: ______________ Route: ______________ Time: ______________
Medication: ______________ Route: ______________ Time: ______________
Medication: ______________ Route: ______________ Time: ______________
Medication: ______________ Route: ______________ Time: ______________
Medication: ______________ Route: ______________ Time: ______________
Medication: ______________ Route: ______________ Time: ______________
Medication: ______________ Route: ______________ Time: ______________
Medication: ______________ Route: ______________ Time: ______________
Medication: ______________ Route: ______________ Time: ______________
Medication: ______________ Route: ______________ Time: ______________
Medication: ______________ Route: ______________ Time: ______________
Medication: ______________ Route: ______________ Time: ______________
Medication: ______________ Route: ______________ Time: ______________
Medication: ______________ Route: ______________ Time: ______________
Medication: ______________ Route: ______________ Time: ______________
Medication: ______________ Route: ______________ Time: ______________
Medication: ______________ Route: ______________ Time: ______________
Medication: ______________ Route: ______________ Time: ______________
Medication: ______________ Route: ______________ Time: ______________
Medication: ______________ Route: ______________ Time: ______________

NOTES FOR DAY NUMBER ______________________________

DATE ______________________________

MEDICAL JOURNAL FOR ______________________________

DATE ____________________, DAY NUMBER ______________

VISITS FROM MY DOCTORS TODAY

Goals for today: ____
____
____.

Things to discuss with my doctor(s): ____________________
____
____

Dr.____________ came in at ____ am/pm. Left at ____ am/pm.
We discussed ____.
Did doctor examine patient: ____ yes, ____ no.
Wash hands before touching patient: ____ yes, ____ no.
Wear gloves: ____ yes, ___ no. Clean stethoscope: ____ yes, ____ no.
Wear gown and mask (precautions only):____ yes, ____ no.
Wash hands before leaving the room: ____ yes, ____ no.

Dr.____________ came in at ____ am/pm. Left at ____ am/pm.
We discussed ____.
Did doctor examine patient: ____ yes, ____ no.
Wash hands before touching patient: ____ yes, ____ no.
Wear gloves: ____ yes, ___ no. Clean stethoscope: ____ yes, ____ no.
Wear gown and mask (precautions only):____ yes, ____ no.
Wash hands before leaving the room: ____ yes, ____ no.

Dr.____________ came in at ____ am/pm. Left at ____ am/pm.
We discussed ____.
Did doctor examine patient: ____ yes, ____ no.
Wash hands before touching patient: ____ yes, ____ no.
Wear gloves: ____ yes, ___ no. Clean stethoscope: ____ yes, ____ no.
Wear gown and mask (precautions only):____ yes, ____ no.
Wash hands before leaving the room: ____ yes, ____ no.

Dr.____________ came in at ____ am/pm. Left at ____ am/pm.
We discussed ____.
Did doctor examine patient: ____ yes, ____ no.
Wash hands before touching patient: ____ yes, ____ no.
Wear gloves: ____ yes, ___ no. Clean stethoscope: ____ yes, ____ no.
Wear gown and mask (precautions only):____ yes, ____ no.
Wash hands before leaving the room: ____ yes, ____ no.

Dr.____________ came in at ____ am/pm. Left at ____ am/pm.
We discussed ____.
Did doctor examine patient: ____ yes, ____ no.
Wash hands before touching patient: ____ yes, ____ no.
Wear gloves: ____ yes, ___ no. Clean stethoscope: ____ yes, ____ no.
Wear gown and mask (precautions only):____ yes, ____ no.
Wash hands before leaving the room: ____ yes, ____ no.

NURSING CARE FOR ______________________________

DATE ____________________, DAY NUMBER ____________________

INITIAL DAY SHIFT EXAM:

My nurse has ______ # of patients. CNA ___yes, ___no. Charge nurse ______________
Nurse ________________ RN/LPN came in at __________ am/pm. Left at __________ am/pm.
Did nurse wash hands and wear gloves before touching patient: _______ yes, _______ no.
Wash hands after touching patient and before leaving the room: _______ yes, _______ no.
Don't hesitate to request staff to wash their hands. This will help decrease the risk of spreading potentially lethal germs.
Did nurse wear protective gear (isolation precautions only): _______ yes, _______ no.
Did nurse provide oral care (to be done every two hours if unable to provide for self, also decreases risk of pneumonia, infections, and aspiration): _______ yes, _______ no.
If able to provide own oral care, then supplies at bedside: _______ yes, _______ no.
Was patient repositioned (every two hours if unable to turn self): _____ yes _____ no.
Head of bed at _________ degrees. This is important for patients on ventilators or on tube feedings. Anything less than thirty degrees places patients at risk for aspiration of stomach contents into the lungs causing aspiration pneumonia.
Checked for incontinence and skin breakdown: _____ yes, _____ no.
Patient's linens wet or soiled: _____ yes, _____ no. Linens changed: ____ yes, ____ no.
Time linens changed: _______ am/pm. Any skin redness or breakdown: ____ yes, ____ no.
If yes, what stage is pressure ulcer: _________. Acquired when: ______________________.
List wounds not associated with pressure ulcers and how acquired: ______________
____.
Mattress type: ____.
Specialty mattresses are important to help prevent pressure ulcers)
If patient on ventilator or has tracheostomy, suction performed: _____ yes, ______ no.
Did nurse listen to lung sounds: _____ yes, _____ no.
Does patient have chest tubes: ____ yes, ____ no. Functioning _____ yes, ______ no.
Bowel sounds: _______ yes, _______ no. Bowel sounds active: ______ yes, ______ no.
Neurological exam: ______ yes, ______ no. Follow commands: ______ yes, ______ no.
Is patient alert and oriented to person, place, time, and events: _____ yes, ____ no.
If confused, patient is not oriented to: ____ person, ___ place, ___ time, ___ event.
Confusion began (time and date): ____.
Glasgow coma scale (checks conscious scale of patient): ____________________________.
Intracranial pressure monitoring: ______ yes, ______ no.
If yes, pressure is at _________ mm mercury. (Normal is one to fifteen).
Moves extremities: ___ yes, ___ no.
Paralysis: (inability to move extremities) ________ yes, _______ no.
If yes, extremities affected and when paralysis began: ____________________________.
Is patient in pain: ____ yes, ____ no. Describe pain and location ________________.
Patient able to eat: ____ yes, ____ no. What type of diet? ______________________.
If patient on tube feedings list type: _____________ at ____________ cc/ml per hour.
Nausea ____, vomiting _____. If so, describe: __________________________________.
Patient has: Nasal gastric tube ______, Dobhoff tube _____, Peg or gastric tube _____.
When was feeding tube placed and what site: ______________________________________.
Catheter for draining urine: ____ yes, ____ no. If so, when placed: _______________.
Find out policy for allowed time to remain in bladder. Too long may cause infections.)
IV site(s) where: ___________________________ when placed: ______________________.
IV fluids (types and rates): ____________________, _____________________________,
_______________________, ___________________________, ___________________________,
Is patient on oxygen: _____ yes, _____ no. If so, how much and route delivered (see oxygen routes): ____.
If patient on ventilator, list settings (see list on ventilator settings): ________
____.
Vital signs: temp _______, pulse _______, resp _______, b/p ______, o2 ______%,
current weight ______ pounds, ______ kg. Glucose level: ______
Insulin coverage: ____ yes, ____ no. Insulin type: ____________, # of units: ______.

NURSING CARE CONTINUED FOR ______________________
DATE ____________________, DAY NUMBER ______________

FOLLOWING EXAMINATIONS FOR DAY SHIFT:

Nurse ____________, CNA ____________, in at _____ am/pm. Left at ______ am/pm.
Wash hands and wear gloves before touching patient: _______ yes, _______ no.
Wash hands before leaving room: ___ yes, ___ no. Wear protective gear: __ yes, __ no.
Clean stethoscope: __ yes, __ no. Oral care: __ yes, __ no. Suctioned: __ yes, __ no.
Repositioned: ___ yes, ___ no. Turned to: ___ left, ___ right, ___ backside ___.
Head of bed at: _______ degrees. Incontinence/skin breakdown: ____ yes, ___ no.
Linens wet or soiled: ____ yes, ____ no. Linens changed: ____ yes, _____ no.
Dressing changed: ____ yes, ____ no. Location: ____________________.
IV site checked: _____ yes, _____ no. IV tubing labeled: _____ yes, ____ no.
IV fluids at: ____.
Pain level (0-10 scale.0-no pain, 10 intolerable): ____________________.
Location of pain: ____________. Medicated for pain: _____ yes, ____ no.
Patient is alert/oriented: ___ yes, __ no. New confusion: ___ yes, ___ no.
Vital signs: temp ____, pulse ____, resp _____, b/p _____, 02 ____ %, ____ liters.
Glucose level: _____. Insulin: ___ yes, ___ no. Type: ____________ # of units ___.

Nurse ____________, CNA ____________, in at _____ am/pm. Left at ______ am/pm.
Wash hands and wear gloves before touching patient: _______ yes, _______ no.
Wash hands before leaving room: ___ yes, ___ no. Wear protective gear: __ yes, __ no.
Clean stethoscope: __ yes, __ no. Oral care: __ yes, __ no. Suctioned: __ yes, __ no.
Repositioned: ___ yes, ___ no. Turned to: ___ left, ___ right, ___ backside ___.
Head of bed at: _______ degrees. Incontinence/skin breakdown: ____ yes, ___ no.
Linens wet or soiled: ____ yes, ____ no. Linens changed: ____ yes, _____ no.
Dressing changed: ____ yes, ____ no. Location: ____________________.
IV site checked: _____ yes, _____ no. IV tubing labeled: _____ yes, ____ no.
IV fluids at: ____.
Pain level (0-10 scale.0-no pain, 10 intolerable): ____________________.
Location of pain: ____________. Medicated for pain: _____ yes, ____ no.
Patient is alert/oriented: ___ yes, __ no. New confusion: ___ yes, ___ no.
Vital signs: temp ____, pulse ____, resp _____, b/p _____, 02 ____ %, ____ liters.
Glucose level: _____. Insulin: ___ yes, ___ no. Type: ____________ # of units ___.

Nurse ____________, CNA ____________, in at _____ am/pm. Left at ______ am/pm.
Wash hands and wear gloves before touching patient: _______ yes, _______ no.
Wash hands before leaving room: ___ yes, ___ no. Wear protective gear: __ yes, __ no.
Clean stethoscope: __ yes, __ no. Oral care: __ yes, __ no. Suctioned: __ yes, __ no.
Repositioned: ___ yes, ___ no. Turned to: ___ left, ___ right, ___ backside ___.
Head of bed at: _______ degrees. Incontinence/skin breakdown: ____ yes, ___ no.
Linens wet or soiled: ____ yes, ____ no. Linens changed: ____ yes, _____ no.
Dressing changed: ____ yes, ____ no. Location: ____________________.
IV site checked: _____ yes, _____ no. IV tubing labeled: _____ yes, ____ no.
IV fluids at: ____.
Pain level (0-10 scale.0-no pain, 10 intolerable): ____________________.
Location of pain: ____________. Medicated for pain: _____ yes, ____ no.
Patient is alert/oriented: ___ yes, __ no. New confusion: ___ yes, ___ no.
Vital signs: temp ____, pulse ____, resp _____, b/p _____, 02 ____ %, ____ liters.
Glucose level: _____. Insulin: ___ yes, ___ no. Type: ____________ # of units ___.

NURSING CARE CONTINUED FOR ______________________
DATE ____________________, DAY NUMBER ______________________

FOLLOWING EXAMINATIONS FOR DAY SHIFT:

Nurse ______________, CNA ______________, in at _____ am/pm. Left at ______ am/pm.
Wash hands and wear gloves before touching patient: _______ yes, _______ no.
Wash hands before leaving room: ___ yes, ___ no. Wear protective gear: __ yes, __ no.
Clean stethoscope: __ yes, __ no. Oral care: __ yes, __ no. Suctioned: __ yes, __ no.
Repositioned: ___ yes, ___ no. Turned to: ___ left, ___ right, ___ backside ___.
Head of bed at: _______ degrees. Incontinence/skin breakdown: ____ yes, ___ no.
Linens wet or soiled: _____ yes, _____ no. Linens changed: _____ yes, ______ no.
Dressing changed: ____ yes, ____ no. Location: ______________________________.
IV site checked: _____ yes, _____ no. IV tubing labeled: _____ yes, _____no.
IV fluids at: ____.
Pain level (0-10 scale.0-no pain, 10 intolerable): __________________________.
Location of pain: _________________. Medicated for pain: _____ yes, ____ no.
Patient is alert/oriented: ____ yes, ____ no. New confusion: ____ yes, ____ no.
Vital signs: temp ____, pulse _____, resp _____, b/p ______, 02 _____ %, ____ liters.
Glucose level: _____. Insulin: ___ yes, ___ no. Type: _______________ # of units ____.

Nurse ______________, CNA ______________, in at _____ am/pm. Left at ______ am/pm.
Wash hands and wear gloves before touching patient: _______ yes, _______ no.
Wash hands before leaving room: ___ yes, ___ no. Wear protective gear: __ yes, __ no.
Clean stethoscope: __ yes, __ no. Oral care: __ yes, __ no. Suctioned: __ yes, __ no.
Repositioned: ___ yes, ___ no. Turned to: ___ left, ___ right, ___ backside ___.
Head of bed at: _______ degrees. Incontinence/skin breakdown: ____ yes, ___ no.
Linens wet or soiled: _____ yes, _____ no. Linens changed: _____ yes, ______ no.
Dressing changed: ____ yes, ____ no. Location: ______________________________.
IV site checked: _____ yes, _____ no. IV tubing labeled: _____ yes, _____no.
IV fluids at: ____.
Pain level (0-10 scale.0-no pain, 10 intolerable): __________________________.
Location of pain: _________________. Medicated for pain: _____ yes, ____ no.
Patient is alert/oriented: ____ yes, ____ no. New confusion: ____ yes, ____ no.
Vital signs: temp ____, pulse _____, resp _____, b/p ______, 02 _____ %, ____ liters.
Glucose level: _____. Insulin: ___ yes, ___ no. Type: _______________ # of units ____.

Nurse ______________, CNA ______________, in at _____ am/pm. Left at ______ am/pm.
Wash hands and wear gloves before touching patient: _______ yes, _______ no.
Wash hands before leaving room: ___ yes, ___ no. Wear protective gear: __ yes, __ no.
Clean stethoscope: __ yes, __ no. Oral care: __ yes, __ no. Suctioned: __ yes, __ no.
Repositioned: ___ yes, ___ no. Turned to: ___ left, ___ right, ___ backside ___.
Head of bed at: _______ degrees. Incontinence/skin breakdown: ____ yes, ___ no.
Linens wet or soiled: _____ yes, _____ no. Linens changed: _____ yes, ______ no.
Dressing changed: ____ yes, ____ no. Location: ______________________________.
IV site checked: _____ yes, _____ no. IV tubing labeled: _____ yes, _____no.
IV fluids at: ____.
Pain level (0-10 scale.0-no pain, 10 intolerable): __________________________.
Location of pain: _________________. Medicated for pain: _____ yes, ____ no.
Patient is alert/oriented: ____ yes, ____ no. New confusion: ____ yes, ____ no.
Vital signs: temp ____, pulse _____, resp _____, b/p ______, 02 _____ %, ____ liters.
Glucose level: _____. Insulin: ___ yes, ___ no. Type: _______________ # of units ____.

NURSING CARE FOR ______________________________

DATE ____________________, DAY NUMBER ____________________

INITIAL NIGHT SHIFT EXAM:

My nurse has _____ # of patients. CNA ___yes, ___no. Charge nurse ____________
Nurse __________ RN/LPN came in at ________ am/pm. Left at ________ am/pm.
Did nurse wash hands and wear gloves before touching patient: ______ yes, ______ no.
Wash hands after touching patient and before leaving the room: ______ yes, ______ no.
Don't hesitate to request staff to wash their hands. This will help decrease the risk of spreading potentially lethal germs.
Did nurse wear protective gear (isolation precautions only): ______ yes, ______ no.
Did nurse provide oral care (to be done every two hours if unable to provide for self, also decreases risk of pneumonia, infections, and aspiration): ______ yes, ______ no.
If able to provide own oral care, then supplies at bedside: ______ yes, ______ no.
Was patient repositioned (every two hours if unable to turn self): _____yes _____ no.
Head of bed at ________ degrees. This is important for patients on ventilators or on tube feedings. Anything less than thirty degrees places patients at risk for aspiration of stomach contents into the lungs causing aspiration pneumonia.
Checked for incontinence and skin breakdown: ____ yes, ____ no.
Patient's linens wet or soiled: ____yes,____ no. Linens changed: ____ yes, ____ no.
Time linens changed: ________ am/pm. Any skin redness or breakdown: ____ yes, ____ no.
If yes, what stage is pressure ulcer: _______. Acquired when: ______________.
List wounds not associated with pressure ulcers and how acquired: ______________
____.
Mattress type: ____.
Specialty mattresses are important to help prevent pressure ulcers)
If patient on ventilator or has tracheostomy, suction performed: _____ yes, _____ no.
Did nurse listen to lung sounds: ____ yes, ____ no.
Does patient have chest tubes: ____ yes, ____ no. Functioning _____ yes, _____ no.
Bowel sounds: _______ yes, ______ no. Bowel sounds active: ______ yes, ______ no.
Neurological exam: ______ yes, ______ no. Follow commands: ______ yes, ______ no.
Is patient alert and oriented to person, place, time, and events: ______ yes, ______ no.
If confused, patient is not oriented to: ___ person, ___ place, ___ time, ___ event.
Confusion began (time and date): ____.
Glasgow coma scale (checks conscious scale of patient): ________________________.
Intracranial pressure monitoring: ______ yes, ______ no.
If yes, pressure is at ________ mm mercury. (Normal is one to fifteen).
Moves extremities: ___ yes, ___ no.
Paralysis: (inability to move extremities) ______ yes, ______ no.
If yes, extremities affected and when paralysis began: __________________________.
Is patient in pain: _____ yes, _____ no. Describe pain and location ______________.
Patient able to eat: _____ yes, _____ no. What type of diet? ____________________.
If patient on tube feedings list type: ____________ at ____________ cc/ml per hour.
Nausea ____, vomiting ____ If so, describe: ____________________________________.
Patient has: Nasal gastric tube ______, Dobhoff tube _____, Peg or gastric tube ____.
When was feeding tube placed and what site: ____________________________________.
Catheter for draining urine: ____ yes, ____ no. If so, when placed: _____________.
Find out policy for allowed time to remain in bladder. Too long may cause infections.)
IV site(s) where: ____________________________ when placed: _____________________.
IV fluids (types and rates): ____,
_____________________________, _____________________________, ____________________,
Is patient on oxygen: _____ yes, _____ no. If so, how much and route delivered (see oxygen routes): ____.
If patient on ventilator, list settings (see list on ventilator settings): __________
____.
Vital signs: temp ______, pulse ______, resp ______, b/p ______, o2 ______%,
current weight ______ pounds, ______ kg. Glucose level: ______
Insulin coverage: ____ yes, ____ no. Insulin type: ____________, # of units: _____.

NURSING CARE CONTINUED FOR ______________________
DATE ____________________, DAY NUMBER ______________

FOLLOWING EXAMINATIONS FOR NIGHT SHIFT:

Nurse ___________, CNA ___________, in at _____ am/pm. Left at ______ am/pm.
Wash hands and wear gloves before touching patient: ______ yes, ______ no.
Wash hands before leaving room: ___ yes, ___ no. Wear protective gear: __ yes, __ no.
Clean stethoscope: __ yes, __ no. Oral care: __ yes, __ no. Suctioned: __ yes, __ no.
Repositioned: ___ yes, ___ no. Turned to: ___ left, ___ right, ___ backside ___.
Head of bed at: _______ degrees. Incontinence/skin breakdown: ____ yes, ____ no.
Linens wet or soiled: _____ yes, _____ no. Linens changed: _____ yes, _____ no.
Dressing changed: ____ yes, ____ no. Location: ______________________.
IV site checked: _____ yes, _____ no. IV tubing labeled: _____ yes, _____no.
IV fluids at: ____.
Pain level (0-10 scale.0-no pain, 10 intolerable): ___________________.
Location of pain: ______________. Medicated for pain: _____ yes, ____ no.
Patient is alert/oriented: ____ yes, ____ no. New confusion: ____ yes, ____ no.
Vital signs: temp ____, pulse ____, resp _____, b/p _____, 02 _____ %, ____ liters.
Glucose level: _____. Insulin: ___ yes, ___ no. Type: ____________ # of units ____.

Nurse ___________, CNA ___________, in at _____ am/pm. Left at ______ am/pm.
Wash hands and wear gloves before touching patient: ______ yes, ______ no.
Wash hands before leaving room: ___ yes, ___ no. Wear protective gear: __ yes, __ no.
Clean stethoscope: __ yes, __ no. Oral care: __ yes, __ no. Suctioned: __ yes, __ no.
Repositioned: ___ yes, ___ no. Turned to: ___ left, ___ right, ___ backside ___.
Head of bed at: _______ degrees. Incontinence/skin breakdown: ____ yes, ____ no.
Linens wet or soiled: _____ yes, _____ no. Linens changed: _____ yes, _____ no.
Dressing changed: ____ yes, ____ no. Location: ______________________.
IV site checked: _____ yes, _____ no. IV tubing labeled: _____ yes, _____no.
IV fluids at: ____.
Pain level (0-10 scale.0-no pain, 10 intolerable): ___________________.
Location of pain: ______________. Medicated for pain: _____ yes, ____ no.
Patient is alert/oriented: ____ yes, ____ no. New confusion: ____ yes, ____ no.
Vital signs: temp ____, pulse ____, resp _____, b/p _____, 02 _____ %, ____ liters.
Glucose level: _____. Insulin: ___ yes, ___ no. Type: ____________ # of units ____.

Nurse ___________, CNA ___________, in at _____ am/pm. Left at ______ am/pm.
Wash hands and wear gloves before touching patient: ______ yes, ______ no.
Wash hands before leaving room: ___ yes, ___ no. Wear protective gear: __ yes, __ no.
Clean stethoscope: __ yes, __ no. Oral care: __ yes, __ no. Suctioned: __ yes, __ no.
Repositioned: ___ yes, ___ no. Turned to: ___ left, ___ right, ___ backside ___.
Head of bed at: _______ degrees. Incontinence/skin breakdown: ____ yes, ____ no.
Linens wet or soiled: _____ yes, _____ no. Linens changed: _____ yes, _____ no.
Dressing changed: ____ yes, ____ no. Location: ______________________.
IV site checked: _____ yes, _____ no. IV tubing labeled: _____ yes, _____no.
IV fluids at: ____.
Pain level (0-10 scale.0-no pain, 10 intolerable): ___________________.
Location of pain: ______________. Medicated for pain: _____ yes, ____ no.
Patient is alert/oriented: ____ yes, ____ no. New confusion: ____ yes, ____ no.
Vital signs: temp ____, pulse ____, resp _____, b/p _____, 02 _____ %, ____ liters.
Glucose level: ____. Insulin: ___ yes, ___ no. Type: ____________ # of units ___.

NURSING CARE CONTINUED FOR ____________________
DATE ____________________, DAY NUMBER ____________________

FOLLOWING EXAMINATIONS FOR NIGHT SHIFT:

Nurse ______________, CNA ______________, in at _____ am/pm. Left at ______ am/pm.
Wash hands and wear gloves before touching patient: _______ yes, _______ no.
Wash hands before leaving room: ___ yes, ___ no. Wear protective gear: __ yes, __ no.
Clean stethoscope: __ yes, __ no. Oral care: __ yes, __ no. Suctioned: __ yes, __ no.
Repositioned: ___ yes, ___ no. Turned to: ___ left, ___ right, ___ backside ___.
Head of bed at: ______ degrees. Incontinence/skin breakdown: ___ yes, ___ no.
Linens wet or soiled: _____ yes, _____ no. Linens changed: _____ yes, _____ no.
Dressing changed: ____ yes, ____ no. Location: ____________________.
IV site checked: _____ yes, _____ no. IV tubing labeled: _____ yes, _____no.
IV fluids at: ____.
Pain level (0-10 scale.0-no pain, 10 intolerable): ______________.
Location of pain: ______________. Medicated for pain: ____ yes, ____ no.
Patient is alert/oriented: ____ yes, ____ no. New confusion: ___ yes, ___ no.
Vital signs: temp ___, pulse ____, resp _____, b/p _____, 02 _____ %, ____ liters.
Glucose level: _____. Insulin: ___ yes, ___ no. Type: _____________ # of units ____.

Nurse ______________, CNA ______________, in at _____ am/pm. Left at ______ am/pm.
Wash hands and wear gloves before touching patient: _______ yes, _______ no.
Wash hands before leaving room: ___ yes, ___ no. Wear protective gear: __ yes, __ no.
Clean stethoscope: __ yes, __ no. Oral care: __ yes, __ no. Suctioned: __ yes, __ no.
Repositioned: ___ yes, ___ no. Turned to: ___ left, ___ right, ___ backside ___.
Head of bed at: ______ degrees. Incontinence/skin breakdown: ___ yes, ___ no.
Linens wet or soiled: _____ yes, _____ no. Linens changed: _____ yes, _____ no.
Dressing changed: ____ yes, ____ no. Location: ____________________.
IV site checked: _____ yes, _____ no. IV tubing labeled: _____ yes, _____no.
IV fluids at: ____.
Pain level (0-10 scale.0-no pain, 10 intolerable): ______________.
Location of pain: ______________. Medicated for pain: ____ yes, ____ no.
Patient is alert/oriented: ____ yes, ____ no. New confusion: ___ yes, ___ no.
Vital signs: temp ___, pulse ____, resp _____, b/p _____, 02 _____ %, ____ liters.
Glucose level: _____. Insulin: ___ yes, ___ no. Type: _____________ # of units ____.

Nurse ______________, CNA ______________, in at _____ am/pm. Left at ______ am/pm.
Wash hands and wear gloves before touching patient: _______ yes, _______ no.
Wash hands before leaving room: ___ yes, ___ no. Wear protective gear: __ yes, __ no.
Clean stethoscope: __ yes, __ no. Oral care: __ yes, __ no. Suctioned: __ yes, __ no.
Repositioned: ___ yes, ___ no. Turned to: ___ left, ___ right, ___ backside ___.
Head of bed at: ______ degrees. Incontinence/skin breakdown: ___ yes, ___ no.
Linens wet or soiled: _____ yes, _____ no. Linens changed: _____ yes, _____ no.
Dressing changed: ____ yes, ____ no. Location: ____________________.
IV site checked: _____ yes, _____ no. IV tubing labeled: _____ yes, _____no.
IV fluids at: ____.
Pain level (0-10 scale.0-no pain, 10 intolerable): ______________.
Location of pain: ______________. Medicated for pain: ____ yes, ____ no.
Patient is alert/oriented: ____ yes, ____ no. New confusion: ___ yes, ___ no.
Vital signs: temp ___, pulse ____, resp _____, b/p _____, 02 _____ %, ____ liters.
Glucose level: _____. Insulin: ___ yes, ___ no. Type: _____________ # of units ____.

MEDICATION ADMINISTRATION LIST FOR ____________________
DATE ______________ DAY NUMBER ____________________

List the medication for each day. Routes of administration: oral, thru feeding tube, intravenous (IV), intramuscular (IM), subcutaneous (SQ), epidural or a catheter in your spinal column, rectal, topical, eye drops, and ear drops.

Medication:		Route:		Time:	
Medication:		Route:		Time:	
Medication:		Route:		Time:	
Medication:		Route:		Time:	
Medication:		Route:		Time:	
Medication:		Route:		Time:	
Medication:		Route:		Time:	
Medication:		Route:		Time:	
Medication:		Route:		Time:	
Medication:		Route:		Time:	
Medication:		Route:		Time:	
Medication:		Route:		Time:	
Medication:		Route:		Time:	
Medication:		Route:		Time:	
Medication:		Route:		Time:	
Medication:		Route:		Time:	
Medication:		Route:		Time:	
Medication:		Route:		Time:	
Medication:		Route:		Time:	
Medication:		Route:		Time:	
Medication:		Route:		Time:	
Medication:		Route:		Time:	
Medication:		Route:		Time:	
Medication:		Route:		Time:	
Medication:		Route:		Time:	
Medication:		Route:		Time:	
Medication:		Route:		Time:	
Medication:		Route:		Time:	
Medication:		Route:		Time:	
Medication:		Route:		Time:	
Medication:		Route:		Time:	
Medication:		Route:		Time:	
Medication:		Route:		Time:	
Medication:		Route:		Time:	
Medication:		Route:		Time:	
Medication:		Route:		Time:	
Medication:		Route:		Time:	
Medication:		Route:		Time:	
Medication:		Route:		Time:	
Medication:		Route:		Time:	
Medication:		Route:		Time:	
Medication:		Route:		Time:	
Medication:		Route:		Time:	
Medication:		Route:		Time:	
Medication:		Route:		Time:	
Medication:		Route:		Time:	
Medication:		Route:		Time:	
Medication:		Route:		Time:	
Medication:		Route:		Time:	
Medication:		Route:		Time:	
Medication:		Route:		Time:	
Medication:		Route:		Time:	
Medication:		Route:		Time:	
Medication:		Route:		Time:	

NOTES FOR DAY NUMBER ____________________

DATE ____________________

MEDICAL JOURNAL FOR ______________________________

DATE ________________, DAY NUMBER ______________

VISITS FROM MY DOCTORS TODAY

Goals for today: ____

____

____.

Things to discuss with my doctor(s): ______________________________

____

____

Dr.____________ came in at ____ am/pm. Left at ____ am/pm.
We discussed ____.
Did doctor examine patient: ____ yes, ____ no.
Wash hands before touching patient: ____ yes, ____ no.
Wear gloves: ___ yes, ___ no. Clean stethoscope: ___ yes, ___ no.
Wear gown and mask (precautions only):___ yes, ____ no.
Wash hands before leaving the room: ____ yes, ____ no.

Dr.____________ came in at ____ am/pm. Left at ____ am/pm.
We discussed ____.
Did doctor examine patient: ____ yes, ____ no.
Wash hands before touching patient: ____ yes, ____ no.
Wear gloves: ___ yes, ___ no. Clean stethoscope: ___ yes, ___ no.
Wear gown and mask (precautions only):___ yes, ____ no.
Wash hands before leaving the room: ____ yes, ____ no.

Dr.____________ came in at ____ am/pm. Left at ____ am/pm.
We discussed ____.
Did doctor examine patient: ____ yes, ____ no.
Wash hands before touching patient: ____ yes, ____ no.
Wear gloves: ___ yes, ___ no. Clean stethoscope: ___ yes, ___ no.
Wear gown and mask (precautions only):___ yes, ____ no.
Wash hands before leaving the room: ____ yes, ____ no.

Dr.____________ came in at ____ am/pm. Left at ____ am/pm.
We discussed ____.
Did doctor examine patient: ____ yes, ____ no.
Wash hands before touching patient: ____ yes, ____ no.
Wear gloves: ___ yes, ___ no. Clean stethoscope: ___ yes, ___ no.
Wear gown and mask (precautions only):___ yes, ____ no.
Wash hands before leaving the room: ____ yes, ____ no.

Dr.____________ came in at ____ am/pm. Left at ____ am/pm.
We discussed ____.
Did doctor examine patient: ____ yes, ____ no.
Wash hands before touching patient: ____ yes, ____ no.
Wear gloves: ___ yes, ___ no. Clean stethoscope: ___ yes, ___ no.
Wear gown and mask (precautions only):___ yes, ____ no.
Wash hands before leaving the room: ____ yes, ____ no.

NURSING CARE FOR ______________________________

DATE ____________________, DAY NUMBER ____________________

INITIAL DAY SHIFT EXAM:

My nurse has ______ # of patients. CNA ___yes, ___no. Charge nurse ________________
Nurse ______________ RN/LPN came in at __________ am/pm. Left at __________ am/pm.
Did nurse wash hands and wear gloves before touching patient: _______ yes, _______ no.
Wash hands after touching patient and before leaving the room: _______ yes, _______ no.
Don't hesitate to request staff to wash their hands. This will help decrease the risk of spreading potentially lethal germs.
Did nurse wear protective gear (isolation precautions only): _______ yes, _______ no.
Did nurse provide oral care (to be done every two hours if unable to provide for self, also decreases risk of pneumonia, infections, and aspiration): _______ yes, _______ no.
If able to provide own oral care, then supplies at bedside: _______ yes, _______ no.
Was patient repositioned (every two hours if unable to turn self): _____ yes _____ no.
Head of bed at _________ degrees. This is important for patients on ventilators or on tube feedings. Anything less than thirty degrees places patients at risk for aspiration of stomach contents into the lungs causing aspiration pneumonia.
Checked for incontinence and skin breakdown: ______ yes, _____ no.
Patient's linens wet or soiled: _____yes, ____ no. Linens changed: ____ yes, ____ no.
Time linens changed: ________ am/pm. Any skin redness or breakdown: ____ yes, ____ no.
If yes, what stage is pressure ulcer: _______. Acquired when: ________________.
List wounds not associated with pressure ulcers and how acquired: ________________
____.
Mattress type: ____
Specialty mattresses are important to help prevent pressure ulcers)
If patient on ventilator or has tracheostomy, suction performed: _____ yes, _____ no.
Did nurse listen to lung sounds: _____ yes, _____ no.
Does patient have chest tubes: _____ yes, _____ no. Functioning _____ yes, _____ no.
Bowel sounds: _______ yes, _______ no. Bowel sounds active: ______ yes, ______ no.
Neurological exam: _____ yes, ______ no. Follow commands: _______ yes, ______ no.
Is patient alert and oriented to person, place, time, and events: ____ yes, _____ no.
If confused, patient is not oriented to: ___ person, ___ place, ___ time, ___ event.
Confusion began (time and date): ____.
Glasgow coma scale (checks conscious scale of patient): __________________________.
Intracranial pressure monitoring: _____ yes, _____ no.
If yes, pressure is at ________ mm mercury. (Normal is one to fifteen).
Moves extremities: ___ yes, ___ no.
Paralysis: (inability to move extremities) ________ yes, ________ no.
If yes, extremities affected and when paralysis began: ___________________________.
Is patient in pain: ____ yes, ____ no. Describe pain and location ________________.
Patient able to eat: ____ yes, ____ no. What type of diet? _____________________.
If patient on tube feedings list type: ____________ at ____________ cc/ml per hour.
Nausea ____, vomiting ____. If so, describe: _____________________________________.
Patient has: Nasal gastric tube ______, Dobhoff tube _____, Peg or gastric tube ____.
When was feeding tube placed and what site: ______________________________________.
Catheter for draining urine: ____ yes, ____ no. If so, when placed: _____________.
Find out policy for allowed time to remain in bladder. Too long may cause infections.)
IV site(s) where: ______________________ when placed: _____________________.
IV fluids (types and rates): ___________, ___________, ___________, ___________,
___________, ___________, ___________, ___________.
Is patient on oxygen: _____ yes, _____ no. If so, how much and route delivered (see oxygen routes): ____.
If patient on ventilator, list settings (see list on ventilator settings): _________
____.
Vital signs: temp ______, pulse ______, resp ______, b/p ______, o2 ______%,
current weight ______ pounds, ______ kg. Glucose level: ______
Insulin coverage: ____ yes, ____ no. Insulin type: ____________, # of units: _____.

NURSING CARE CONTINUED FOR ____________________________
DATE ____________________, DAY NUMBER ____________________

FOLLOWING EXAMINATIONS FOR DAY SHIFT:

Nurse ______________, CNA ______________, in at ______ am/pm. Left at ______ am/pm.
Wash hands and wear gloves before touching patient: ______ yes, ______ no.
Wash hands before leaving room: ___ yes, ___ no. Wear protective gear: __ yes, __ no.
Clean stethoscope: __ yes, __ no. Oral care: __ yes, __ no. Suctioned: __ yes, __ no.
Repositioned: ___ yes, ___ no. Turned to: ___ left, ___ right, ___ backside ___.
Head of bed at: _______ degrees. Incontinence/skin breakdown: ____ yes, ____ no.
Linens wet or soiled: _____ yes, _____ no. Linens changed: _____ yes, ______ no.
Dressing changed: ____ yes, ____ no. Location: ______________________________.
IV site checked: _____ yes, _____ no. IV tubing labeled: _____ yes, _____no.
IV fluids at: ____.
Pain level (0-10 scale.0-no pain, 10 intolerable): ____________________________.
Location of pain: ____________________. Medicated for pain: _____ yes, ____ no.
Patient is alert/oriented: ____ yes, ____ no. New confusion: ____ yes, ____ no.
Vital signs: temp ____, pulse _____, resp ______, b/p ______, 02 _____ %, ____ liters.
Glucose level: _____. Insulin: ___ yes, ___ no. Type: ______________ # of units ____.

Nurse ______________, CNA ______________, in at ______ am/pm. Left at ______ am/pm.
Wash hands and wear gloves before touching patient: ______ yes, ______ no.
Wash hands before leaving room: ___ yes, ___ no. Wear protective gear: __ yes, __ no.
Clean stethoscope: __ yes, __ no. Oral care: __ yes, __ no. Suctioned: __ yes, __ no.
Repositioned: ___ yes, ___ no. Turned to: ___ left, ___ right, ___ backside ___.
Head of bed at: _______ degrees. Incontinence/skin breakdown: ____ yes, ____ no.
Linens wet or soiled: _____ yes, _____ no. Linens changed: _____ yes, ______ no.
Dressing changed: ____ yes, ____ no. Location: ______________________________.
IV site checked: _____ yes, _____ no. IV tubing labeled: _____ yes, _____no.
IV fluids at: ____.
Pain level (0-10 scale.0-no pain, 10 intolerable): ____________________________.
Location of pain: ____________________. Medicated for pain: _____ yes, ____ no.
Patient is alert/oriented: ____ yes, ____ no. New confusion: ____ yes, ____ no.
Vital signs: temp ____, pulse _____, resp ______, b/p ______, 02 _____ %, ____ liters.
Glucose level: _____. Insulin: ___ yes, ___ no. Type: ______________ # of units ____.

Nurse ______________, CNA ______________, in at ______ am/pm. Left at ______ am/pm.
Wash hands and wear gloves before touching patient: ______ yes, ______ no.
Wash hands before leaving room: ___ yes, ___ no. Wear protective gear: __ yes, __ no.
Clean stethoscope: __ yes, __ no. Oral care: __ yes, __ no. Suctioned: __ yes, __ no.
Repositioned: ___ yes, ___ no. Turned to: ___ left, ___ right, ___ backside ___.
Head of bed at: _______ degrees. Incontinence/skin breakdown: ____ yes, ____ no.
Linens wet or soiled: _____ yes, _____ no. Linens changed: _____ yes, ______ no.
Dressing changed:____ yes, ____ no. Location: ______________________________.
IV site checked: _____ yes, _____ no. IV tubing labeled: _____ yes, _____no.
IV fluids at: ____.
Pain level (0-10 scale.0-no pain, 10 intolerable): ____________________________.
Location of pain: ____________________. Medicated for pain: _____ yes, ____ no.
Patient is alert/oriented: ____ yes, ____ no. New confusion: ____ yes, ____ no.
Vital signs: temp ____, pulse _____, resp ______, b/p ______, 02 _____ %, ____ liters.
Glucose level: _____. Insulin: ___ yes, ___ no. Type: ______________ # of units ____.

NURSING CARE CONTINUED FOR ______________________
DATE ____________________, DAY NUMBER _________________

FOLLOWING EXAMINATIONS FOR DAY SHIFT:

Nurse _____________, CNA _____________, in at ______ am/pm. Left at ______ am/pm.
Wash hands and wear gloves before touching patient: _______ yes, _______ no.
Wash hands before leaving room: ___ yes, ___ no. Wear protective gear: __ yes, __ no.
Clean stethoscope: __ yes, __ no. Oral care: __ yes, __ no. Suctioned: __ yes, __ no.
Repositioned: ___ yes, ___ no. Turned to: ___ left, ___ right, ___ backside ___.
Head of bed at: ________ degrees. Incontinence/skin breakdown: ____ yes, ____ no.
Linens wet or soiled: _____ yes, _____ no. Linens changed: _____ yes, ______ no.
Dressing changed: ____ yes, ____ no. Location: ____________________________.
IV site checked: _____ yes, _____ no. IV tubing labeled: _____ yes, _____no.
IV fluids at: ____.
Pain level (0-10 scale.0-no pain, 10 intolerable): __________________________.
Location of pain: _______________. Medicated for pain: ____ yes, ____ no.
Patient is alert/oriented: ____ yes, ____ no. New confusion: ____ yes, ____ no.
Vital signs: temp ____, pulse ____, resp _____, b/p _____, 02 ____ %, ____ liters.
Glucose level: _____. Insulin: ___ yes, ___ no. Type: ___________ # of units ___.

Nurse _____________, CNA _____________, in at ______ am/pm. Left at ______ am/pm.
Wash hands and wear gloves before touching patient: _______ yes, _______ no.
Wash hands before leaving room: ___ yes, ___ no. Wear protective gear: __ yes, __ no.
Clean stethoscope: __ yes, __ no. Oral care: __ yes, __ no. Suctioned: __ yes, __ no.
Repositioned: ___ yes, ___ no. Turned to: ___ left, ___ right, ___ backside ___.
Head of bed at: ________ degrees. Incontinence/skin breakdown: ____ yes, ____ no.
Linens wet or soiled: _____ yes, _____ no. Linens changed: _____ yes, ______ no.
Dressing changed: ____ yes, ____ no. Location: ____________________________.
IV site checked: _____ yes, _____ no. IV tubing labeled: _____ yes, _____no.
IV fluids at: ____.
Pain level (0-10 scale.0-no pain, 10 intolerable): __________________________.
Location of pain: _______________. Medicated for pain: ____ yes, ____ no.
Patient is alert/oriented: ____ yes, ____ no. New confusion: ____ yes, ____ no.
Vital signs: temp ____, pulse ____, resp _____, b/p _____, 02 ____ %, ____ liters.
Glucose level: _____. Insulin: ___ yes, ___ no. Type: ___________ # of units ___.

Nurse _____________, CNA _____________, in at ______ am/pm. Left at ______ am/pm.
Wash hands and wear gloves before touching patient: _______ yes, _______ no.
Wash hands before leaving room: ___ yes, ___ no. Wear protective gear: __ yes, __ no.
Clean stethoscope: __ yes, __ no. Oral care: __ yes, __ no. Suctioned: __ yes, __ no.
Repositioned: ___ yes, ___ no. Turned to: ___ left, ___ right, ___ backside ___.
Head of bed at: ________ degrees. Incontinence/skin breakdown: ____ yes, ____ no.
Linens wet or soiled: _____ yes, _____ no. Linens changed: _____ yes, ______ no.
Dressing changed: ____ yes, ____ no. Location: ____________________________.
IV site checked: _____ yes, _____ no. IV tubing labeled: _____ yes, _____no.
IV fluids at: ____.
Pain level (0-10 scale.0-no pain, 10 intolerable): __________________________.
Location of pain: _______________. Medicated for pain: ____ yes, ____ no.
Patient is alert/oriented: ____ yes, ____ no. New confusion: ____ yes, ____ no.
Vital signs: temp ____, pulse ____, resp _____, b/p _____, 02 ____ %, ____ liters.
Glucose level: _____. Insulin: ___ yes, ___ no. Type: ___________ # of units ___.

NURSING CARE FOR ______________________________

DATE ____________________, DAY NUMBER ____________________

INITIAL NIGHT SHIFT EXAM:

My nurse has ______ # of patients. CNA ___yes, ___no. Charge nurse ________________
Nurse ______________ RN/LPN came in at __________ am/pm. Left at __________ am/pm.
Did nurse wash hands and wear gloves before touching patient: _______ yes, _______ no.
Wash hands after touching patient and before leaving the room: _______ yes, _______ no.
Don't hesitate to request staff to wash their hands. This will help decrease the risk of spreading potentially lethal germs.
Did nurse wear protective gear (isolation precautions only): _______ yes, _______ no.
Did nurse provide oral care (to be done every two hours if unable to provide for self, also decreases risk of pneumonia, infections, and aspiration): _______ yes, _______ no.
If able to provide own oral care, then supplies at bedside: _______ yes, _______ no.
Was patient repositioned (every two hours if unable to turn self): _____ yes _____ no.
Head of bed at ________ degrees. This is important for patients on ventilators or on tube feedings. Anything less than thirty degrees places patients at risk for aspiration of stomach contents into the lungs causing aspiration pneumonia.
Checked for incontinence and skin breakdown: _____ yes, _____ no.
Patient's linens wet or soiled: _____ yes, _____ no. Linens changed: ____ yes, ____ no.
Time linens changed: _______ am/pm. Any skin redness or breakdown: _____ yes, ____ no.
If yes, what stage is pressure ulcer: ________. Acquired when: ________________.
List wounds not associated with pressure ulcers and how acquired: ________________
____.
Mattress type: ____.
Specialty mattresses are important to help prevent pressure ulcers)
If patient on ventilator or has tracheostomy, suction performed: _____ yes, ______ no.
Did nurse listen to lung sounds: _____ yes, _____ no.
Does patient have chest tubes: ____ yes, ____ no. Functioning _____ yes, ______ no.
Bowel sounds: _______ yes, _______ no. Bowel sounds active: ______ yes, ______ no.
Neurological exam: _____ yes, ______ no. Follow commands: _______ yes, ______ no.
Is patient alert and oriented to person, place, time, and events: _____ yes, _____ no.
If confused, patient is not oriented to: ____ person, ___ place, ___ time, ___ event.
Confusion began (time and date): ______________________________________.
Glasgow coma scale (checks conscious scale of patient): ____________________.
Intracranial pressure monitoring: ______ yes, ______ no.
If yes, pressure is at ________ mm mercury. (Normal is one to fifteen).
Moves extremities: ___ yes, ___ no.
Paralysis: (inability to move extremities) ________ yes, ________ no.
If yes, extremities affected and when paralysis began: ____________________.
Is patient in pain: ____ yes, ____ no. Describe pain and location ______________
Patient able to eat: ____ yes, ____ no. What type of diet? ____________________
If patient on tube feedings list type: ____________ at __________ cc/ml per hour.
Nausea ____, vomiting _____. If so, describe: _____________________________.
Patient has: Nasal gastric tube ______, Dobhoff tube _____, Peg or gastric tube _____.
When was feeding tube placed and what site: _________________________________.
Catheter for draining urine: ____ yes, ____ no. If so, when placed: ____________
Find out policy for allowed time to remain in bladder. Too long may cause infections.)
IV site(s) where: ______________________________ when placed: ____________.
IV fluids (types and rates): ______________________, ______________________,
______________________, ______________________, ______________________,
Is patient on oxygen: _____ yes, _____ no. If so, how much and route delivered (see oxygen routes): ____.
If patient on ventilator, list settings (see list on ventilator settings): __________
____.
Vital signs: temp ______, pulse ______, resp ______, b/p ______, o2 ______%,
current weight ______ pounds, _____ kg. Glucose level: ______
Insulin coverage: ____ yes, ____ no. Insulin type: ____________, # of units: ______.

NURSING CARE CONTINUED FOR ____________________
DATE ____________________, DAY NUMBER ____________________

FOLLOWING EXAMINATIONS FOR NIGHT SHIFT:

Nurse ____________, CNA ____________, in at ______ am/pm. Left at _______ am/pm.
Wash hands and wear gloves before touching patient: ______ yes, ______ no.
Wash hands before leaving room: ___ yes, ___ no. Wear protective gear: __ yes, __ no.
Clean stethoscope: __ yes, __ no. Oral care: __ yes, __ no. Suctioned: __ yes, __ no.
Repositioned: ___ yes, ___ no. Turned to: ___ left, ___ right, ___ backside ___.
Head of bed at: ______ degrees. Incontinence/skin breakdown: ____ yes, ___ no.
Linens wet or soiled: ____ yes, ____ no. Linens changed: ____ yes, ____ no.
Dressing changed: ____ yes, ____ no. Location: ______________.
IV site checked: _____ yes, _____ no. IV tubing labeled: _____ yes, _____no.
IV fluids at: ____.
Pain level (0-10 scale.0-no pain, 10 intolerable): _______________.
Location of pain: ____________. Medicated for pain: ____ yes, ____ no.
Patient is alert/oriented: ____ yes, ____ no. New confusion: ____ yes, ____ no.
Vital signs: temp ____, pulse ____, resp ____, b/p ______, 02 _____%, ____ liters.
Glucose level: _____. Insulin: ___ yes, ___ no. Type: ___________ # of units ____.

Nurse ____________, CNA ____________, in at ______ am/pm. Left at _______ am/pm.
Wash hands and wear gloves before touching patient: ______ yes, ______ no.
Wash hands before leaving room: ___ yes, ___ no. Wear protective gear: __ yes, __ no.
Clean stethoscope: __ yes, __ no. Oral care: __ yes, __ no. Suctioned: __ yes, __ no.
Repositioned: ___ yes, ___ no. Turned to: ___ left, ___ right, ___ backside ___.
Head of bed at: ______ degrees. Incontinence/skin breakdown: ____ yes, ___ no.
Linens wet or soiled: ____ yes, ____ no. Linens changed: ____ yes, ____ no.
Dressing changed: ____ yes, ____ no. Location: ______________.
IV site checked: _____ yes, _____ no. IV tubing labeled: _____ yes, _____no.
IV fluids at: ____.
Pain level (0-10 scale.0-no pain, 10 intolerable): _______________.
Location of pain: ____________. Medicated for pain: ____ yes, ____ no.
Patient is alert/oriented: ____ yes, ____ no. New confusion: ____ yes, ____ no.
Vital signs: temp ____, pulse ____, resp ____, b/p ______, 02 _____%, ____ liters.
Glucose level: _____. Insulin: ___ yes, ___ no. Type: ___________ # of units ____.

Nurse ____________, CNA ____________, in at ______ am/pm. Left at _______ am/pm.
Wash hands and wear gloves before touching patient: ______ yes, ______ no.
Wash hands before leaving room: ___ yes, ___ no. Wear protective gear: __ yes, __ no.
Clean stethoscope: __ yes, __ no. Oral care: __ yes, __ no. Suctioned: __ yes, __ no.
Repositioned: ___ yes, ___ no. Turned to: ___ left, ___ right, ___ backside ___.
Head of bed at: ______ degrees. Incontinence/skin breakdown: ____ yes, ___ no.
Linens wet or soiled: ____ yes, ____ no. Linens changed: ____ yes, ____ no.
Dressing changed: ____ yes, ____ no. Location: ______________.
IV site checked: _____ yes, _____ no. IV tubing labeled: _____ yes, _____no.
IV fluids at: ____.
Pain level (0-10 scale.0-no pain, 10 intolerable): _______________.
Location of pain: ____________. Medicated for pain: ____ yes, ____ no.
Patient is alert/oriented: ____ yes, ____ no. New confusion: ____ yes, ____ no.
Vital signs: temp ____, pulse ____, resp ____, b/p ______, 02 _____%, ____ liters.
Glucose level: _____. Insulin: ___ yes, ___ no. Type: ___________ # of units ____.

NURSING CARE CONTINUED FOR ____________________________
DATE ____________________, DAY NUMBER ____________________

FOLLOWING EXAMINATIONS FOR NIGHT SHIFT:

Nurse ____________, CNA ____________, in at _____ am/pm. Left at ______ am/pm.
Wash hands and wear gloves before touching patient: ______ yes, ______ no.
Wash hands before leaving room: ___ yes, ___ no. Wear protective gear: __ yes, __ no.
Clean stethoscope: __ yes, __ no. Oral care: __ yes, __ no. Suctioned: __ yes, __ no.
Repositioned: ___ yes, ___ no. Turned to: ___ left, ___ right, ___ backside ___.
Head of bed at: _______ degrees. Incontinence/skin breakdown: ____ yes, ____ no.
Linens wet or soiled: ____ yes, ____ no. Linens changed: ____ yes, _____ no.
Dressing changed: ____ yes, ____ no. Location: ______________________.
IV site checked: _____ yes, _____ no. IV tubing labeled: _____ yes, _____no.
IV fluids at: ____.
Pain level (0-10 scale.0-no pain, 10 intolerable): ________________.
Location of pain: ________________. Medicated for pain: _____ yes, ____ no.
Patient is alert/oriented: ____ yes, ____ no. New confusion: ____ yes, ____ no.
Vital signs: temp ____, pulse _____, resp ______, b/p ______, 02 _____ %, ____ liters.
Glucose level: _____. Insulin: ___ yes, ___ no. Type: ____________ # of units ____.

Nurse ____________, CNA ____________, in at _____ am/pm. Left at ______ am/pm.
Wash hands and wear gloves before touching patient: ______ yes, ______ no.
Wash hands before leaving room: ___ yes, ___ no. Wear protective gear: __ yes, __ no.
Clean stethoscope: __ yes, __ no. Oral care: __ yes, __ no. Suctioned: __ yes, __ no.
Repositioned: ___ yes, ___ no. Turned to: ___ left, ___ right, ___ backside ___.
Head of bed at: _______ degrees. Incontinence/skin breakdown: ____ yes, ____ no.
Linens wet or soiled: ____ yes, ____ no. Linens changed: ____ yes, _____ no.
Dressing changed: ____ yes, ____ no. Location: ______________________.
IV site checked: _____ yes, _____ no. IV tubing labeled: _____ yes, _____no.
IV fluids at: ____.
Pain level (0-10 scale.0-no pain, 10 intolerable): ________________.
Location of pain: ________________. Medicated for pain: _____ yes, ____ no.
Patient is alert/oriented: ____ yes, ____ no. New confusion: ____ yes, ____ no.
Vital signs: temp ____, pulse _____, resp ______, b/p ______, 02 _____ %, ____ liters.
Glucose level: _____. Insulin: ___ yes, ___ no. Type: ____________ # of units ____.

Nurse ____________, CNA ____________, in at _____ am/pm. Left at ______ am/pm.
Wash hands and wear gloves before touching patient: ______ yes, ______ no.
Wash hands before leaving room: ___ yes, ___ no. Wear protective gear: __ yes, __ no.
Clean stethoscope: __ yes, __ no. Oral care: __ yes, __ no. Suctioned: __ yes, __ no.
Repositioned: ___ yes, ___ no. Turned to: ___ left, ___ right, ___ backside ___.
Head of bed at: _______ degrees. Incontinence/skin breakdown: ____ yes, ____ no.
Linens wet or soiled: ____ yes, ____ no. Linens changed: ____ yes, _____ no.
Dressing changed: ____ yes, ____ no. Location: ______________________.
IV site checked: _____ yes, _____ no. IV tubing labeled: _____ yes, _____no.
IV fluids at: ____.
Pain level (0-10 scale.0-no pain, 10 intolerable): ________________.
Location of pain: ________________. Medicated for pain: _____ yes, ____ no.
Patient is alert/oriented: ____ yes, ____ no. New confusion: ____ yes, ____ no.
Vital signs: temp ____, pulse _____, resp ______, b/p ______, 02 _____ %, ____ liters.
Glucose level: _____. Insulin: ___ yes, ___ no. Type: ____________ # of units ____.

MEDICATION ADMINISTRATION LIST FOR ______________________
DATE ________________ DAY NUMBER ________________________

List the medication for each day. Routes of administration: oral, thru feeding tube, intravenous (IV), intramuscular (IM), subcutaneous (SQ), epidural or a catheter in your spinal column, rectal, topical, eye drops, and ear drops.

Medication: ________________ Route: ________________ Time: ____________
Medication: ________________ Route: ________________ Time: ____________
Medication: ________________ Route: ________________ Time: ____________
Medication: ________________ Route: ________________ Time: ____________
Medication: ________________ Route: ________________ Time: ____________
Medication: ________________ Route: ________________ Time: ____________
Medication: ________________ Route: ________________ Time: ____________
Medication: ________________ Route: ________________ Time: ____________
Medication: ________________ Route: ________________ Time: ____________
Medication: ________________ Route: ________________ Time: ____________
Medication: ________________ Route: ________________ Time: ____________
Medication: ________________ Route: ________________ Time: ____________
Medication: ________________ Route: ________________ Time: ____________
Medication: ________________ Route: ________________ Time: ____________
Medication: ________________ Route: ________________ Time: ____________
Medication: ________________ Route: ________________ Time: ____________
Medication: ________________ Route: ________________ Time: ____________
Medication: ________________ Route: ________________ Time: ____________
Medication: ________________ Route: ________________ Time: ____________
Medication: ________________ Route: ________________ Time: ____________
Medication: ________________ Route: ________________ Time: ____________
Medication: ________________ Route: ________________ Time: ____________
Medication: ________________ Route: ________________ Time: ____________
Medication: ________________ Route: ________________ Time: ____________
Medication: ________________ Route: ________________ Time: ____________
Medication: ________________ Route: ________________ Time: ____________
Medication: ________________ Route: ________________ Time: ____________
Medication: ________________ Route: ________________ Time: ____________
Medication: ________________ Route: ________________ Time: ____________
Medication: ________________ Route: ________________ Time: ____________
Medication: ________________ Route: ________________ Time: ____________
Medication: ________________ Route: ________________ Time: ____________
Medication: ________________ Route: ________________ Time: ____________
Medication: ________________ Route: ________________ Time: ____________
Medication: ________________ Route: ________________ Time: ____________
Medication: ________________ Route: ________________ Time: ____________
Medication: ________________ Route: ________________ Time: ____________
Medication: ________________ Route: ________________ Time: ____________
Medication: ________________ Route: ________________ Time: ____________
Medication: ________________ Route: ________________ Time: ____________
Medication: ________________ Route: ________________ Time: ____________
Medication: ________________ Route: ________________ Time: ____________
Medication: ________________ Route: ________________ Time: ____________
Medication: ________________ Route: ________________ Time: ____________
Medication: ________________ Route: ________________ Time: ____________
Medication: ________________ Route: ________________ Time: ____________
Medication: ________________ Route: ________________ Time: ____________
Medication: ________________ Route: ________________ Time: ____________
Medication: ________________ Route: ________________ Time: ____________
Medication: ________________ Route: ________________ Time: ____________
Medication: ________________ Route: ________________ Time: ____________
Medication: ________________ Route: ________________ Time: ____________
Medication: ________________ Route: ________________ Time: ____________
Medication: ________________ Route: ________________ Time: ____________

NOTES FOR DAY NUMBER ______________________________

DATE ______________________________________

MEDICAL JOURNAL FOR ______________________________

DATE ____________________, DAY NUMBER ____________

VISITS FROM MY DOCTORS TODAY

Goals for today: ____

____

____.

Things to discuss with my doctor(s): ____________________________

____

____

Dr.__________ came in at ____ am/pm. Left at ____ am/pm.
We discussed ____.
Did doctor examine patient: ____ yes, ____ no.
Wash hands before touching patient: ____ yes, ____ no.
Wear gloves: ____ yes, ___ no. Clean stethoscope: ____ yes, ____ no.
Wear gown and mask (precautions only):____ yes, _____ no.
Wash hands before leaving the room: _____ yes, _____ no.

Dr.__________ came in at ____ am/pm. Left at ____ am/pm.
We discussed ____.
Did doctor examine patient: ____ yes, ____ no.
Wash hands before touching patient: ____ yes, ____ no.
Wear gloves: ____ yes, ___ no. Clean stethoscope: ____ yes, ____ no.
Wear gown and mask (precautions only):____ yes, _____ no.
Wash hands before leaving the room: _____ yes, _____ no.

Dr.__________ came in at ____ am/pm. Left at ____ am/pm.
We discussed ____.
Did doctor examine patient: ____ yes, ____ no.
Wash hands before touching patient: ____ yes, ____ no.
Wear gloves: ____ yes, ___ no. Clean stethoscope: ____ yes, ____ no.
Wear gown and mask (precautions only):____ yes, _____ no.
Wash hands before leaving the room: _____ yes, _____ no.

Dr.__________ came in at ____ am/pm. Left at ____ am/pm.
We discussed ____.
Did doctor examine patient: ____ yes, ____ no.
Wash hands before touching patient: ____ yes, ____ no.
Wear gloves: ____ yes, ___ no. Clean stethoscope: ____ yes, ____ no.
Wear gown and mask (precautions only):____ yes, _____ no.
Wash hands before leaving the room: _____ yes, _____ no.

Dr.__________ came in at ____ am/pm. Left at ____ am/pm.
We discussed ____.
Did doctor examine patient: ____ yes, ____ no.
Wash hands before touching patient: ____ yes, ____ no.
Wear gloves: ____ yes, ___ no. Clean stethoscope: ____ yes, ____ no.
Wear gown and mask (precautions only):____ yes, _____ no.
Wash hands before leaving the room: _____ yes, _____ no.

NURSING CARE FOR ____

DATE ____________________, DAY NUMBER ____________________

INITIAL DAY SHIFT EXAM:

My nurse has ______ # of patients. CNA ___yes, ___no. Charge nurse ____________
Nurse ________________ RN/LPN came in at __________ am/pm. Left at __________ am/pm.
Did nurse wash hands and wear gloves before touching patient: _______ yes, _______ no.
Wash hands after touching patient and before leaving the room: ______ yes, _______ no.
Don't hesitate to request staff to wash their hands. This will help decrease the risk of spreading potentially lethal germs.
Did nurse wear protective gear (isolation precautions only): _______ yes, _______ no.
Did nurse provide oral care (to be done every two hours if unable to provide for self, also decreases risk of pneumonia, infections, and aspiration): ______ yes, ______ no.
If able to provide own oral care, then supplies at bedside: _______ yes, _______ no.
Was patient repositioned (every two hours if unable to turn self): _____ yes _____ no.
Head of bed at ________ degrees. This is important for patients on ventilators or on tube feedings. Anything less than thirty degrees places patients at risk for aspiration of stomach contents into the lungs causing aspiration pneumonia.
Checked for incontinence and skin breakdown: _____ yes, _____ no.
Patient's linens wet or soiled: _____ yes, ____ no. Linens changed: ____ yes, ____ no.
Time linens changed: ________ am/pm. Any skin redness or breakdown: ____ yes, ____ no.
If yes, what stage is pressure ulcer: ________. Acquired when: ________________.
List wounds not associated with pressure ulcers and how acquired: ______________
____.
Mattress type: ____.
Specialty mattresses are important to help prevent pressure ulcers)
If patient on ventilator or has tracheostomy, suction performed: _____ yes, ______ no.
Did nurse listen to lung sounds: _____ yes, _____ no.
Does patient have chest tubes: ____ yes, ____ no. Functioning _____ yes, _____ no.
Bowel sounds: _______ yes, _______ no. Bowel sounds active: _____ yes, _____ no.
Neurological exam: ______ yes, ______ no. Follow commands: _____ yes, _____ no.
Is patient alert and oriented to person, place, time, and events: _____ yes, _____ no.
If confused, patient is not oriented to: ____ person, ___ place, ___ time, ___ event.
Confusion began (time and date): ____.
Glasgow coma scale (checks conscious scale of patient): _______________________.
Intracranial pressure monitoring: ______ yes, ______ no.
If yes, pressure is at _________ mm mercury. (Normal is one to fifteen).
Moves extremities: ___ yes, ___ no.
Paralysis: (inability to move extremities) ________ yes, ________ no.
If yes, extremities affected and when paralysis began: _________________________.
Is patient in pain: ____ yes, ____ no. Describe pain and location ______________.
Patient able to eat: ____ yes, ____ no. What type of diet? _____________________.
If patient on tube feedings list type: _______________ at ____________ cc/ml per hour.
Nausea ____, vomiting _____. If so, describe: ________________________________.
Patient has: Nasal gastric tube ______, Dobhoff tube _____, Peg or gastric tube _____.
When was feeding tube placed and what site: ____________________________________.
Catheter for draining urine: ___ yes, ___ no. If so, when placed: ______________.
Find out policy for allowed time to remain in bladder. Too long may cause infections.)
IV site(s) where: ______________________ when placed: __________________________.
IV fluids (types and rates): ________________________, __________________________,
____________________________, _______________________, ___________________________,
Is patient on oxygen: _____ yes, _____ no. If so, how much and route delivered (see oxygen routes): ____.
If patient on ventilator, list settings (see list on ventilator settings): __________
____.
Vital signs: temp _____, pulse _____, resp _____, b/p _____, o2 _____%,
current weight ______ pounds, ______ kg. Glucose level: _____
Insulin coverage: ____ yes, ____ no. Insulin type: ____________, # of units: _____.

NURSING CARE CONTINUED FOR ______________________
DATE ____________________, DAY NUMBER ________________

FOLLOWING EXAMINATIONS FOR DAY SHIFT:

Nurse __________, CNA __________, in at _____ am/pm. Left at ______ am/pm.
Wash hands and wear gloves before touching patient: _____yes, _____ no.
Wash hands before leaving room: ___ yes, ___ no. Wear protective gear: __ yes, __ no.
Clean stethoscope: __ yes, __ no. Oral care: __ yes, __ no. Suctioned: __ yes, __ no.
Repositioned: ___ yes, ___ no. Turned to: ___left, ___ right, ___ backside ___.
Head of bed at: _______ degrees. Incontinence/skin breakdown: ____ yes, ___ no.
Linens wet or soiled: _____ yes, _____ no. Linens changed: _____ yes, _____ no.
Dressing changed: ____ yes, ____ no. Location: _______________________.
IV site checked: _____ yes, _____ no. IV tubing labeled: _____ yes, _____no.
IV fluids at: ____.
Pain level (0-10 scale.0-no pain, 10 intolerable): _____________________.
Location of pain: __________. Medicated for pain: _____ yes, ____ no.
Patient is alert/oriented: ____ yes, ___ no. New confusion: ____yes, ____ no.
Vital signs: temp ____, pulse ____, resp ______, b/p _____, 02 _____%, ____ liters.
Glucose level: _____. Insulin: ___ yes, ___ no. Type: ____________ # of units ____.

Nurse __________, CNA __________, in at _____ am/pm. Left at ______ am/pm.
Wash hands and wear gloves before touching patient: _____yes, _____ no.
Wash hands before leaving room: ___ yes, ___ no. Wear protective gear: __ yes, __ no.
Clean stethoscope: __ yes, __ no. Oral care: __ yes, __ no. Suctioned: __ yes, __ no.
Repositioned: ___ yes, ___ no. Turned to: ___left, ___ right, ___ backside ___.
Head of bed at: _______ degrees. Incontinence/skin breakdown: ____ yes, ___ no.
Linens wet or soiled: _____ yes, _____ no. Linens changed: _____ yes, _____ no.
Dressing changed: ____ yes, ____ no. Location: _______________________.
IV site checked: _____ yes, _____ no. IV tubing labeled: _____ yes, _____no.
IV fluids at: ____.
Pain level (0-10 scale.0-no pain, 10 intolerable): _____________________.
Location of pain: __________. Medicated for pain: _____ yes, ____ no.
Patient is alert/oriented: ____ yes, ___ no. New confusion: ____yes, ____ no.
Vital signs: temp ____, pulse ____, resp ______, b/p _____, 02 _____%, ____ liters.
Glucose level: _____. Insulin: ___ yes, ___ no. Type: ____________ # of units ____.

Nurse __________, CNA __________, in at _____ am/pm. Left at ______ am/pm.
Wash hands and wear gloves before touching patient: _____yes, _____ no.
Wash hands before leaving room: ___ yes, ___ no. Wear protective gear: __ yes, __ no.
Clean stethoscope: __ yes, __ no. Oral care: __ yes, __ no. Suctioned: __ yes, __ no.
Repositioned: ___ yes, ___ no. Turned to: ___left, ___ right, ___ backside ___.
Head of bed at: _______ degrees. Incontinence/skin breakdown: ____ yes, ___ no.
Linens wet or soiled: _____ yes, _____ no. Linens changed: _____ yes, _____ no.
Dressing changed: ____ yes, ____ no. Location: _______________________.
IV site checked: _____ yes, _____ no. IV tubing labeled: _____ yes, _____no.
IV fluids at: ____.
Pain level (0-10 scale.0-no pain, 10 intolerable): _____________________.
Location of pain: __________. Medicated for pain: _____ yes, ____ no.
Patient is alert/oriented: ____ yes, ___ no. New confusion: ____yes, ____ no.
Vital signs: temp ____, pulse ____, resp ______, b/p _____, 02 _____%, ____ liters.
Glucose level: _____. Insulin: ___ yes, ___ no. Type: ____________ # of units ____.

NURSING CARE CONTINUED FOR ______________________________
DATE ___________________, DAY NUMBER ____________________

FOLLOWING EXAMINATIONS FOR DAY SHIFT:

Nurse ____________, CNA ____________, in at _____ am/pm. Left at ______ am/pm.
Wash hands and wear gloves before touching patient: ________ yes, ________ no.
Wash hands before leaving room: ___ yes, ___ no. Wear protective gear: __ yes, __ no.
Clean stethoscope: __ yes, __ no. Oral care: __ yes, __ no. Suctioned: __ yes, __ no.
Repositioned: ___ yes, ___ no. Turned to: ___ left, ___ right, ___ backside ___.
Head of bed at: _______ degrees. Incontinence/skin breakdown: ____ yes, ____ no.
Linens wet or soiled: _____ yes, _____ no. Linens changed: _____ yes, ______ no.
Dressing changed: ____ yes, ____ no. Location: ______________________________.
IV site checked: _____ yes, _____ no. IV tubing labeled: _____ yes, _____no.
IV fluids at: ____.
Pain level (0-10 scale.0-no pain, 10 intolerable): ____________________________.
Location of pain: ______________. Medicated for pain: _____ yes, ____ no.
Patient is alert/oriented: ____ yes, ____ no. New confusion: ____ yes, ____ no.
Vital signs: temp ____, pulse ____, resp _____, b/p ______, 02 _____ %, ____ liters.
Glucose level: _____. Insulin: ___ yes, ___ no. Type: _____________ # of units ____.

Nurse ____________, CNA ____________, in at _____ am/pm. Left at ______ am/pm.
Wash hands and wear gloves before touching patient: ________ yes, ________ no.
Wash hands before leaving room: ___ yes, ___ no. Wear protective gear: __ yes, __ no.
Clean stethoscope: __ yes, __ no. Oral care: __ yes, __ no. Suctioned: __ yes, __ no.
Repositioned: ___ yes, ___ no. Turned to: ___ left, ___ right, ___ backside ___.
Head of bed at: _______ degrees. Incontinence/skin breakdown: ____ yes, ____ no.
Linens wet or soiled: _____ yes, _____ no. Linens changed: _____ yes, ______ no.
Dressing changed: ____ yes, ____ no. Location: ______________________________.
IV site checked: _____ yes, _____ no. IV tubing labeled: _____ yes, _____no.
IV fluids at: ____.
Pain level (0-10 scale.0-no pain, 10 intolerable): ____________________________.
Location of pain: ______________. Medicated for pain: _____ yes, ____ no.
Patient is alert/oriented: ____ yes, ____ no. New confusion: ____ yes, ____ no.
Vital signs: temp ____, pulse ____, resp _____, b/p ______, 02 _____ %, ____ liters.
Glucose level: _____. Insulin: ___ yes, ___ no. Type: _____________ # of units ____.

Nurse ____________, CNA ____________, in at _____ am/pm. Left at ______ am/pm.
Wash hands and wear gloves before touching patient: ________ yes, ________ no.
Wash hands before leaving room: ___ yes, ___ no. Wear protective gear: __ yes, __ no.
Clean stethoscope: __ yes, __ no. Oral care: __ yes, __ no. Suctioned: __ yes, __ no.
Repositioned: ___ yes, ___ no. Turned to: ___ left, ___ right, ___ backside ___.
Head of bed at: _______ degrees. Incontinence/skin breakdown: ____ yes, ____ no.
Linens wet or soiled: _____ yes, _____ no. Linens changed: _____ yes, ______ no.
Dressing changed: ____ yes, ____ no. Location: ______________________________.
IV site checked: _____ yes, _____ no. IV tubing labeled: _____ yes, _____no.
IV fluids at: ____.
Pain level (0-10 scale.0-no pain, 10 intolerable): ____________________________.
Location of pain: ______________. Medicated for pain: _____ yes, ____ no.
Patient is alert/oriented: ____ yes, ____ no. New confusion: ____ yes, ____ no.
Vital signs: temp ____, pulse ____, resp _____, b/p ______, 02 _____ %, ____ liters.
Glucose level: _____. Insulin: ___ yes, ___ no. Type: _____________ # of units ____.

NURSING CARE FOR ______________________________________

DATE ____________________, DAY NUMBER ____________________

INITIAL NIGHT SHIFT EXAM:

My nurse has ______ # of patients. CNA ___yes, ___no. Charge nurse ______________
Nurse ______________ RN/LPN came in at __________ am/pm. Left at __________ am/pm.
Did nurse wash hands and wear gloves before touching patient: ______ yes, ______ no.
Wash hands after touching patient and before leaving the room: ______ yes, ______ no.
Don't hesitate to request staff to wash their hands. This will help decrease the risk of spreading potentially lethal germs.
Did nurse wear protective gear (isolation precautions only): ______ yes, ______ no.
Did nurse provide oral care (to be done every two hours if unable to provide for self, also decreases risk of pneumonia, infections, and aspiration): ______ yes, ______ no.
If able to provide own oral care, then supplies at bedside: ______ yes, ______ no.
Was patient repositioned (every two hours if unable to turn self): ______ yes ______ no.
Head of bed at ________ degrees. This is important for patients on ventilators or on tube feedings. Anything less than thirty degrees places patients at risk for aspiration of stomach contents into the lungs causing aspiration pneumonia.
Checked for incontinence and skin breakdown: ____ yes, ____ no.
Patient's linens wet or soiled: ____ yes, ____ no. Linens changed: ____ yes, ____ no.
Time linens changed: ________ am/pm. Any skin redness or breakdown: ____ yes, ____ no.
If yes, what stage is pressure ulcer: ________. Acquired when: ______________
List wounds not associated with pressure ulcers and how acquired: ______________
____.
Mattress type: ____
Specialty mattresses are important to help prevent pressure ulcers)
If patient on ventilator or has tracheostomy, suction performed: ____ yes, ____ no.
Did nurse listen to lung sounds: ____ yes, ____ no.
Does patient have chest tubes: ____ yes, ____ no. Functioning _____ yes, _____ no.
Bowel sounds: ______ yes, ______ no. Bowel sounds active: ______ yes, ______ no.
Neurological exam: ______ yes, ______ no. Follow commands: ______ yes, ______ no.
Is patient alert and oriented to person, place, time, and events: ____ yes, ____ no.
If confused, patient is not oriented to: ____ person, ___ place, ___ time, ___ event.
Confusion began (time and date): ____.
Glasgow coma scale (checks conscious scale of patient): __________________________.
Intracranial pressure monitoring: _____ yes, _____ no.
If yes, pressure is at ________ mm mercury. (Normal is one to fifteen).
Moves extremities: ___ yes, ___ no.
Paralysis: (inability to move extremities) ______ yes, ______ no.
If yes, extremities affected and when paralysis began: __________________________.
Is patient in pain: ____ yes, ____ no. Describe pain and location ________________.
Patient able to eat: ____ yes, ____ no. What type of diet? _______________________.
If patient on tube feedings list type: ____________ at ____________ cc/ml per hour.
Nausea ____, vomiting ____. If so, describe: _____________________________________.
Patient has: Nasal gastric tube ______, Dobhoff tube ____, Peg or gastric tube ____.
When was feeding tube placed and what site: _____________________________________.
Catheter for draining urine: ____ yes, ____ no. If so, when placed: ______________.
Find out policy for allowed time to remain in bladder. Too long may cause infections.)
IV site(s) where: ____________________ when placed: ______________________________.
IV fluids (types and rates): ____________________, ____________________,
____________________, ____________________, ____________________,
Is patient on oxygen: ____ yes, ____ no. If so, how much and route delivered
(see oxygen routes): ____.
If patient on ventilator, list settings (see list on ventilator settings): ___________
____.
Vital signs: temp ______, pulse ______, resp ______, b/p ______, o2 ______%,
current weight ______ pounds, ______ kg. Glucose level: ______
Insulin coverage: ____ yes, ____ no. Insulin type: ____________, # of units: ______.

NURSING CARE CONTINUED FOR ______________________
DATE ______________, DAY NUMBER ______________

FOLLOWING EXAMINATIONS FOR NIGHT SHIFT:

Nurse __________, CNA __________, in at _____ am/pm. Left at _____ am/pm.
Wash hands and wear gloves before touching patient: _____ yes, _____ no.
Wash hands before leaving room: ___ yes, ___ no. Wear protective gear: __ yes, __ no.
Clean stethoscope: __ yes, __ no. Oral care: __ yes, __ no. Suctioned: __ yes, __ no.
Repositioned: ___ yes, ___ no. Turned to: ___ left, ___ right, ___ backside ___.
Head of bed at: ______ degrees. Incontinence/skin breakdown: ____ yes, ____ no.
Linens wet or soiled: _____ yes, _____ no. Linens changed: _____ yes, _____ no.
Dressing changed: ____ yes, ____ no. Location: ______________________.
IV site checked: _____ yes, _____ no. IV tubing labeled: _____ yes, _____no.
IV fluids at: ______________________________________.
Pain level (0-10 scale.0-no pain, 10 intolerable): ______________.
Location of pain: ______________. Medicated for pain: ____ yes, ____ no.
Patient is alert/oriented: ____ yes, ____ no. New confusion: ____ yes, ____ no.
Vital signs: temp ____, pulse ____, resp _____, b/p _____, 02 _____%, ____ liters.
Glucose level: _____. Insulin: ___ yes, ___ no. Type: __________ # of units ___.

Nurse __________, CNA __________, in at _____ am/pm. Left at _____ am/pm.
Wash hands and wear gloves before touching patient: _____ yes, _____ no.
Wash hands before leaving room: ___ yes, ___ no. Wear protective gear: __ yes, __ no.
Clean stethoscope: __ yes, __ no. Oral care: __ yes, __ no. Suctioned: __ yes, __ no.
Repositioned: ___ yes, ___ no. Turned to: ___ left, ___ right, ___ backside ___.
Head of bed at: ______ degrees. Incontinence/skin breakdown: ____ yes, ____ no.
Linens wet or soiled: _____ yes, _____ no. Linens changed: _____ yes, _____ no.
Dressing changed: ____ yes, ____ no. Location: ______________________.
IV site checked: _____ yes, _____ no. IV tubing labeled: _____ yes, _____no.
IV fluids at: ______________________________________.
Pain level (0-10 scale.0-no pain, 10 intolerable): ______________.
Location of pain: ______________. Medicated for pain: ____ yes, ____ no.
Patient is alert/oriented: ____ yes, ____ no. New confusion: ____ yes, ____ no.
Vital signs: temp ____, pulse ____, resp _____, b/p _____, 02 _____%, ____ liters.
Glucose level: _____. Insulin: ___ yes, ___ no. Type: __________ # of units ___.

Nurse __________, CNA __________, in at _____ am/pm. Left at _____ am/pm.
Wash hands and wear gloves before touching patient: _____ yes, _____ no.
Wash hands before leaving room: ___ yes, ___ no. Wear protective gear: __ yes, __ no.
Clean stethoscope: __ yes, __ no. Oral care: __ yes, __ no. Suctioned: __ yes, __ no.
Repositioned: ___ yes, ___ no. Turned to: ___ left, ___ right, ___ backside ___.
Head of bed at: ______ degrees. Incontinence/skin breakdown: ____ yes, ____ no.
Linens wet or soiled: _____ yes, _____ no. Linens changed: _____ yes, _____ no.
Dressing changed: ____ yes, ____ no. Location: ______________________.
IV site checked: _____ yes, _____ no. IV tubing labeled: _____ yes, _____no.
IV fluids at: ______________________________________.
Pain level (0-10 scale.0-no pain, 10 intolerable): ______________.
Location of pain: ______________. Medicated for pain: ____ yes, ____ no.
Patient is alert/oriented: ____ yes, ____ no. New confusion: ____ yes, ____ no.
Vital signs: temp ____, pulse ____, resp _____, b/p _____, 02 _____%, ____ liters.
Glucose level: _____. Insulin: ___ yes, ___ no. Type: __________ # of units ___.

NURSING CARE CONTINUED FOR ____________________
DATE ____________________, DAY NUMBER ____________________

FOLLOWING EXAMINATIONS FOR NIGHT SHIFT:

Nurse ______________, CNA ______________, in at _____ am/pm. Left at ______ am/pm.
Wash hands and wear gloves before touching patient: _______ yes, ______ no.
Wash hands before leaving room: ___ yes, ___ no. Wear protective gear: __ yes, __ no.
Clean stethoscope: __ yes, __ no. Oral care: __ yes, __ no. Suctioned: __ yes, __ no.
Repositioned: ___ yes, ___ no. Turned to: ___ left, ___ right, ___ backside ___.
Head of bed at: _______ degrees. Incontinence/skin breakdown: ____ yes, ____ no.
Linens wet or soiled: _____ yes, _____ no. Linens changed: _____ yes, _____ no.
Dressing changed: ____ yes, ____ no. Location: ____________________.
IV site checked: _____ yes, _____ no. IV tubing labeled: _____ yes, _____no.
IV fluids at: ____.
Pain level (0-10 scale.0-no pain, 10 intolerable): ____________________.
Location of pain: ______________. Medicated for pain: ____ yes, ____ no.
Patient is alert/oriented: ____ yes, ____ no. New confusion: ____ yes, ____ no.
Vital signs: temp ____, pulse _____, resp ______, b/p ______, 02 _____ %, ____ liters.
Glucose level: _____. Insulin: ___ yes, ___ no. Type: ______________ # of units ____.

Nurse ______________, CNA ______________, in at _____ am/pm. Left at ______ am/pm.
Wash hands and wear gloves before touching patient: _______ yes, ______ no.
Wash hands before leaving room: ___ yes, ___ no. Wear protective gear: __ yes, __ no.
Clean stethoscope: __ yes, __ no. Oral care: __ yes, __ no. Suctioned: __ yes, __ no.
Repositioned: ___ yes, ___ no. Turned to: ___ left, ___ right, ___ backside ___.
Head of bed at: _______ degrees. Incontinence/skin breakdown: ____ yes, ____ no.
Linens wet or soiled: _____ yes, _____ no. Linens changed: _____ yes, _____ no.
Dressing changed: ____ yes, ____ no. Location: ____________________.
IV site checked: _____ yes, _____ no. IV tubing labeled: _____ yes, _____no.
IV fluids at: ____.
Pain level (0-10 scale.0-no pain, 10 intolerable): ____________________.
Location of pain: ______________. Medicated for pain: ____ yes, ____ no.
Patient is alert/oriented: ____ yes, ____ no. New confusion: ____ yes, ____ no.
Vital signs: temp ____, pulse _____, resp ______, b/p ______, 02 _____ %, ____ liters.
Glucose level: _____. Insulin: ___ yes, ___ no. Type: ______________ # of units ____.

Nurse ______________, CNA ______________, in at _____ am/pm. Left at ______ am/pm.
Wash hands and wear gloves before touching patient: _______ yes, ______ no.
Wash hands before leaving room: ___ yes, ___ no. Wear protective gear: __ yes, __ no.
Clean stethoscope: __ yes, __ no. Oral care: __ yes, __ no. Suctioned: __ yes, __ no.
Repositioned: ___ yes, ___ no. Turned to: ___ left, ___ right, ___ backside ___.
Head of bed at: _______ degrees. Incontinence/skin breakdown: ____ yes, ____ no.
Linens wet or soiled: _____ yes, _____ no. Linens changed: _____ yes, _____ no.
Dressing changed: ____ yes, ____ no. Location: ____________________.
IV site checked: _____ yes, _____ no. IV tubing labeled: _____ yes, _____no.
IV fluids at: ____.
Pain level (0-10 scale.0-no pain, 10 intolerable): ____________________.
Location of pain: ______________. Medicated for pain: ____ yes, ____ no.
Patient is alert/oriented: ____ yes, ____ no. New confusion: ____ yes, ____ no.
Vital signs: temp ____, pulse _____, resp ______, b/p ______, 02 _____ %, ____ liters.
Glucose level: _____. Insulin: ___ yes, ___ no. Type: ______________ # of units ____.

MEDICATION ADMINISTRATION LIST FOR ____________________
DATE ________________ DAY NUMBER ____________________

List the medication for each day. Routes of administration: oral, thru feeding tube, intravenous (IV), intramuscular (IM), subcutaneous (SQ), epidural or a catheter in your spinal column, rectal, topical, eye drops, and ear drops.

Medication: ________________ Route: ________________ Time: ____________
Medication: ________________ Route: ________________ Time: ____________
Medication: ________________ Route: ________________ Time: ____________
Medication: ________________ Route: ________________ Time: ____________
Medication: ________________ Route: ________________ Time: ____________
Medication: ________________ Route: ________________ Time: ____________
Medication: ________________ Route: ________________ Time: ____________
Medication: ________________ Route: ________________ Time: ____________
Medication: ________________ Route: ________________ Time: ____________
Medication: ________________ Route: ________________ Time: ____________
Medication: ________________ Route: ________________ Time: ____________
Medication: ________________ Route: ________________ Time: ____________
Medication: ________________ Route: ________________ Time: ____________
Medication: ________________ Route: ________________ Time: ____________
Medication: ________________ Route: ________________ Time: ____________
Medication: ________________ Route: ________________ Time: ____________
Medication: ________________ Route: ________________ Time: ____________
Medication: ________________ Route: ________________ Time: ____________
Medication: ________________ Route: ________________ Time: ____________
Medication: ________________ Route: ________________ Time: ____________
Medication: ________________ Route: ________________ Time: ____________
Medication: ________________ Route: ________________ Time: ____________
Medication: ________________ Route: ________________ Time: ____________
Medication: ________________ Route: ________________ Time: ____________
Medication: ________________ Route: ________________ Time: ____________
Medication: ________________ Route: ________________ Time: ____________
Medication: ________________ Route: ________________ Time: ____________
Medication: ________________ Route: ________________ Time: ____________
Medication: ________________ Route: ________________ Time: ____________
Medication: ________________ Route: ________________ Time: ____________
Medication: ________________ Route: ________________ Time: ____________
Medication: ________________ Route: ________________ Time: ____________
Medication: ________________ Route: ________________ Time: ____________
Medication: ________________ Route: ________________ Time: ____________
Medication: ________________ Route: ________________ Time: ____________
Medication: ________________ Route: ________________ Time: ____________
Medication: ________________ Route: ________________ Time: ____________
Medication: ________________ Route: ________________ Time: ____________
Medication: ________________ Route: ________________ Time: ____________
Medication: ________________ Route: ________________ Time: ____________
Medication: ________________ Route: ________________ Time: ____________
Medication: ________________ Route: ________________ Time: ____________
Medication: ________________ Route: ________________ Time: ____________
Medication: ________________ Route: ________________ Time: ____________
Medication: ________________ Route: ________________ Time: ____________
Medication: ________________ Route: ________________ Time: ____________
Medication: ________________ Route: ________________ Time: ____________
Medication: ________________ Route: ________________ Time: ____________
Medication: ________________ Route: ________________ Time: ____________
Medication: ________________ Route: ________________ Time: ____________
Medication: ________________ Route: ________________ Time: ____________
Medication: ________________ Route: ________________ Time: ____________
Medication: ________________ Route: ________________ Time: ____________
Medication: ________________ Route: ________________ Time: ____________

NOTES FOR DAY NUMBER ______________________________

DATE ______________________________

MEDICAL JOURNAL FOR ______________________________

DATE ________________, DAY NUMBER ______________

VISITS FROM MY DOCTORS TODAY

Goals for today: ____

____

____.

Things to discuss with my doctor(s): ______________________________

____

____

Dr.____________ came in at ____ am/pm. Left at ____ am/pm.
We discussed ____.
Did doctor examine patient: _____ yes, _____ no.
Wash hands before touching patient: _____ yes, _____ no.
Wear gloves: ____ yes, ___ no. Clean stethoscope: ____ yes, ____ no.
Wear gown and mask (precautions only):____ yes, _____ no.
Wash hands before leaving the room: _____ yes, _____ no.

Dr.____________ came in at ____ am/pm. Left at ____ am/pm.
We discussed ____.
Did doctor examine patient: _____ yes, _____ no.
Wash hands before touching patient: _____ yes, _____ no.
Wear gloves: ____ yes, ___ no. Clean stethoscope: ____ yes, ____ no.
Wear gown and mask (precautions only):____ yes, _____ no.
Wash hands before leaving the room: _____ yes, _____ no.

Dr.____________ came in at ____ am/pm. Left at ____ am/pm.
We discussed ____.
Did doctor examine patient: _____ yes, _____ no.
Wash hands before touching patient: _____ yes, _____ no.
Wear gloves: ____ yes, ___ no. Clean stethoscope: ____ yes, ____ no.
Wear gown and mask (precautions only):____ yes, _____ no.
Wash hands before leaving the room: _____ yes, _____ no.

Dr.____________ came in at ____ am/pm. Left at ____ am/pm.
We discussed ____.
Did doctor examine patient: _____ yes, _____ no.
Wash hands before touching patient: _____ yes, _____ no.
Wear gloves: ____ yes, ___ no. Clean stethoscope: ____ yes, ____ no.
Wear gown and mask (precautions only):____ yes, _____ no.
Wash hands before leaving the room: _____ yes, _____ no.

Dr.____________ came in at ____ am/pm. Left at ____ am/pm.
We discussed ____.
Did doctor examine patient: _____ yes, _____ no.
Wash hands before touching patient: _____ yes, _____ no.
Wear gloves: ____ yes, ___ no. Clean stethoscope: ____ yes, ____ no.
Wear gown and mask (precautions only):____ yes, _____ no.
Wash hands before leaving the room: _____ yes, _____ no.

NURSING CARE FOR ______________________________

DATE ____________________, DAY NUMBER ____________________

INITIAL DAY SHIFT EXAM:

My nurse has ______ # of patients. CNA ___yes, ___no. Charge nurse _______________
Nurse ____________ RN/LPN came in at _________ am/pm. Left at __________ am/pm.
Did nurse wash hands and wear gloves before touching patient: ______ yes, _______ no.
Wash hands after touching patient and before leaving the room: ______ yes, _______ no.
Don't hesitate to request staff to wash their hands. This will help decrease the risk of spreading potentially lethal germs.
Did nurse wear protective gear (isolation precautions only): _______ yes, _______ no.
Did nurse provide oral care (to be done every two hours if unable to provide for self, also decreases risk of pneumonia, infections, and aspiration): _______ yes, ______ no.
If able to provide own oral care, then supplies at bedside: _______ yes, ______ no.
Was patient repositioned (every two hours if unable to turn self): _____ yes _____ no.
Head of bed at _________ degrees. This is important for patients on ventilators or on tube feedings. Anything less than thirty degrees places patients at risk for aspiration of stomach contents into the lungs causing aspiration pneumonia.
Checked for incontinence and skin breakdown: ____ yes, _____ no.
Patient's linens wet or soiled: _____ yes, ____ no. Linens changed: ____ yes, ____ no.
Time linens changed: ________ am/pm. Any skin redness or breakdown: ____ yes, ____ no.
If yes, what stage is pressure ulcer: __________. Acquired when: ________________
List wounds not associated with pressure ulcers and how acquired: ________________
____.
Mattress type: ____
Specialty mattresses are important to help prevent pressure ulcers)
If patient on ventilator or has tracheostomy, suction performed: ______ yes, ______ no.
Did nurse listen to lung sounds: ______ yes, ______ no.
Does patient have chest tubes: ____ yes, ____ no. Functioning _____ yes, _____ no.
Bowel sounds: ________ yes, _______ no. Bowel sounds active: ______ yes, ______ no.
Neurological exam: ______ yes, _______ no. Follow commands: ______ yes, ______ no.
Is patient alert and oriented to person, place, time, and events: _____ yes, _____ no.
If confused, patient is not oriented to: ___ person, ___ place, ___ time, ___ event.
Confusion began (time and date): ____.
Glasgow coma scale (checks conscious scale of patient): ___________________________.
Intracranial pressure monitoring: _____ yes, _____ no.
If yes, pressure is at ________ mm mercury. (Normal is one to fifteen).
Moves extremities: ___ yes, ___ no.
Paralysis: (inability to move extremities) _______ yes, _______ no.
If yes, extremities affected and when paralysis began: ____________________________.
Is patient in pain: ____ yes, ____ no. Describe pain and location ________________.
Patient able to eat: ___ yes, ___ no. What type of diet? ________________________
If patient on tube feedings list type: ____________ at ___________ cc/ml per hour.
Nausea ____, vomiting ____ If so, describe: _____________________________________
Patient has: Nasal gastric tube ______, Dobhoff tube _____, Peg or gastric tube _____
When was feeding tube placed and what site: ______________________________________.
Catheter for draining urine: ____ yes, ____ no. If so, when placed: ______________.
Find out policy for allowed time to remain in bladder. Too long may cause infections.)
IV site(s) where: ___________________ when placed: _______________________________.
IV fluids (types and rates): ______________, ______________, ______________________,
_________________, ________________, ________________, ____________________________,
Is patient on oxygen: _____ yes, _____ no. If so, how much and route delivered (see oxygen routes): ____.
If patient on ventilator, list settings (see list on ventilator settings): __________
____.
Vital signs: temp ______, pulse ______, resp ______, b/p ______, o2 ______%,
current weight ______ pounds, ______ kg. Glucose level: ______
Insulin coverage: ____ yes, ____ no. Insulin type: _____________, # of units: ______.

NURSING CARE CONTINUED FOR ______________________
DATE ______________, DAY NUMBER ______________

FOLLOWING EXAMINATIONS FOR DAY SHIFT:

Nurse ____________, CNA ____________, in at ______ am/pm. Left at ______ am/pm.
Wash hands and wear gloves before touching patient: ______ yes, ______ no.
Wash hands before leaving room: ___ yes, ___ no. Wear protective gear: __ yes, __ no.
Clean stethoscope: __ yes, __ no. Oral care: __ yes, __ no. Suctioned: __ yes, __ no.
Repositioned: ___ yes, ___ no. Turned to: ___ left, ___ right, ___ backside ___.
Head of bed at: ______ degrees. Incontinence/skin breakdown: ____ yes, ____ no.
Linens wet or soiled: _____ yes, _____ no. Linens changed: _____ yes, ______ no.
Dressing changed: ____ yes, ____ no. Location: ______________________.
IV site checked: _____ yes, _____ no. IV tubing labeled: _____ yes, _____no.
IV fluids at: ______________________________________.
Pain level (0-10 scale.0-no pain, 10 intolerable): ______________________.
Location of pain: ____________. Medicated for pain: _____ yes, ___ no.
Patient is alert/oriented: ____ yes, ____ no. New confusion: ____ yes, ____ no.
Vital signs: temp ____, pulse _____, resp _____, b/p ______, 02 _____ %, ____ liters.
Glucose level: _____. Insulin: ___ yes, ___ no. Type: ____________ # of units ____.

Nurse ____________, CNA ____________, in at ______ am/pm. Left at ______ am/pm.
Wash hands and wear gloves before touching patient: ______ yes, ______ no.
Wash hands before leaving room: ___ yes, ___ no. Wear protective gear: __ yes, __ no.
Clean stethoscope: __ yes, __ no. Oral care: __ yes, __ no. Suctioned: __ yes, __ no.
Repositioned: ___ yes, ___ no. Turned to: ___ left, ___ right, ___ backside ___.
Head of bed at: ______ degrees. Incontinence/skin breakdown: ____ yes, ____ no.
Linens wet or soiled: _____ yes, _____ no. Linens changed: _____ yes, ______ no.
Dressing changed: ____ yes, ____ no. Location: ______________________.
IV site checked: _____ yes, _____ no. IV tubing labeled: _____ yes, _____no.
IV fluids at: ______________________________________.
Pain level (0-10 scale.0-no pain, 10 intolerable): ______________________.
Location of pain: ____________. Medicated for pain: _____ yes, ___ no.
Patient is alert/oriented: ____ yes, ____ no. New confusion: ____ yes, ____ no.
Vital signs: temp ____, pulse _____, resp _____, b/p ______, 02 _____ %, ____ liters.
Glucose level: _____. Insulin: ___ yes, ___ no. Type: ____________ # of units ____.

Nurse ____________, CNA ____________, in at ______ am/pm. Left at ______ am/pm.
Wash hands and wear gloves before touching patient: ______ yes, ______ no.
Wash hands before leaving room: ___ yes, ___ no. Wear protective gear: __ yes, __ no.
Clean stethoscope: __ yes, __ no. Oral care: __ yes, __ no. Suctioned: __ yes, __ no.
Repositioned: ___ yes, ___ no. Turned to: ___ left, ___ right, ___ backside ___.
Head of bed at: ______ degrees. Incontinence/skin breakdown: ____ yes, ____ no.
Linens wet or soiled: _____ yes, _____ no. Linens changed: _____ yes, ______ no.
Dressing changed: ____ yes, ____ no. Location: ______________________.
IV site checked: _____ yes, _____ no. IV tubing labeled: _____ yes, _____no.
IV fluids at: ______________________________________.
Pain level (0-10 scale.0-no pain, 10 intolerable): ______________________.
Location of pain: ____________. Medicated for pain: _____ yes, ___ no.
Patient is alert/oriented: ____ yes, ____ no. New confusion: ____ yes, ____ no.
Vital signs: temp ____, pulse _____, resp _____, b/p ______, 02 _____ %, ____ liters.
Glucose level: _____. Insulin: ___ yes, ___ no. Type: ____________ # of units ____.

NURSING CARE CONTINUED FOR ______________________
DATE ____________________, DAY NUMBER ____________________

FOLLOWING EXAMINATIONS FOR DAY SHIFT:

Nurse ______________, CNA ______________, in at ______ am/pm. Left at ______ am/pm.
Wash hands and wear gloves before touching patient: ______ yes, ______ no.
Wash hands before leaving room: ___ yes, ___ no. Wear protective gear: __ yes, __ no.
Clean stethoscope: __ yes, __ no. Oral care: __ yes, __ no. Suctioned: __ yes, __ no.
Repositioned: ___ yes, ___ no. Turned to: ___ left, ___ right, ___ backside ___.
Head of bed at: ________ degrees. Incontinence/skin breakdown: ___ yes, ___ no.
Linens wet or soiled: _____ yes, _____ no. Linens changed: ____ yes, ____ no.
Dressing changed: ____ yes, ____ no. Location: ______________________________.
IV site checked: _____ yes, _____ no. IV tubing labeled: _____ yes, _____ no.
IV fluids at: ____.
Pain level (0-10 scale.0-no pain, 10 intolerable): ____________________________.
Location of pain: _____________________. Medicated for pain: ____ yes, ____ no.
Patient is alert/oriented: ____ yes, ____ no. New confusion: ____ yes, ____ no.
Vital signs: temp ____, pulse ____, resp ____, b/p ______, O2 ____ %, ____ liters.
Glucose level: _____. Insulin: ___ yes, ___ no. Type: _________ # of units ____.

Nurse ______________, CNA ______________, in at ______ am/pm. Left at ______ am/pm.
Wash hands and wear gloves before touching patient: ______ yes, ______ no.
Wash hands before leaving room: ___ yes, ___ no. Wear protective gear: __ yes, __ no.
Clean stethoscope: __ yes, __ no. Oral care: __ yes, __ no. Suctioned: __ yes, __ no.
Repositioned: ___ yes, ___ no. Turned to: ___ left, ___ right, ___ backside ___.
Head of bed at: ________ degrees. Incontinence/skin breakdown: ___ yes, ___ no.
Linens wet or soiled: _____ yes, _____ no. Linens changed: ____ yes, ____ no.
Dressing changed: ____ yes, ____ no. Location: ______________________________.
IV site checked: _____ yes, _____ no. IV tubing labeled: _____ yes, _____ no.
IV fluids at: ____.
Pain level (0-10 scale.0-no pain, 10 intolerable): ____________________________.
Location of pain: _____________________. Medicated for pain: ____ yes, ____ no.
Patient is alert/oriented: ____ yes, ____ no. New confusion: ____ yes, ____ no.
Vital signs: temp ____, pulse ____, resp ____, b/p ______, O2 ____ %, ____ liters.
Glucose level: _____. Insulin: ___ yes, ___ no. Type: _________ # of units ____.

Nurse ______________, CNA ______________, in at ______ am/pm. Left at ______ am/pm.
Wash hands and wear gloves before touching patient: ______ yes, ______ no.
Wash hands before leaving room: ___ yes, ___ no. Wear protective gear: __ yes, __ no.
Clean stethoscope: __ yes, __ no. Oral care: __ yes, __ no. Suctioned: __ yes, __ no.
Repositioned: ___ yes, ___ no. Turned to: ___ left, ___ right, ___ backside ___.
Head of bed at: ________ degrees. Incontinence/skin breakdown: ___ yes, ___ no.
Linens wet or soiled: _____ yes, _____ no. Linens changed: ____ yes, ____ no.
Dressing changed: ____ yes, ____ no. Location: ______________________________.
IV site checked: _____ yes, _____ no. IV tubing labeled: _____ yes, _____ no.
IV fluids at: ____.
Pain level (0-10 scale.0-no pain, 10 intolerable): ____________________________.
Location of pain: _____________________. Medicated for pain: ____ yes, ____ no.
Patient is alert/oriented: ____ yes, ____ no. New confusion: ____ yes, ____ no.
Vital signs: temp ____, pulse ____, resp ____, b/p ______, O2 ____ %, ____ liters.
Glucose level: _____. Insulin: ___ yes, ___ no. Type: _________ # of units ____.

NURSING CARE FOR ______________________________

DATE __________________, DAY NUMBER _____________________

INITIAL NIGHT SHIFT EXAM:

My nurse has _____ # of patients. CNA ___yes, ___no. Charge nurse _______________
Nurse _____________ RN/LPN came in at ________ am/pm. Left at _________ am/pm.
Did nurse wash hands and wear gloves before touching patient: ______ yes, ______ no.
Wash hands after touching patient and before leaving the room: ______ yes, ______ no.
Don't hesitate to request staff to wash their hands. This will help decrease the risk of spreading potentially lethal germs.
Did nurse wear protective gear (isolation precautions only): ______ yes, ______ no.
Did nurse provide oral care (to be done every two hours if unable to provide for self, also decreases risk of pneumonia, infections, and aspiration): ______ yes, _____ no.
If able to provide own oral care, then supplies at bedside: ______ yes, ______ no.
Was patient repositioned (every two hours if unable to turn self): ____ yes ____ no.
Head of bed at _______ degrees. This is important for patients on ventilators or on tube feedings. Anything less than thirty degrees places patients at risk for aspiration of stomach contents into the lungs causing aspiration pneumonia.
Checked for incontinence and skin breakdown: ____ yes, ____ no.
Patient's linens wet or soiled: _____ yes, ____ no. Linens changed: ____ yes, ____ no.
Time linens changed: _______ am/pm. Any skin redness or breakdown: ____ yes, ____ no.
If yes, what stage is pressure ulcer: _______. Acquired when: _______________.
List wounds not associated with pressure ulcers and how acquired: _____________
____.
Mattress type: ____.
Specialty mattresses are important to help prevent pressure ulcers)
If patient on ventilator or has tracheostomy, suction performed: _____ yes, _____ no.
Did nurse listen to lung sounds: ____ yes, _____ no.
Does patient have chest tubes: ____ yes, ____ no. Functioning _____ yes, _____ no.
Bowel sounds: ______ yes, ______ no. Bowel sounds active: ______ yes, ______ no.
Neurological exam: _____ yes, ______ no. Follow commands: ______ yes, ______ no.
Is patient alert and oriented to person, place, time, and events: _____ yes, _____ no.
If confused, patient is not oriented to: ____ person, ___ place, ___ time, ___ event.
Confusion began (time and date): _____________________________________.
Glasgow coma scale (checks conscious scale of patient): __________________.
Intracranial pressure monitoring: _____ yes, _____ no.
If yes, pressure is at ________ mm mercury. (Normal is one to fifteen).
Moves extremities: ___ yes, ___ no.
Paralysis: (inability to move extremities) ______ yes, ______ no.
If yes, extremities affected and when paralysis began: _________________.
Is patient in pain: ____ yes, ____ no. Describe pain and location ____________.
Patient able to eat: ____ yes, ____ no. What type of diet? ________________.
If patient on tube feedings list type: __________ at __________ cc/ml per hour.
Nausea ____, vomiting ____. If so, describe: ____________________________.
Patient has: Nasal gastric tube _____, Dobhoff tube _____, Peg or gastric tube _____.
When was feeding tube placed and what site: ________________________________.
Catheter for draining urine: ____ yes, ____ no. If so, when placed: __________
Find out policy for allowed time to remain in bladder. Too long may cause infections.)
IV site(s) where: ___________________________ when placed: ______________.
IV fluids (types and rates): ____________________, ___________________,
_______________, ___________________, ____________________.
Is patient on oxygen: _____ yes, _____ no. If so, how much and route delivered
(see oxygen routes): ____.
If patient on ventilator, list settings (see list on ventilator settings): _______
____.
Vital signs: temp _____, pulse _____, resp _____, b/p _____, o2 _____%,
current weight _____ pounds, _____ kg. Glucose level: _____
Insulin coverage: ____ yes, ____ no. Insulin type: ___________, # of units: _____.

NURSING CARE CONTINUED FOR ____________________
DATE ____________________, DAY NUMBER ____________________

FOLLOWING EXAMINATIONS FOR NIGHT SHIFT:

Nurse ____________, CNA ____________, in at _____ am/pm. Left at ______ am/pm.
Wash hands and wear gloves before touching patient: ______ yes, ______ no.
Wash hands before leaving room: ___ yes, ___ no. Wear protective gear: __ yes, __ no.
Clean stethoscope: __ yes, __ no. Oral care: __ yes, __ no. Suctioned: __ yes, __ no.
Repositioned: ___ yes, ___ no. Turned to: __ left, __ right, __ backside ___.
Head of bed at: ______ degrees. Incontinence/skin breakdown: ____ yes, ___ no.
Linens wet or soiled: _____ yes, _____ no. Linens changed: _____ yes, _____ no.
Dressing changed: ____ yes, ____ no. Location: ____________________.
IV site checked: _____ yes, _____ no. IV tubing labeled: _____ yes, _____ no.
IV fluids at: ____.
Pain level (0-10 scale.0-no pain, 10 intolerable): ____________.
Location of pain: ____________. Medicated for pain: ____ yes, ___ no.
Patient is alert/oriented: ___ yes, ___ no. New confusion: ____ yes, ___ no.
Vital signs: temp ____, pulse ____, resp ____, b/p ____, 02 ____%, ____ liters.
Glucose level: _____. Insulin: ___ yes, ___ no. Type: __________ # of units ____.

Nurse ____________, CNA ____________, in at _____ am/pm. Left at ______ am/pm.
Wash hands and wear gloves before touching patient: ______ yes, ______ no.
Wash hands before leaving room: ___ yes, ___ no. Wear protective gear: __ yes, __ no.
Clean stethoscope: __ yes, __ no. Oral care: __ yes, __ no. Suctioned: __ yes, __ no.
Repositioned: ___ yes, ___ no. Turned to: __ left, __ right, __ backside ___.
Head of bed at: ______ degrees. Incontinence/skin breakdown: ____ yes, ___ no.
Linens wet or soiled: _____ yes, _____ no. Linens changed: _____ yes, _____ no.
Dressing changed: ____ yes, ____ no. Location: ____________________.
IV site checked: _____ yes, _____ no. IV tubing labeled: _____ yes, _____ no.
IV fluids at: ____.
Pain level (0-10 scale.0-no pain, 10 intolerable): ____________.
Location of pain: ____________. Medicated for pain: ____ yes, ___ no.
Patient is alert/oriented: ___ yes, ___ no. New confusion: ____ yes, ___ no.
Vital signs: temp ____, pulse ____, resp ____, b/p ____, 02 ____%, ____ liters.
Glucose level: _____. Insulin: ___ yes, ___ no. Type: __________ # of units ____.

Nurse ____________, CNA ____________, in at _____ am/pm. Left at ______ am/pm.
Wash hands and wear gloves before touching patient: ______ yes, ______ no.
Wash hands before leaving room: ___ yes, ___ no. Wear protective gear: __ yes, __ no.
Clean stethoscope: __ yes, __ no. Oral care: __ yes, __ no. Suctioned: __ yes, __ no.
Repositioned: ___ yes, ___ no. Turned to: __ left, __ right, __ backside ___.
Head of bed at: ______ degrees. Incontinence/skin breakdown: ____ yes, ___ no.
Linens wet or soiled: _____ yes, _____ no. Linens changed: _____ yes, _____ no.
Dressing changed: ____ yes, ____ no. Location: ____________________.
IV site checked: _____ yes, _____ no. IV tubing labeled: _____ yes, _____ no.
IV fluids at: ____.
Pain level (0-10 scale.0-no pain, 10 intolerable): ____________.
Location of pain: ____________. Medicated for pain: ____ yes, ___ no.
Patient is alert/oriented: ___ yes, ___ no. New confusion: ____ yes, ___ no.
Vital signs: temp ____, pulse ____, resp ____, b/p ____, 02 ____%, ____ liters.
Glucose level: _____. Insulin: ___ yes, ___ no. Type: __________ # of units ____.

NURSING CARE CONTINUED FOR ____________________
DATE __________________, DAY NUMBER ____________________

FOLLOWING EXAMINATIONS FOR NIGHT SHIFT:

Nurse ____________, CNA ____________, in at _____ am/pm. Left at ______ am/pm.
Wash hands and wear gloves before touching patient: ______ yes, ______ no.
Wash hands before leaving room: ___ yes, ___ no. Wear protective gear: __ yes, __ no.
Clean stethoscope: __ yes, __ no. Oral care: __ yes, __ no. Suctioned: __ yes, __ no.
Repositioned: ___ yes, ___ no. Turned to: ___ left, ___ right, ___ backside ___.
Head of bed at: ______ degrees. Incontinence/skin breakdown: ____ yes, ____ no.
Linens wet or soiled: ____ yes, ____ no. Linens changed: _____ yes, _____ no.
Dressing changed: ____ yes, ____ no. Location: ____________________.
IV site checked: _____ yes, _____ no. IV tubing labeled: _____ yes, _____no.
IV fluids at: ______________________________________.
Pain level (0-10 scale.0-no pain, 10 intolerable): ____________________.
Location of pain: ____________. Medicated for pain: _____ yes, ____ no.
Patient is alert/oriented: ____ yes, ____ no. New confusion: ____ yes, ____ no.
Vital signs: temp ____, pulse _____, resp _____, b/p _____, 02 _____ %, ____ liters.
Glucose level: _____. Insulin: ___ yes, ___ no. Type: ____________ # of units ____.

Nurse ____________, CNA ____________, in at _____ am/pm. Left at ______ am/pm.
Wash hands and wear gloves before touching patient: ______ yes, ______ no.
Wash hands before leaving room: ___ yes, ___ no. Wear protective gear: __ yes, __ no.
Clean stethoscope: __ yes, __ no. Oral care: __ yes, __ no. Suctioned: __ yes, __ no.
Repositioned: ___ yes, ___ no. Turned to: ___ left, ___ right, ___ backside ___.
Head of bed at: ______ degrees. Incontinence/skin breakdown: ____ yes, ____ no.
Linens wet or soiled: ____ yes, ____ no. Linens changed: _____ yes, _____ no.
Dressing changed: ____ yes, ____ no. Location: ____________________.
IV site checked: _____ yes, _____ no. IV tubing labeled: _____ yes, _____no.
IV fluids at: ______________________________________.
Pain level (0-10 scale.0-no pain, 10 intolerable): ____________________.
Location of pain: ____________. Medicated for pain: _____ yes, ____ no.
Patient is alert/oriented: ____ yes, ____ no. New confusion: ____ yes, ____ no.
Vital signs: temp ____, pulse _____, resp _____, b/p _____, 02 _____ %, ____ liters.
Glucose level: _____. Insulin: ___ yes, ___ no. Type: ____________ # of units ____.

Nurse ____________, CNA ____________, in at _____ am/pm. Left at ______ am/pm.
Wash hands and wear gloves before touching patient: ______ yes, ______ no.
Wash hands before leaving room: ___ yes, ___ no. Wear protective gear: __ yes, __ no.
Clean stethoscope: __ yes, __ no. Oral care: __ yes, __ no. Suctioned: __ yes, __ no.
Repositioned: ___ yes, ___ no. Turned to: ___ left, ___ right, ___ backside ___.
Head of bed at: ______ degrees. Incontinence/skin breakdown: ____ yes, ____ no.
Linens wet or soiled: ____ yes, ____ no. Linens changed: _____ yes, _____ no.
Dressing changed: ____ yes, ____ no. Location: ____________________.
IV site checked: _____ yes, _____ no. IV tubing labeled: _____ yes, _____no.
IV fluids at: ______________________________________.
Pain level (0-10 scale.0-no pain, 10 intolerable): ____________________.
Location of pain: ____________. Medicated for pain: _____ yes, ____ no.
Patient is alert/oriented: ____ yes, ____ no. New confusion: ____ yes, ____ no.
Vital signs: temp ____, pulse _____, resp _____, b/p _____, 02 _____ %, ____ liters.
Glucose level: _____. Insulin: ___ yes, ___ no. Type: ____________ # of units ____.

MEDICATION ADMINISTRATION LIST FOR ______________________

DATE ________________ DAY NUMBER ________________________

List the medication for each day. Routes of administration: oral, thru feeding tube, intravenous (IV), intramuscular (IM), subcutaneous (SQ), epidural or a catheter in your spinal column, rectal, topical, eye drops, and ear drops.

Medication:	Route:	Time:
________________	________________	____________
________________	________________	____________
________________	________________	____________
________________	________________	____________
________________	________________	____________
________________	________________	____________
________________	________________	____________
________________	________________	____________
________________	________________	____________
________________	________________	____________
________________	________________	____________
________________	________________	____________
________________	________________	____________
________________	________________	____________
________________	________________	____________
________________	________________	____________
________________	________________	____________
________________	________________	____________
________________	________________	____________
________________	________________	____________
________________	________________	____________
________________	________________	____________
________________	________________	____________
________________	________________	____________
________________	________________	____________
________________	________________	____________
________________	________________	____________
________________	________________	____________
________________	________________	____________
________________	________________	____________
________________	________________	____________
________________	________________	____________
________________	________________	____________
________________	________________	____________
________________	________________	____________
________________	________________	____________
________________	________________	____________
________________	________________	____________
________________	________________	____________
________________	________________	____________
________________	________________	____________
________________	________________	____________
________________	________________	____________
________________	________________	____________
________________	________________	____________
________________	________________	____________
________________	________________	____________
________________	________________	____________
________________	________________	____________
________________	________________	____________
________________	________________	____________
________________	________________	____________
________________	________________	____________
________________	________________	____________

NOTES FOR DAY NUMBER ______________________________

DATE ______________________________

MEDICAL JOURNAL FOR ______________________________

DATE ____________________, DAY NUMBER ______________

VISITS FROM MY DOCTORS TODAY

Goals for today: ____

____

____.

Things to discuss with my doctor(s): ______________________

____

____

Dr.____________ came in at ____ am/pm. Left at ____ am/pm.
We discussed ____.
Did doctor examine patient: ____ yes, ____ no.
Wash hands before touching patient: ____ yes, ____ no.
Wear gloves: ____ yes, ___ no. Clean stethoscope: ____ yes, ___ no.
Wear gown and mask (precautions only):____ yes, ____ no.
Wash hands before leaving the room: ____ yes, ____ no.

Dr.____________ came in at ____ am/pm. Left at ____ am/pm.
We discussed ____.
Did doctor examine patient: ____ yes, ____ no.
Wash hands before touching patient: ____ yes, ____ no.
Wear gloves: ____ yes, ___ no. Clean stethoscope: ____ yes, ___ no.
Wear gown and mask (precautions only):____ yes, ____ no.
Wash hands before leaving the room: ____ yes, ____ no.

Dr.____________ came in at ____ am/pm. Left at ____ am/pm.
We discussed ____.
Did doctor examine patient: ____ yes, ____ no.
Wash hands before touching patient: ____ yes, ____ no.
Wear gloves: ____ yes, ___ no. Clean stethoscope: ____ yes, ___ no.
Wear gown and mask (precautions only):____ yes, ____ no.
Wash hands before leaving the room: ____ yes, ____ no.

Dr.____________ came in at ____ am/pm. Left at ____ am/pm.
We discussed ____.
Did doctor examine patient: ____ yes, ____ no.
Wash hands before touching patient: ____ yes, ____ no.
Wear gloves: ____ yes, ___ no. Clean stethoscope: ____ yes, ___ no.
Wear gown and mask (precautions only):____ yes, ____ no.
Wash hands before leaving the room: ____ yes, ____ no.

Dr.____________ came in at ____ am/pm. Left at ____ am/pm.
We discussed ____.
Did doctor examine patient: ____ yes, ____ no.
Wash hands before touching patient: ____ yes, ____ no.
Wear gloves: ____ yes, ___ no. Clean stethoscope: ____ yes, ___ no.
Wear gown and mask (precautions only):____ yes, ____ no.
Wash hands before leaving the room: ____ yes, ____ no.

NURSING CARE FOR ____

DATE ____________________, DAY NUMBER ____________________

INITIAL DAY SHIFT EXAM:

My nurse has ______ # of patients. CNA ___yes, ___no. Charge nurse ______________
Nurse ________________ RN/LPN came in at __________ am/pm. Left at ___________ am/pm.
Did nurse wash hands and wear gloves before touching patient: _______ yes, _______ no.
Wash hands after touching patient and before leaving the room: _______ yes, _______ no.
Don't hesitate to request staff to wash their hands. This will help decrease the risk of spreading potentially lethal germs.
Did nurse wear protective gear (isolation precautions only): _______ yes, _______ no.
Did nurse provide oral care (to be done every two hours if unable to provide for self, also decreases risk of pneumonia, infections, and aspiration): _______ yes, ______ no.
If able to provide own oral care, then supplies at bedside: ________ yes, ________ no.
Was patient repositioned (every two hours if unable to turn self): _____ yes _____ no.
Head of bed at _________ degrees. This is important for patients on ventilators or on tube feedings. Anything less than thirty degrees places patients at risk for aspiration of stomach contents into the lungs causing aspiration pneumonia.
Checked for incontinence and skin breakdown: _____ yes, _____ no.
Patient's linens wet or soiled: _____ yes, ____ no. Linens changed: ____ yes, ____ no.
Time linens changed: ________ am/pm. Any skin redness or breakdown: ____ yes, ____ no.
If yes, what stage is pressure ulcer: ________. Acquired when: ________________.
List wounds not associated with pressure ulcers and how acquired: ______________
____.
Mattress type: ____.
Specialty mattresses are important to help prevent pressure ulcers)
If patient on ventilator or has tracheostomy, suction performed: _____ yes, ______ no.
Did nurse listen to lung sounds: _____ yes, _____ no.
Does patient have chest tubes: ____ yes, ____ no. Functioning _____ yes, ______ no.
Bowel sounds: _______ yes, _______ no. Bowel sounds active: _______ yes, _______ no.
Neurological exam: ______ yes, ______ no. Follow commands: _______ yes, _______ no.
Is patient alert and oriented to person, place, time, and events: _____ yes, _____ no.
If confused, patient is not oriented to: ____ person, ___ place, ___ time, ___ event.
Confusion began (time and date): ____.
Glasgow coma scale (checks conscious scale of patient): _________________________.
Intracranial pressure monitoring: ______ yes, ______ no.
If yes, pressure is at _________ mm mercury. (Normal is one to fifteen).
Moves extremities: ___ yes, ___ no.
Paralysis: (inability to move extremities) ______ yes, _______ no.
If yes, extremities affected and when paralysis began: _______________________.
Is patient in pain: ___ yes, ____ no. Describe pain and location ______________.
Patient able to eat: ____ yes, ____ no. What type of diet? ______________________.
If patient on tube feedings list type: _______________ at _____________ cc/ml per hour.
Nausea ____, vomiting _____. If so, describe: ______________________________.
Patient has: Nasal gastric tube ______, Dobhoff tube _____, Peg or gastric tube _____.
When was feeding tube placed and what site: _________________________________.
Catheter for draining urine: ____ yes, ____ no. If so, when placed: _____________.
Find out policy for allowed time to remain in bladder. Too long may cause infections.)
IV site(s) where: _______________________________ when placed: _____________.
IV fluids (types and rates): _______________________, _______________________,
______________________________, ______________________, _____________________,
Is patient on oxygen: _____ yes, _____ no. If so, how much and route delivered (see oxygen routes): ____.
If patient on ventilator, list settings (see list on ventilator settings): __________
____.
Vital signs: temp _____, pulse ______, resp ______, b/p ______, o2 ______%,
current weight ______ pounds, ______ kg. Glucose level: ______
Insulin coverage: ____ yes, ____ no. Insulin type: _____________, # of units: ______.

NURSING CARE CONTINUED FOR ____________________
DATE ____________________, DAY NUMBER ____________________

FOLLOWING EXAMINATIONS FOR DAY SHIFT:

Nurse ____________, CNA ____________, in at ______ am/pm. Left at _______ am/pm.
Wash hands and wear gloves before touching patient: _______ yes, _______ no.
Wash hands before leaving room: ___ yes, ___ no. Wear protective gear: __ yes, __ no.
Clean stethoscope: __ yes, no. Oral care: __ yes, __ no. Suctioned: __ yes, __ no.
Repositioned: ___ yes, ___ no. Turned to: ___ left, ___ right, ___ backside ___.
Head of bed at: _______ degrees. Incontinence/skin breakdown: ____ yes, ____ no.
Linens wet or soiled: _____ yes, _____ no. Linens changed: _____ yes, _____ no.
Dressing changed: ____ yes, ____ no. Location: ____________________.
IV site checked: _____ yes, _____ no. IV tubing labeled: _____ yes, _____no.
IV fluids at: ____.
Pain level (0-10 scale.0-no pain, 10 intolerable): ____________________.
Location of pain: ____________. Medicated for pain: ____ yes, ____ no.
Patient is alert/oriented: ____ yes, ____ no. New confusion: ____ yes, ____ no.
Vital signs: temp ____, pulse ____, resp ____, b/p ____, 02 ____ %, ____ liters.
Glucose level: _____. Insulin: ___ yes, ___ no. Type: ____________ # of units ____.

Nurse ____________, CNA ____________, in at ______ am/pm. Left at _______ am/pm.
Wash hands and wear gloves before touching patient: _______ yes, _______ no.
Wash hands before leaving room: ___ yes, ___ no. Wear protective gear: __ yes, __ no.
Clean stethoscope: __ yes, no. Oral care: __ yes, __ no. Suctioned: __ yes, __ no.
Repositioned: ___ yes, ___ no. Turned to: ___ left, ___ right, ___ backside ___.
Head of bed at: _______ degrees. Incontinence/skin breakdown: ____ yes, ____ no.
Linens wet or soiled: _____ yes, _____ no. Linens changed: _____ yes, _____ no.
Dressing changed: ____ yes, ____ no. Location: ____________________.
IV site checked: _____ yes, _____ no. IV tubing labeled: _____ yes, _____no.
IV fluids at: ____.
Pain level (0-10 scale.0-no pain, 10 intolerable): ____________________.
Location of pain: ____________. Medicated for pain: ____ yes, ____ no.
Patient is alert/oriented: ____ yes, ____ no. New confusion: ____ yes, ____ no.
Vital signs: temp ____, pulse ____, resp ____, b/p ____, 02 ____ %, ____ liters.
Glucose level: _____. Insulin: ___ yes, ___ no. Type: ____________ # of units ____.

Nurse ____________, CNA ____________, in at ______ am/pm. Left at _______ am/pm.
Wash hands and wear gloves before touching patient: _______ yes, _______ no.
Wash hands before leaving room: ___ yes, ___ no. Wear protective gear: __ yes, __ no.
Clean stethoscope: __ yes, __ no. Oral care: __ yes, __ no. Suctioned: __ yes, __ no.
Repositioned: ___ yes, ___ no. Turned to: ___ left, ___ right, ___ backside ___.
Head of bed at: _______ degrees. Incontinence/skin breakdown: ____ yes, ____ no.
Linens wet or soiled: _____ yes, _____ no. Linens changed: _____ yes, _____ no.
Dressing changed: ____ yes, ____ no. Location: ____________________.
IV site checked: _____ yes, _____ no. IV tubing labeled: _____ yes, _____no.
IV fluids at: ____.
Pain level (0-10 scale.0-no pain, 10 intolerable): ____________________.
Location of pain: ____________. Medicated for pain: ____ yes, ____ no.
Patient is alert/oriented: ____ yes, ____ no. New confusion: ____ yes, ____ no.
Vital signs: temp ____, pulse ____, resp ____, b/p ____, 02 ____ %, ____ liters.
Glucose level: _____. Insulin: ___ yes, ___ no. Type: ____________ # of units ____.

NURSING CARE CONTINUED FOR ____________________
DATE ____________________, DAY NUMBER ____________________

FOLLOWING EXAMINATIONS FOR DAY SHIFT:

Nurse ____________, CNA ____________, in at _____ am/pm. Left at ______ am/pm.
Wash hands and wear gloves before touching patient: ______ yes, ______ no.
Wash hands before leaving room: ___ yes, ___ no. Wear protective gear: __ yes, __ no.
Clean stethoscope: __ yes, __ no. Oral care: __ yes, __ no. Suctioned: __ yes, __ no.
Repositioned: ___ yes, ___ no. Turned to: ___ left, ___ right, ___ backside ___.
Head of bed at: ______ degrees. Incontinence/skin breakdown: ____ yes, ___ no.
Linens wet or soiled: ____ yes, ____ no. Linens changed: ____ yes, _____ no.
Dressing changed: ___ yes, ___ no. Location: ____________________.
IV site checked: ____ yes, ____ no. IV tubing labeled: ____ yes, ____no.
IV fluids at: ____________________.
Pain level (0-10 scale.0-no pain, 10 intolerable): ____________.
Location of pain: ____________. Medicated for pain: ____ yes, ___ no.
Patient is alert/oriented: ___ yes, ___ no. New confusion: ___ yes, ___ no.
Vital signs: temp ____, pulse ____, resp _____, b/p _____, 02 _____ %, ____ liters.
Glucose level: _____. Insulin: ___ yes, ___ no. Type: ____________ # of units ___.

Nurse ____________, CNA ____________, in at _____ am/pm. Left at ______ am/pm.
Wash hands and wear gloves before touching patient: ______ yes, ______ no.
Wash hands before leaving room: ___ yes, ___ no. Wear protective gear: __ yes, __ no.
Clean stethoscope: __ yes, __ no. Oral care: __ yes, __ no. Suctioned: __ yes, __ no.
Repositioned: ___ yes, ___ no. Turned to: ___ left, ___ right, ___ backside ___.
Head of bed at: ______ degrees. Incontinence/skin breakdown: ____ yes, ___ no.
Linens wet or soiled: ____ yes, ____ no. Linens changed: ____ yes, _____ no.
Dressing changed: ___ yes, ___ no. Location: ____________________.
IV site checked: ____ yes, ____ no. IV tubing labeled: ____ yes, ____no.
IV fluids at: ____________________.
Pain level (0-10 scale.0-no pain, 10 intolerable): ____________.
Location of pain: ____________. Medicated for pain: ____ yes, ___ no.
Patient is alert/oriented: ___ yes, ___ no. New confusion: ___ yes, ___ no.
Vital signs: temp ____, pulse ____, resp _____, b/p _____, 02 _____ %, ____ liters.
Glucose level: _____. Insulin: ___ yes, ___ no. Type: ____________ # of units ____.

Nurse ____________, CNA ____________, in at _____ am/pm. Left at ______ am/pm.
Wash hands and wear gloves before touching patient: ______ yes, ______ no.
Wash hands before leaving room: ___ yes, ___ no. Wear protective gear: __ yes, __ no.
Clean stethoscope: __ yes, __ no. Oral care: __ yes, __ no. Suctioned: __ yes,__ no.
Repositioned: ___ yes, ___ no. Turned to: ___ left, ___ right, ___ backside ___.
Head of bed at: ______ degrees. Incontinence/skin breakdown: ____ yes, ___ no.
Linens wet or soiled: ____ yes, ____ no. Linens changed: ____ yes, _____ no.
Dressing changed: ___ yes, ___ no. Location: ____________________.
IV site checked: ____ yes, ____ no. IV tubing labeled: ____ yes, ____no.
IV fluids at: ____________________.
Pain level (0-10 scale.0-no pain, 10 intolerable): ____________.
Location of pain: ____________. Medicated for pain: ____ yes, ___ no.
Patient is alert/oriented: ___ yes, ___ no. New confusion: ___ yes, ___ no.
Vital signs: temp ____, pulse ____, resp _____, b/p _____, 02 _____ %, ____ liters.
Glucose level: _____. Insulin: ___ yes, ___ no. Type: ____________ # of units ____.

NURSING CARE FOR ______________________________

DATE ____________________, DAY NUMBER ____________________

INITIAL NIGHT SHIFT EXAM:

My nurse has _____ # of patients. CNA ___yes, ___no. Charge nurse ____________
Nurse ____________ RN/LPN came in at _________ am/pm. Left at __________ am/pm.
Did nurse wash hands and wear gloves before touching patient: _____ yes, _____ no.
Wash hands after touching patient and before leaving the room: _____ yes, _____ no.
Don't hesitate to request staff to wash their hands. This will help decrease the risk of spreading potentially lethal germs.
Did nurse wear protective gear (isolation precautions only): _____ yes, _____ no.
Did nurse provide oral care (to be done every two hours if unable to provide for self, also decreases risk of pneumonia, infections, and aspiration): _____yes, _____ no.
If able to provide own oral care, then supplies at bedside: _____ yes, _____ no.
Was patient repositioned (every two hours if unable to turn self): ____ yes ____ no.
Head of bed at ________ degrees. This is important for patients on ventilators or on tube feedings. Anything less than thirty degrees places patients at risk for aspiration of stomach contents into the lungs causing aspiration pneumonia.
Checked for incontinence and skin breakdown: ____ yes, ____ no.
Patient's linens wet or soiled: ____ yes, ____ no. Linens changed: ____ yes, ____ no.
Time linens changed: ________ am/pm. Any skin redness or breakdown: ____ yes, ____ no.
If yes, what stage is pressure ulcer: ________. Acquired when: ______________.
List wounds not associated with pressure ulcers and how acquired: ______________
____.
Mattress type: ____
Specialty mattresses are important to help prevent pressure ulcers)
If patient on ventilator or has tracheostomy, suction performed: ____ yes, ____ no.
Did nurse listen to lung sounds: ____ yes, ____ no.
Does patient have chest tubes: ____ yes, ____ no. Functioning _____ yes, _____ no.
Bowel sounds: _____ yes, _____ no. Bowel sounds active: _____ yes, _____ no.
Neurological exam: _____ yes, _____ no. Follow commands: _____ yes, _____ no.
Is patient alert and oriented to person, place, time, and events: ____ yes, ____ no.
If confused, patient is not oriented to: ___ person, ___ place, ___ time, ___ event.
Confusion began (time and date): ______________________________________.
Glasgow coma scale (checks conscious scale of patient): ____________________.
Intracranial pressure monitoring: ____ yes, ____ no.
If yes, pressure is at ________ mm mercury. (Normal is one to fifteen).
Moves extremities: ___ yes, ___ no.
Paralysis: (inability to move extremities) _____ yes, _____ no.
If yes, extremities affected and when paralysis began: ______________________
Is patient in pain: ____ yes, ____ no. Describe pain and location ____________
Patient able to eat: ____ yes, ____ no. What type of diet? ___________________
If patient on tube feedings list type: __________ at __________ cc/ml per hour.
Nausea ____, vomiting _____. If so, describe: _______________________________
Patient has: Nasal gastric tube _____, Dobhoff tube _____, Peg or gastric tube ____.
When was feeding tube placed and what site: ________________________________
Catheter for draining urine: ____ yes, ____ no. If so, when placed: __________.
Find out policy for allowed time to remain in bladder. Too long may cause infections.)
IV site(s) where: ________________________ when placed: _______________.
IV fluids (types and rates): ____,
______________________, ______________________, ______________________.
Is patient on oxygen: _____ yes, _____ no. If so, how much and route delivered (see oxygen routes): ____.
If patient on ventilator, list settings (see list on ventilator settings): _________
____.
Vital signs: temp _____, pulse _____, resp _____, b/p _____, o2 _____%,
current weight _____ pounds, _____ kg. Glucose level: _____
Insulin coverage: ____ yes, ____ no. Insulin type: ____________, # of units: _____.

NURSING CARE CONTINUED FOR ______________________________
DATE ____________________, DAY NUMBER ______________________

FOLLOWING EXAMINATIONS FOR NIGHT SHIFT:

Nurse ______________, CNA ______________, in at ____ am/pm. Left at ______ am/pm.
Wash hands and wear gloves before touching patient: ______ yes, ______ no.
Wash hands before leaving room: ___ yes, ___ no. Wear protective gear: __ yes, __ no.
Clean stethoscope: __ yes, __ no. Oral care: __ yes, __ no. Suctioned: __ yes, __ no.
Repositioned: ___ yes, ___ no. Turned to: ___ left, ___ right, ___ backside ___.
Head of bed at: _______ degrees. Incontinence/skin breakdown: ____ yes, ____ no.
Linens wet or soiled: _____ yes, _____ no. Linens changed: _____ yes, _____ no.
Dressing changed: ____ yes, ____ no. Location: _____________________________.
IV site checked: _____ yes, _____ no. IV tubing labeled: _____ yes, _____no.
IV fluids ____.
Pain level (0-10 scale.0-no pain, 10 intolerable): __________________________.
Location of pain: ______________. Medicated for pain: _____ yes, ____ no.
Patient is alert/oriented: ____ yes, ____ no. New confusion: ____ yes, ____ no.
Vital signs: temp ____, pulse _____, resp _____, b/p _____, 02 _____ %, ____ liters.
Glucose level: _____. Insulin: ___ yes, ___ no. Type: ______________ # of units ____.

Nurse ______________, CNA ______________, in at ____ am/pm. Left at ______ am/pm.
Wash hands and wear gloves before touching patient: ______ yes, ______ no.
Wash hands before leaving room: ___ yes, ___ no. Wear protective gear: __ yes, __ no.
Clean stethoscope: __ yes, __ no. Oral care: __ yes, __ no. Suctioned: __ yes, __ no.
Repositioned: ___ yes, ___ no. Turned to: ___ left, ___ right, ___ backside ___.
Head of bed at: _______ degrees. Incontinence/skin breakdown: ____ yes, ____ no.
Linens wet or soiled: _____ yes, _____ no. Linens changed: _____ yes, _____ no.
Dressing changed: ____ yes, ____ no. Location: _____________________________.
IV site checked: _____ yes, _____ no. IV tubing labeled: _____ yes, _____no.
IV fluids at: ____.
Pain level (0-10 scale.0-no pain, 10 intolerable): __________________________.
Location of pain: ______________. Medicated for pain: _____ yes, ____ no.
Patient is alert/oriented: ____ yes, ____ no. New confusion: ____ yes, ____ no.
Vital signs: temp ____, pulse _____, resp _____, b/p _____, 02 _____ %, ____ liters.
Glucose level: _____. Insulin: ___ yes, ___ no. Type: ______________ # of units ____.

Nurse ______________, CNA ______________, in at ____ am/pm. Left at ______ am/pm.
Wash hands and wear gloves before touching patient: ______ yes, ______ no.
Wash hands before leaving room: ___ yes, ___ no. Wear protective gear: __ yes, __ no.
Clean stethoscope: __ yes, __ no. Oral care: __ yes, __ no. Suctioned: __ yes, __ no.
Repositioned: ___ yes, ___ no. Turned to: ___ left, ___ right, ___ backside ___.
Head of bed at: _______ degrees. Incontinence/skin breakdown: ____ yes, ____ no.
Linens wet or soiled: _____ yes, _____ no. Linens changed: _____ yes, _____ no.
Dressing changed: ____ yes, ____ no. Location: _____________________________.
IV site checked: _____ yes, _____ no. IV tubing labeled: _____ yes, _____no.
IV fluids at: ____.
Pain level (0-10 scale.0-no pain, 10 intolerable): __________________________.
Location of pain: ______________. Medicated for pain: _____ yes, ____ no.
Patient is alert/oriented: ____ yes, ____ no. New confusion: ____ yes, ____ no.
Vital signs: temp ____, pulse _____, resp _____, b/p _____, 02 _____ %, ____ liters.
Glucose level: _____. Insulin: ___ yes, ___ no. Type: ______________ # of units ____.

NURSING CARE CONTINUED FOR
DATE , DAY NUMBER

FOLLOWING EXAMINATIONS FOR NIGHT SHIFT:

Nurse , CNA , in at am/pm. Left at am/pm.
Wash hands and wear gloves before touching patient: yes, no.
Wash hands before leaving room: yes, no. Wear protective gear: yes, no.
Clean stethoscope: yes, no. Oral care: yes, no. Suctioned: yes, no.
Repositioned: yes, no. Turned to: left, right, backside .
Head of bed at: degrees. Incontinence/skin breakdown: yes, no.
Linens wet or soiled: yes, no. Linens changed: yes, no.
Dressing changed: yes, no. Location: .
IV site checked: yes, no. IV tubing labeled: yes, no.
IV fluids at: .
Pain level (0-10 scale.0-no pain, 10 intolerable): .
Location of pain: . Medicated for pain: yes, no.
Patient is alert/oriented: yes, no. New confusion: yes, no.
Vital signs: temp , pulse , resp , b/p , 02 %, liters.
Glucose level: . Insulin: yes, no. Type: # of units .

Nurse , CNA , in at am/pm. Left at am/pm.
Wash hands and wear gloves before touching patient: yes, no.
Wash hands before leaving room: yes, no. Wear protective gear: yes, no.
Clean stethoscope: yes, no. Oral care: yes, no. Suctioned: yes, no.
Repositioned: yes, no. Turned to: left, right, backside .
Head of bed at: degrees. Incontinence/skin breakdown: yes, no.
Linens wet or soiled: yes, no. Linens changed: yes, no.
Dressing changed: yes, no. Location: .
IV site checked: yes, no. IV tubing labeled: yes, no.
IV fluids at: .
Pain level (0-10 scale.0-no pain, 10 intolerable): .
Location of pain: . Medicated for pain: yes, no.
Patient is alert/oriented: yes, no. New confusion: yes, no.
Vital signs: temp , pulse , resp , b/p , 02 %, liters.
Glucose level: . Insulin: yes, no. Type: # of units .

Nurse , CNA , in at am/pm. Left at am/pm.
Wash hands and wear gloves before touching patient: yes, no.
Wash hands before leaving room: yes, no. Wear protective gear: yes, no.
Clean stethoscope: yes, no. Oral care: yes, no. Suctioned: yes, no.
Repositioned: yes, no. Turned to: left, right, backside .
Head of bed at: degrees. Incontinence/skin breakdown: yes, no.
Linens wet or soiled: yes, no. Linens changed: yes, no.
Dressing changed: yes, no. Location: .
IV site checked: yes, no. IV tubing labeled: yes, no.
IV fluids at: .
Pain level (0-10 scale.0-no pain, 10 intolerable): .
Location of pain: . Medicated for pain: yes, no.
Patient is alert/oriented: yes, no. New confusion: yes, no.
Vital signs: temp , pulse , resp , b/p , 02 %, liters.
Glucose level: . Insulin: yes, no. Type: # of units .

MEDICATION ADMINISTRATION LIST FOR ____________________
DATE ____________________ DAY NUMBER ____________________

List the medication for each day. Routes of administration: oral, thru feeding tube, intravenous (IV), intramuscular (IM), subcutaneous (SQ), epidural or a catheter in your spinal column, rectal, topical, eye drops, and ear drops.

Medication: ____________________ Route: ____________________ Time: ____________
Medication: ____________________ Route: ____________________ Time: ____________
Medication: ____________________ Route: ____________________ Time: ____________
Medication: ____________________ Route: ____________________ Time: ____________
Medication: ____________________ Route: ____________________ Time: ____________
Medication: ____________________ Route: ____________________ Time: ____________
Medication: ____________________ Route: ____________________ Time: ____________
Medication: ____________________ Route: ____________________ Time: ____________
Medication: ____________________ Route: ____________________ Time: ____________
Medication: ____________________ Route: ____________________ Time: ____________
Medication: ____________________ Route: ____________________ Time: ____________
Medication: ____________________ Route: ____________________ Time: ____________
Medication: ____________________ Route: ____________________ Time: ____________
Medication: ____________________ Route: ____________________ Time: ____________
Medication: ____________________ Route: ____________________ Time: ____________
Medication: ____________________ Route: ____________________ Time: ____________
Medication: ____________________ Route: ____________________ Time: ____________
Medication: ____________________ Route: ____________________ Time: ____________
Medication: ____________________ Route: ____________________ Time: ____________
Medication: ____________________ Route: ____________________ Time: ____________
Medication: ____________________ Route: ____________________ Time: ____________
Medication: ____________________ Route: ____________________ Time: ____________
Medication: ____________________ Route: ____________________ Time: ____________
Medication: ____________________ Route: ____________________ Time: ____________
Medication: ____________________ Route: ____________________ Time: ____________
Medication: ____________________ Route: ____________________ Time: ____________
Medication: ____________________ Route: ____________________ Time: ____________
Medication: ____________________ Route: ____________________ Time: ____________
Medication: ____________________ Route: ____________________ Time: ____________
Medication: ____________________ Route: ____________________ Time: ____________
Medication: ____________________ Route: ____________________ Time: ____________
Medication: ____________________ Route: ____________________ Time: ____________
Medication: ____________________ Route: ____________________ Time: ____________
Medication: ____________________ Route: ____________________ Time: ____________
Medication: ____________________ Route: ____________________ Time: ____________
Medication: ____________________ Route: ____________________ Time: ____________
Medication: ____________________ Route: ____________________ Time: ____________
Medication: ____________________ Route: ____________________ Time: ____________
Medication: ____________________ Route: ____________________ Time: ____________
Medication: ____________________ Route: ____________________ Time: ____________
Medication: ____________________ Route: ____________________ Time: ____________
Medication: ____________________ Route: ____________________ Time: ____________
Medication: ____________________ Route: ____________________ Time: ____________
Medication: ____________________ Route: ____________________ Time: ____________
Medication: ____________________ Route: ____________________ Time: ____________
Medication: ____________________ Route: ____________________ Time: ____________
Medication: ____________________ Route: ____________________ Time: ____________
Medication: ____________________ Route: ____________________ Time: ____________
Medication: ____________________ Route: ____________________ Time: ____________
Medication: ____________________ Route: ____________________ Time: ____________
Medication: ____________________ Route: ____________________ Time: ____________
Medication: ____________________ Route: ____________________ Time: ____________
Medication: ____________________ Route: ____________________ Time: ____________
Medication: ____________________ Route: ____________________ Time: ____________

NOTES FOR DAY NUMBER ______________________________

DATE ______________________________

MEDICAL JOURNAL FOR ______________________________

DATE ____________________, DAY NUMBER _______________

VISITS FROM MY DOCTORS TODAY

Goals for today: ____

____

____.

Things to discuss with my doctor(s): ______________________________

____

____

Dr.____________ came in at ____ am/pm. Left at ____ am/pm.
We discussed ____.
Did doctor examine patient: _____ yes, _____ no.
Wash hands before touching patient: _____ yes, _____ no.
Wear gloves: ____ yes, ___ no. Clean stethoscope: ____ yes, ____ no.
Wear gown and mask (precautions only):____ yes, _____ no.
Wash hands before leaving the room: _____ yes, _____ no.

Dr.____________ came in at ____ am/pm. Left at ____ am/pm.
We discussed ____.
Did doctor examine patient: _____ yes, _____ no.
Wash hands before touching patient: _____ yes, _____ no.
Wear gloves: ____ yes, ___ no. Clean stethoscope: ____ yes, ____ no.
Wear gown and mask (precautions only):____ yes, _____ no.
Wash hands before leaving the room: _____ yes, _____ no.

Dr.____________ came in at ____ am/pm. Left at ____ am/pm.
We discussed ____.
Did doctor examine patient: _____ yes, _____ no.
Wash hands before touching patient: _____ yes, _____ no.
Wear gloves: ____ yes, ___ no. Clean stethoscope: ____ yes, ____ no.
Wear gown and mask (precautions only):____ yes, _____ no.
Wash hands before leaving the room: _____ yes, _____ no.

Dr.____________ came in at ____ am/pm. Left at ____ am/pm.
We discussed ____.
Did doctor examine patient: _____ yes, _____ no.
Wash hands before touching patient: _____ yes, _____ no.
Wear gloves: ____ yes, ___ no. Clean stethoscope: ____ yes, ____ no.
Wear gown and mask (precautions only):____ yes, _____ no.
Wash hands before leaving the room: _____ yes, _____ no.

Dr.____________ came in at ____ am/pm. Left at ____ am/pm.
We discussed ____.
Did doctor examine patient: _____ yes, _____ no.
Wash hands before touching patient: _____ yes, _____ no.
Wear gloves: ____ yes, ___ no. Clean stethoscope: ____ yes, ____ no.
Wear gown and mask (precautions only):____ yes, _____ no.
Wash hands before leaving the room: _____ yes, _____ no.

NURSING CARE FOR ______________________________

DATE ____________________, DAY NUMBER ____________________

INITIAL DAY SHIFT EXAM:

My nurse has ______ # of patients. CNA ___yes, ___no. Charge nurse ______________
Nurse ______________ RN/LPN came in at _________ am/pm. Left at __________ am/pm.
Did nurse wash hands and wear gloves before touching patient: ______ yes, ______ no.
Wash hands after touching patient and before leaving the room: ______ yes, ______ no.
Don't hesitate to request staff to wash their hands. This will help decrease the risk of spreading potentially lethal germs.
Did nurse wear protective gear (isolation precautions only): ______ yes, ______ no.
Did nurse provide oral care (to be done every two hours if unable to provide for self, also decreases risk of pneumonia, infections, and aspiration): _______yes, _____ no.
If able to provide own oral care, then supplies at bedside: ________ yes, ______ no.
Was patient repositioned (every two hours if unable to turn self): _____ yes _____ no.
Head of bed at ________ degrees. This is important for patients on ventilators or on tube feedings. Anything less than thirty degrees places patients at risk for aspiration of stomach contents into the lungs causing aspiration pneumonia.
Checked for incontinence and skin breakdown: ___ yes, ___ no.
Patient's linens wet or soiled: ____ yes,____ no. Linens changed: ____ yes, ____ no.
Time linens changed: ________ am/pm. Any skin redness or breakdown: ____ yes, ____ no.
If yes, what stage is pressure ulcer: _______. Acquired when: __________________.
List wounds not associated with pressure ulcers and how acquired: ______________
____.
Mattress type: ____.
Specialty mattresses are important to help prevent pressure ulcers)
If patient on ventilator or has tracheostomy, suction performed: _____ yes, _____ no.
Did nurse listen to lung sounds: _____ yes, _____ no.
Does patient have chest tubes: ____ yes, ____ no. Functioning _____ yes, _____ no.
Bowel sounds: ______ yes, ______ no. Bowel sounds active: ______ yes, ______ no.
Neurological exam: ______ yes, ______ no. Follow commands: ______ yes, ______ no.
Is patient alert and oriented to person, place, time, and events: _____ yes, _____ no.
If confused, patient is not oriented to: ____ person, ___ place, ___ time, ___ event.
Confusion began (time and date): ____.
Glasgow coma scale (checks conscious scale of patient): ________________________.
Intracranial pressure monitoring: _____ yes, _____ no.
If yes, pressure is at ________ mm mercury. (Normal is one to fifteen).
Moves extremities: ___ yes, ___ no.
Paralysis: (inability to move extremities) _____ yes, _____ no.
If yes, extremities affected and when paralysis began: _________________________.
Is patient in pain: ____ yes, ____ no. Describe pain and location ______________.
Patient able to eat: ____ yes, ____ no. What type of diet? ____________________.
If patient on tube feedings list type: __________ at __________ cc/ml per hour.
Nausea ____, vomiting ____. If so, describe: _____________________________________.
Patient has: Nasal gastric tube _____, Dobhoff tube _____, Peg or gastric tube _____.
When was feeding tube placed and what site: ______________________________________.
Catheter for draining urine: ____ yes, ____ no. If so, when placed: _____________.
Find out policy for allowed time to remain in bladder. Too long may cause infections.)
IV site(s) where: ___________________________ when placed: ______________________.
IV fluids (types and rates): _____________________, _______________, ____________,
___________________________, ___________________, _____________, _______________.
Is patient on oxygen: _____ yes, _____ no. If so, how much and route delivered (see oxygen routes): ____.
If patient on ventilator, list settings (see list on ventilator settings): _________
____.
Vital signs: temp ______, pulse ______, resp ______, b/p ______, o2 ______%,
current weight ______ pounds, ______ kg. Glucose level: ______
Insulin coverage: ____ yes, ____ no. Insulin type: ____________, # of units: _____.

NURSING CARE CONTINUED FOR ______________________
DATE ____________________, DAY NUMBER __________________

FOLLOWING EXAMINATIONS FOR DAY SHIFT:

Nurse ______________, CNA ______________, in at _____ am/pm. Left at ______ am/pm.
Wash hands and wear gloves before touching patient: _______ yes, _______ no.
Wash hands before leaving room: ___ yes, ___ no. Wear protective gear: __ yes, __ no.
Clean stethoscope: __ yes, __ no. Oral care: __ yes, __ no. Suctioned: __ yes, __ no.
Repositioned: ___ yes, ___ no. Turned to: ___ left, ___ right, ___ backside ___.
Head of bed at: _______ degrees. Incontinence/skin breakdown: ____ yes, ___ no.
Linens wet or soiled: _____ yes, _____ no. Linens changed: _____ yes, ______ no.
Dressing changed: ____ yes, ____ no. Location: _______________________________.
IV site checked: _____ yes, _____ no. IV tubing labeled: ____ yes, _____no.
IV fluids at: ____.
Pain level (0-10 scale.0-no pain, 10 intolerable): ______________________.
Location of pain: _______________. Medicated for pain: ____ yes, ____ no.
Patient is alert/oriented: ____ yes, ____ no. New confusion: ____ yes, ____ no.
Vital signs: temp ____, pulse _____, resp ______, b/p ______, 02 _____ %, ____ liters.
Glucose level: _____. Insulin: ___ yes, ___ no. Type: _____________ # of units ___.

Nurse ______________, CNA ______________, in at _____ am/pm. Left at ______ am/pm.
Wash hands and wear gloves before touching patient: _______ yes, _______ no.
Wash hands before leaving room: ___ yes, ___ no. Wear protective gear: __ yes, __ no.
Clean stethoscope: __ yes, __ no. Oral care: __ yes, __ no. Suctioned: __ yes, __ no.
Repositioned: ___ yes, ___ no. Turned to: ___ left, ___ right, ___ backside ___.
Head of bed at: _______ degrees. Incontinence/skin breakdown: ____ yes, ___ no.
Linens wet or soiled: _____ yes, _____ no. Linens changed: _____ yes, ______ no.
Dressing changed: ____ yes, ____ no. Location: _______________________________.
IV site checked: _____ yes, _____ no. IV tubing labeled: ____ yes, _____no.
IV fluids at: ____.
Pain level (0-10 scale.0-no pain, 10 intolerable): ______________________.
Location of pain: _______________. Medicated for pain: ____ yes, ____ no.
Patient is alert/oriented: ____ yes, ____ no. New confusion: ____ yes, ____ no.
Vital signs: temp ____, pulse _____, resp ______, b/p ______, 02 _____ %, ____ liters.
Glucose level: _____. Insulin: ___ yes, ___ no. Type: _____________ # of units ___.

Nurse ______________, CNA ______________, in at _____ am/pm. Left at ______ am/pm.
Wash hands and wear gloves before touching patient: _______ yes, _______ no.
Wash hands before leaving room: ___ yes, ___ no. Wear protective gear: __ yes, __ no.
Clean stethoscope: __ yes, __ no. Oral care: __ yes, __ no. Suctioned: __ yes, __ no.
Repositioned: ___ yes, ___ no. Turned to: ___ left, ___ right, ___ backside ___.
Head of bed at: _______ degrees. Incontinence/skin breakdown: ____ yes, ___ no.
Linens wet or soiled: _____ yes, _____ no. Linens changed: _____ yes, ______ no.
Dressing changed: ____ yes, ____ no. Location: _______________________________.
IV site checked: _____ yes, _____ no. IV tubing labeled: ____ yes, _____no.
IV fluids at: ____.
Pain level (0-10 scale.0-no pain, 10 intolerable): ______________________.
Location of pain: _______________. Medicated for pain: ____ yes, ____ no.
Patient is alert/oriented: ____ yes, ____ no. New confusion: ____ yes, ____ no.
Vital signs: temp ____, pulse _____, resp ______, b/p ______, 02 _____ %, ____ liters.
Glucose level: _____. Insulin: ___ yes, ___ no. Type: _____________ # of units ___.

NURSING CARE CONTINUED FOR ______________________
DATE ______________________, DAY NUMBER ______________

FOLLOWING EXAMINATIONS FOR DAY SHIFT:

Nurse ______________, CNA ______________, in at _____ am/pm. Left at _______ am/pm.
Wash hands and wear gloves before touching patient: _______ yes, _______ no.
Wash hands before leaving room: ___ yes, ___ no. Wear protective gear: __ yes, __ no.
Clean stethoscope: __ yes, __ no. Oral care: __ yes, __ no. Suctioned: __ yes, __ no.
Repositioned: ___ yes, ___ no. Turned to: ___ left, ___ right, ___ backside ___.
Head of bed at: ________ degrees. Incontinence/skin breakdown: ___ yes, ___ no.
Linens wet or soiled: _____ yes, _____ no. Linens changed: _____ yes, _____ no.
Dressing changed: ____ yes, ____ no. Location: ______________________________.
IV site checked: _____ yes, _____ no. IV tubing labeled: _____ yes, _____no.
IV fluids at: ____.
Pain level (0-10 scale.0-no pain, 10 intolerable): _____________________________.
Location of pain: ______________. Medicated for pain: ____ yes, ____ no.
Patient is alert/oriented: ___ yes, ___ no. New confusion: ___ yes, ___ no.
Vital signs: temp ____, pulse ____, resp _____, b/p ______, 02 _____ %, _____ liters.
Glucose level: _____. Insulin: ___ yes, ___ no. Type: __________ # of units ___.

Nurse ______________, CNA ______________, in at _____ am/pm. Left at _______ am/pm.
Wash hands and wear gloves before touching patient: _______ yes, _______ no.
Wash hands before leaving room: ___ yes, ___ no. Wear protective gear: __ yes, __ no.
Clean stethoscope: __ yes, __ no. Oral care: __ yes, __ no. Suctioned: __ yes, __ no.
Repositioned: ___ yes, ___ no. Turned to: ___ left, ___ right, ___ backside ___.
Head of bed at: ________ degrees. Incontinence/skin breakdown: ___ yes, ___ no.
Linens wet or soiled: _____ yes, _____ no. Linens changed: _____ yes, _____ no.
Dressing changed: ____ yes, ____ no. Location: ______________________________.
IV site checked: _____ yes, _____ no. IV tubing labeled: _____ yes, _____no.
IV fluids at: ____.
Pain level (0-10 scale.0-no pain, 10 intolerable): _____________________________.
Location of pain: ______________. Medicated for pain: ____ yes, ____ no.
Patient is alert/oriented: ___ yes, ___ no. New confusion: ___ yes, ___ no.
Vital signs: temp ____, pulse ____, resp _____, b/p ______, 02 _____ %, _____ liters.
Glucose level: _____. Insulin: ___ yes, ___ no. Type: __________ # of units ___.

Nurse ______________, CNA ______________, in at _____ am/pm. Left at _______ am/pm.
Wash hands and wear gloves before touching patient: _______ yes, _______ no.
Wash hands before leaving room: ___ yes, ___ no. Wear protective gear: __ yes, __ no.
Clean stethoscope: __ yes, __ no. Oral care: __ yes, __ no. Suctioned: __ yes, __ no.
Repositioned: ___ yes, ___ no. Turned to: ___ left, ___ right, ___ backside ___.
Head of bed at: ________ degrees. Incontinence/skin breakdown: ___ yes, ___ no.
Linens wet or soiled: _____ yes, _____ no. Linens changed: _____ yes, _____ no.
Dressing changed: ____ yes, ____ no. Location: ______________________________.
IV site checked: _____ yes, _____ no. IV tubing labeled: _____ yes, _____no.
IV fluids at: ____.
Pain level (0-10 scale.0-no pain, 10 intolerable): _____________________________.
Location of pain: ______________. Medicated for pain: ____ yes, ____ no.
Patient is alert/oriented: ___ yes, ___ no. New confusion: ___ yes, ___ no.
Vital signs: temp ____, pulse ____, resp _____, b/p ______, 02 _____ %, _____ liters.
Glucose level: _____. Insulin: ___ yes, ___ no. Type: __________ # of units ___.

NURSING CARE FOR ______________________________

DATE ____________________, DAY NUMBER ______________________

INITIAL NIGHT SHIFT EXAM:

My nurse has _____ # of patients. CNA ___yes, ___no. Charge nurse ______________
Nurse _____________ RN/LPN came in at _________ am/pm. Left at _________ am/pm.
Did nurse wash hands and wear gloves before touching patient: ______ yes, ______ no.
Wash hands after touching patient and before leaving the room: ______ yes, ______ no.
Don't hesitate to request staff to wash their hands. This will help decrease the risk of spreading potentially lethal germs.
Did nurse wear protective gear (isolation precautions only): ______ yes, ______ no.
Did nurse provide oral care (to be done every two hours if unable to provide for self, also decreases risk of pneumonia, infections, and aspiration): ______ yes, _____ no.
If able to provide own oral care, then supplies at bedside: ______ yes, ______ no.
Was patient repositioned (every two hours if unable to turn self): ____ yes ____ no.
Head of bed at ________ degrees. This is important for patients on ventilators or on tube feedings. Anything less than thirty degrees places patients at risk for aspiration of stomach contents into the lungs causing aspiration pneumonia.
Checked for incontinence and skin breakdown: ____ yes, ____ no.
Patient's linens wet or soiled: ____ yes, ____ no. Linens changed: ____ yes, ____ no.
Time linens changed: _______ am/pm. Any skin redness or breakdown: ____ yes, ____ no.
If yes, what stage is pressure ulcer: ________. Acquired when: ________________.
List wounds not associated with pressure ulcers and how acquired: ________________
____.
Mattress type: ____.
Specialty mattresses are important to help prevent pressure ulcers)
If patient on ventilator or has tracheostomy, suction performed: _____ yes, _____ no.
Did nurse listen to lung sounds: _____ yes, _____ no.
Does patient have chest tubes: ____ yes, ____ no. Functioning _____ yes, _____ no.
Bowel sounds: ______ yes, ______ no. Bowel sounds active: ______ yes, ______ no.
Neurological exam: _____ yes, _____ no. Follow commands: ______ yes, ______ no.
Is patient alert and oriented to person, place, time, and events: ____ yes, ____ no.
If confused, patient is not oriented to: ____ person, ___ place, ___ time, ___ event.
Confusion began (time and date): ____.
Glasgow coma scale (checks conscious scale of patient): __________________________.
Intracranial pressure monitoring: _____ yes, _____ no.
If yes, pressure is at ________ mm mercury. (Normal is one to fifteen).
Moves extremities: ___ yes, ___ no.
Paralysis: (inability to move extremities) _______ yes, _______ no.
If yes, extremities affected and when paralysis began: ___________________________.
Is patient in pain: ____ yes, ____ no. Describe pain and location ______________.
Patient able to eat: ____ yes, ____ no. What type of diet? _______________________.
If patient on tube feedings list type: __________ at __________ cc/ml per hour.
Nausea ____, vomiting ____. If so, describe: _____________________________________.
Patient has: Nasal gastric tube _____, Dobhoff tube _____, Peg or gastric tube _____.
When was feeding tube placed and what site: ______________________________________.
Catheter for draining urine: ____ yes, ____ no. If so, when placed: _____________.
Find out policy for allowed time to remain in bladder. Too long may cause infections.)
IV site(s) where: ________________________ when placed: __________________________.
IV fluids (types and rates): ________________________, ___________________________,
__________________________, ________________________, ___________________________.
Is patient on oxygen: _____ yes, _____ no. If so, how much and route delivered (see oxygen routes): ____.
If patient on ventilator, list settings (see list on ventilator settings): __________
____.
Vital signs: temp _____, pulse _____, resp _____, b/p _____, o2 _____%,
current weight _____ pounds, _____ kg. Glucose level: _____
Insulin coverage: ____ yes, ____ no. Insulin type: ___________, # of units: _____.

NURSING CARE CONTINUED FOR ____________________
DATE ____________________, DAY NUMBER ____________________

FOLLOWING EXAMINATIONS FOR NIGHT SHIFT:

Nurse ____________, CNA ____________, in at _____ am/pm. Left at _______ am/pm.
Wash hands and wear gloves before touching patient: _______ yes, _______ no.
Wash hands before leaving room: ___ yes, ___ no. Wear protective gear: __ yes, __ no.
Clean stethoscope: __ yes, __ no. Oral care: __ yes, __ no. Suctioned: __ yes, __ no.
Repositioned: ___ yes, ___ no. Turned to: ___ left, ___ right, ___ backside ___.
Head of bed at: _______ degrees. Incontinence/skin breakdown: ____ yes, ___ no.
Linens wet or soiled: _____ yes, _____ no. Linens changed: _____ yes, _____ no.
Dressing changed: ____ yes, ____ no. Location: ____________________.
IV site checked: _____ yes, _____ no. IV tubing labeled: _____ yes, _____ no.
IV fluids at: ____.
Pain level (0-10 scale.0-no pain, 10 intolerable): ____________________.
Location of pain: ____________. Medicated for pain: ____ yes, ____ no.
Patient is alert/oriented: ____ yes, ____ no. New confusion: ____ yes, ____ no.
Vital signs: temp ____, pulse ____, resp _____, b/p _____, 02 _____ %, _____ liters.
Glucose level: _____. Insulin: ___ yes, ___ no. Type: __________ # of units ____.

Nurse ____________, CNA ____________, in at _____ am/pm. Left at _______ am/pm.
Wash hands and wear gloves before touching patient: _______ yes, _______ no.
Wash hands before leaving room: ___ yes, ___ no. Wear protective gear: __ yes, __ no.
Clean stethoscope: __ yes, __ no. Oral care: __ yes, __ no. Suctioned: __ yes, __ no.
Repositioned: ___ yes, ___ no. Turned to: ___ left, ___ right, ___ backside ___.
Head of bed at: _______ degrees. Incontinence/skin breakdown: ____ yes, ___ no.
Linens wet or soiled: _____ yes, _____ no. Linens changed: _____ yes, _____ no.
Dressing changed: ____ yes, ____ no. Location: ____________________.
IV site checked: _____ yes, _____ no. IV tubing labeled: _____ yes, _____ no.
IV fluids at: ____.
Pain level (0-10 scale.0-no pain, 10 intolerable): ____________________.
Location of pain: ____________. Medicated for pain: ____ yes, ____ no.
Patient is alert/oriented: ____ yes, ____ no. New confusion: ____ yes, ____ no.
Vital signs: temp ____, pulse ____, resp _____, b/p _____, 02 _____ %, _____ liters.
Glucose level: _____. Insulin: ___ yes, ___ no. Type: __________ # of units ____.

Nurse ____________, CNA ____________, in at _____ am/pm. Left at _______ am/pm.
Wash hands and wear gloves before touching patient: _______ yes, _______ no.
Wash hands before leaving room: ___ yes, ___ no. Wear protective gear: __ yes, __ no.
Clean stethoscope: __ yes, __ no. Oral care: __ yes, __ no. Suctioned: __ yes, __ no.
Repositioned: ___ yes, ___ no. Turned to: ___ left, ___ right, ___ backside ___.
Head of bed at: _______ degrees. Incontinence/skin breakdown: ____ yes, ___ no.
Linens wet or soiled: _____ yes, _____ no. Linens changed: _____ yes, _____ no.
Dressing changed: ____ yes, ____ no. Location: ____________________.
IV site checked: _____ yes, _____ no. IV tubing labeled: _____ yes, _____ no.
IV fluids at: ____.
Pain level (0-10 scale.0-no pain, 10 intolerable): ____________________.
Location of pain: ____________. Medicated for pain: ____ yes, ____ no.
Patient is alert/oriented: ____ yes, ____ no. New confusion: ____ yes, ____ no.
Vital signs: temp ____, pulse ____, resp _____, b/p _____, 02 _____ %, _____ liters.
Glucose level: _____. Insulin: ___ yes, ___ no. Type: __________ # of units ____.

NURSING CARE CONTINUED FOR ______________________
DATE ______________________, DAY NUMBER ______________________

FOLLOWING EXAMINATIONS FOR NIGHT SHIFT:

Nurse ____________, CNA ____________, in at _____ am/pm. Left at ______ am/pm.
Wash hands and wear gloves before touching patient: _______ yes, _______ no.
Wash hands before leaving room: ___ yes, ___ no. Wear protective gear: __ yes, __ no.
Clean stethoscope: __ yes, __ no. Oral care: __ yes, __ no. Suctioned: __ yes, __ no.
Repositioned: ___ yes, ___ no. Turned to: ___ left, ___ right, ___ backside ___.
Head of bed at: _______ degrees. Incontinence/skin breakdown: ____ yes, ___ no.
Linens wet or soiled: ____ yes, _____ no. Linens changed: _____ yes, _____ no.
Dressing changed: ____ yes, ____ no. Location: ______________________.
IV site checked: _____ yes, _____ no. IV tubing labeled: _____ yes, _____ no.
IV fluids at: ____.
Pain level (0-10 scale.0-no pain, 10 intolerable): ______________________.
Location of pain: ______________. Medicated for pain: _____ yes, ____ no.
Patient is alert/oriented: ____ yes, ____ no. New confusion: ____ yes, ____ no.
Vital signs: temp ____, pulse ____, resp _____, b/p _____, 02 _____ %, ____ liters.
Glucose level: _____. Insulin: ___ yes, ___ no. Type: __________ # of units ____.

Nurse ____________, CNA ____________, in at _____ am/pm. Left at ______ am/pm.
Wash hands and wear gloves before touching patient: _______ yes, _______ no.
Wash hands before leaving room: ___ yes, ___ no. Wear protective gear: __ yes, __ no.
Clean stethoscope: __ yes, __ no. Oral care: __ yes, __ no. Suctioned: __ yes, __ no.
Repositioned: ___ yes, ___ no. Turned to: ___ left, ___ right, ___ backside ___.
Head of bed at: _______ degrees. Incontinence/skin breakdown: ____ yes, ___ no.
Linens wet or soiled: ____ yes, _____ no. Linens changed: _____ yes, _____ no.
Dressing changed: ____ yes, ____ no. Location: ______________________.
IV site checked: _____ yes, _____ no. IV tubing labeled: _____ yes, _____ no.
IV fluids at: ____.
Pain level (0-10 scale.0-no pain, 10 intolerable): ______________________.
Location of pain: ______________. Medicated for pain: _____ yes, ____ no.
Patient is alert/oriented: ____ yes, ____ no. New confusion: ____ yes, ____ no.
Vital signs: temp ____, pulse ____, resp _____, b/p _____, 02 _____ %, ____ liters.
Glucose level: _____. Insulin: ___ yes, ___ no. Type: __________ # of units ____.

Nurse ____________, CNA ____________, in at _____ am/pm. Left at ______ am/pm.
Wash hands and wear gloves before touching patient: _______ yes, _______ no.
Wash hands before leaving room: ___ yes, ___ no. Wear protective gear: __ yes, __ no.
Clean stethoscope: __ yes, __ no. Oral care: __ yes, __ no. Suctioned: __ yes, __ no.
Repositioned: ___ yes, ___ no. Turned to: ___ left, ___ right, ___ backside ___.
Head of bed at: _______ degrees. Incontinence/skin breakdown: ____ yes, ___ no.
Linens wet or soiled: ____ yes, _____ no. Linens changed: _____ yes, _____ no.
Dressing changed: ____ yes, ____ no. Location: ______________________.
IV site checked: _____ yes, _____ no. IV tubing labeled: _____ yes, _____ no.
IV fluids at: ____.
Pain level (0-10 scale.0-no pain, 10 intolerable): ______________________.
Location of pain: ______________. Medicated for pain: _____ yes, ____ no.
Patient is alert/oriented: ____ yes, ____ no. New confusion: ____ yes, ____ no.
Vital signs: temp ____, pulse ____, resp _____, b/p _____, 02 _____ %, ____ liters.
Glucose level: _____. Insulin: ___ yes, ___ no. Type: __________ # of units ____.

MEDICATION ADMINISTRATION LIST FOR ____________
DATE ____________ DAY NUMBER ____________

List the medication for each day. Routes of administration: oral, thru feeding tube, intravenous (IV), intramuscular (IM), subcutaneous (SQ), epidural or a catheter in your spinal column, rectal, topical, eye drops, and ear drops.

Medication:		Route:		Time:	
Medication:		Route:		Time:	
Medication:		Route:		Time:	
Medication:		Route:		Time:	
Medication:		Route:		Time:	
Medication:		Route:		Time:	
Medication:		Route:		Time:	
Medication:		Route:		Time:	
Medication:		Route:		Time:	
Medication:		Route:		Time:	
Medication:		Route:		Time:	
Medication:		Route:		Time:	
Medication:		Route:		Time:	
Medication:		Route:		Time:	
Medication:		Route:		Time:	
Medication:		Route:		Time:	
Medication:		Route:		Time:	
Medication:		Route:		Time:	
Medication:		Route:		Time:	
Medication:		Route:		Time:	
Medication:		Route:		Time:	
Medication:		Route:		Time:	
Medication:		Route:		Time:	
Medication:		Route:		Time:	
Medication:		Route:		Time:	
Medication:		Route:		Time:	
Medication:		Route:		Time:	
Medication:		Route:		Time:	
Medication:		Route:		Time:	
Medication:		Route:		Time:	
Medication:		Route:		Time:	
Medication:		Route:		Time:	
Medication:		Route:		Time:	
Medication:		Route:		Time:	
Medication:		Route:		Time:	
Medication:		Route:		Time:	
Medication:		Route:		Time:	
Medication:		Route:		Time:	
Medication:		Route:		Time:	
Medication:		Route:		Time:	
Medication:		Route:		Time:	
Medication:		Route:		Time:	
Medication:		Route:		Time:	
Medication:		Route:		Time:	
Medication:		Route:		Time:	
Medication:		Route:		Time:	
Medication:		Route:		Time:	
Medication:		Route:		Time:	
Medication:		Route:		Time:	
Medication:		Route:		Time:	
Medication:		Route:		Time:	
Medication:		Route:		Time:	
Medication:		Route:		Time:	
Medication:		Route:		Time:	

NOTES FOR DAY NUMBER ______________________________

DATE ______________________________

MEDICAL JOURNAL FOR ______________________

DATE ______________________, DAY NUMBER ______________

VISITS FROM MY DOCTORS TODAY

Goals for today: ______________________

____

______________________.

Things to discuss with my doctor(s): ______________________

____

____

Dr.__________ came in at _____ am/pm. Left at _____ am/pm.
We discussed ______________________.
Did doctor examine patient: _____ yes, _____ no.
Wash hands before touching patient: _____ yes, _____ no.
Wear gloves: _____ yes, ___ no. Clean stethoscope: ____ yes, ____ no.
Wear gown and mask (precautions only):_____ yes, _____ no.
Wash hands before leaving the room: _____ yes, _____ no.

Dr.__________ came in at _____ am/pm. Left at _____ am/pm.
We discussed ______________________.
Did doctor examine patient: _____ yes, _____ no.
Wash hands before touching patient: _____ yes, _____ no.
Wear gloves: _____ yes, ___ no. Clean stethoscope: ____ yes, ____ no.
Wear gown and mask (precautions only):_____ yes, _____ no.
Wash hands before leaving the room: _____ yes, _____ no.

Dr.__________ came in at _____ am/pm. Left at _____ am/pm.
We discussed ______________________.
Did doctor examine patient: _____ yes, _____ no.
Wash hands before touching patient: _____ yes, _____ no.
Wear gloves: _____ yes, ___ no. Clean stethoscope: ____ yes, ____ no.
Wear gown and mask (precautions only):_____ yes, _____ no.
Wash hands before leaving the room: _____ yes, _____ no.

Dr.__________ came in at _____ am/pm. Left at _____ am/pm.
We discussed ______________________.
Did doctor examine patient: _____ yes, _____ no.
Wash hands before touching patient: _____ yes, _____ no.
Wear gloves: _____ yes, ___ no. Clean stethoscope: ____ yes, ____ no.
Wear gown and mask (precautions only):_____ yes, _____ no.
Wash hands before leaving the room: _____ yes, _____ no.

Dr.__________ came in at _____ am/pm. Left at _____ am/pm.
We discussed ______________________.
Did doctor examine patient: _____ yes, _____ no.
Wash hands before touching patient: _____ yes, _____ no.
Wear gloves: _____ yes, ___ no. Clean stethoscope: ____ yes, ____ no.
Wear gown and mask (precautions only):_____ yes, _____ no.
Wash hands before leaving the room: _____ yes, _____ no.

NURSING CARE FOR ______________________________

DATE ______________, DAY NUMBER ______________

INITIAL DAY SHIFT EXAM:

My nurse has ______ # of patients. CNA ___yes, ___no. Charge nurse __________
Nurse ____________ RN/LPN came in at ________ am/pm. Left at ________ am/pm.
Did nurse wash hands and wear gloves before touching patient: ______ yes, ______ no.
Wash hands after touching patient and before leaving the room: ______ yes, ______ no.
Don't hesitate to request staff to wash their hands. This will help decrease the risk of spreading potentially lethal germs.
Did nurse wear protective gear (isolation precautions only): ______ yes, ______ no.
Did nurse provide oral care (to be done every two hours if unable to provide for self, also decreases risk of pneumonia, infections, and aspiration): ______ yes, ______ no.
If able to provide own oral care, then supplies at bedside: ______ yes, ______ no.
Was patient repositioned (every two hours if unable to turn self): _____ yes _____ no.
Head of bed at ________ degrees. This is important for patients on ventilators or on tube feedings. Anything less than thirty degrees places patients at risk for aspiration of stomach contents into the lungs causing aspiration pneumonia.
Checked for incontinence and skin breakdown: _____ yes, _____ no.
Patient's linens wet or soiled: _____ yes, ____ no. Linens changed: ____ yes, ____ no.
Time linens changed: _______ am/pm. Any skin redness or breakdown: ____ yes, ____ no.
If yes, what stage is pressure ulcer: ________. Acquired when: ______________.
List wounds not associated with pressure ulcers and how acquired: ______________
____.
Mattress type: ____.
Specialty mattresses are important to help prevent pressure ulcers)
If patient on ventilator or has tracheostomy, suction performed: _____ yes, ______ no.
Did nurse listen to lung sounds: _____ yes, _____ no.
Does patient have chest tubes: ____ yes, ____ no. Functioning _____ yes, ______ no.
Bowel sounds: _______ yes, _______ no. Bowel sounds active: _____ yes, ______ no.
Neurological exam: ______ yes, ______ no. Follow commands: _____ yes, ______ no.
Is patient alert and oriented to person, place, time, and events: _____ yes, _____ no.
If confused, patient is not oriented to: ____ person, ___ place, ___ time, ___ event.
Confusion began (time and date): ______________________________________.
Glasgow coma scale (checks conscious scale of patient): ______________________.
Intracranial pressure monitoring: ______ yes, ______ no.
If yes, pressure is at ________ mm mercury. (Normal is one to fifteen).
Moves extremities: ___ yes, ___ no.
Paralysis: (inability to move extremities) _________ yes, ______ no.
If yes, extremities affected and when paralysis began: ______________________.
Is patient in pain: ____ yes, ____ no. Describe pain and location ______________.
Patient able to eat: ____ yes, ____ no. What type of diet? ____________________.
If patient on tube feedings list type: ______________ at ___________ cc/ml per hour.
Nausea ____, vomiting _____. If so, describe: ______________________________.
Patient has: Nasal gastric tube ______, Dobhoff tube _____, Peg or gastric tube _____.
When was feeding tube placed and what site: ____________________________________.
Catheter for draining urine: ___ yes, ____ no. If so, when placed: ______________.
Find out policy for allowed time to remain in bladder. Too long may cause infections.)
IV site(s) where: ________________________ when placed: ____________.
IV fluids (types and rates): __________________, __________________,
__________________, __________________, __________________,
Is patient on oxygen: _____ yes, _____ no. If so, how much and route delivered (see oxygen routes): ____.
If patient on ventilator, list settings (see list on ventilator settings): ________
____.
Vital signs: temp ______, pulse ______, resp ______, b/p ______, o2 ______%,
current weight ____ pounds, ____ kg. Glucose level: ______________________.
Insulin coverage: ____ yes, ____ no. Insulin type: __________, # of units: ______.

NURSING CARE CONTINUED FOR ____________________
DATE ____________________, DAY NUMBER ____________________

FOLLOWING EXAMINATIONS FOR DAY SHIFT:

Nurse ____________, CNA ____________, in at ______ am/pm. Left at _______ am/pm.
Wash hands and wear gloves before touching patient: _______ yes, _______ no.
Wash hands before leaving room: ___ yes, ___ no. Wear protective gear: __ yes, __ no.
Clean stethoscope: __ yes, __ no. Oral care: __ yes, __ no. Suctioned: __ yes, __ no.
Repositioned: ___ yes, ___ no. Turned to: ___ left, ___ right, ___ backside ___.
Head of bed at: _______ degrees. Incontinence/skin breakdown: ____ yes, ____ no.
Linens wet or soiled: _____ yes, _____ no. Linens changed: _____ yes, _____ no.
Dressing changed: ____ yes, ____ no. Location: ____________________.
IV site checked: _____ yes, _____ no. IV tubing labeled: _____ yes, _____ no.
IV fluids at: ____________________.
Pain level (0-10 scale.0-no pain, 10 intolerable): ____________________.
Location of pain: ____________. Medicated for pain: _____ yes, ____ no.
Patient is alert/oriented: ___ yes, ___ no. New confusion: ___ yes, ___ no.
Vital signs: temp ____, pulse ____, resp ____, b/p ____, 02 ____ %, ____ liters.
Glucose level: _____. Insulin: ___ yes, ___ no. Type: ____________ # of units ____.

Nurse ____________, CNA ____________, in at ______ am/pm. Left at _______ am/pm.
Wash hands and wear gloves before touching patient: _______ yes, _______ no.
Wash hands before leaving room: ___ yes, ___ no. Wear protective gear: __ yes, __ no.
Clean stethoscope: __ yes, __ no. Oral care: __ yes, __ no. Suctioned: __ yes, __ no.
Repositioned: ___ yes, ___ no. Turned to: ___ left, ___ right, ___ backside ___.
Head of bed at: _______ degrees. Incontinence/skin breakdown: ____ yes, ____ no.
Linens wet or soiled: _____ yes, _____ no. Linens changed: _____ yes, _____ no.
Dressing changed: ____ yes, ____ no. Location: ____________________.
IV site checked: _____ yes, _____ no. IV tubing labeled: _____ yes, _____ no.
IV fluids at: ____________________.
Pain level (0-10 scale.0-no pain, 10 intolerable): ____________________.
Location of pain: ____________. Medicated for pain: _____ yes, ____ no.
Patient is alert/oriented: ___ yes, ___ no. New confusion: ___ yes, ___ no.
Vital signs: temp ____, pulse ____, resp ____, b/p ____, 02 ____ %, ____ liters.
Glucose level: _____. Insulin: ___ yes, ___ no. Type: ____________ # of units ____.

Nurse ____________, CNA ____________, in at ______ am/pm. Left at _______ am/pm.
Wash hands and wear gloves before touching patient: _______ yes, _______ no.
Wash hands before leaving room: ___ yes, ___ no. Wear protective gear: __ yes, __ no.
Clean stethoscope: __ yes, __ no. Oral care: __ yes, __ no. Suctioned: __ yes, __ no.
Repositioned: ___ yes, ___ no. Turned to: ___ left, ___ right, ___ backside ___.
Head of bed at: _______ degrees. Incontinence/skin breakdown: ____ yes, ____ no.
Linens wet or soiled: _____ yes, _____ no. Linens changed: _____ yes, _____ no.
Dressing changed: ____ yes, ____ no. Location: ____________________.
IV site checked: _____ yes, _____ no. IV tubing labeled: _____ yes, _____ no.
IV fluids at: ____________________.
Pain level (0-10 scale.0-no pain, 10 intolerable): ____________________.
Location of pain: ____________. Medicated for pain: _____ yes, ____ no.
Patient is alert/oriented: ___ yes, ___ no. New confusion: ___ yes, ___ no.
Vital signs: temp ____, pulse ____, resp ____, b/p ____, 02 ____ %, ____ liters.
Glucose level: _____. Insulin: ___ yes, ___ no. Type: ____________ # of units ____.

NURSING CARE CONTINUED FOR ____________________
DATE ________________, DAY NUMBER ________________

FOLLOWING EXAMINATIONS FOR DAY SHIFT:

Nurse ____________, CNA ____________, in at _____ am/pm. Left at ______ am/pm.
Wash hands and wear gloves before touching patient: ______ yes, ______ no.
Wash hands before leaving room: ___ yes, ___ no. Wear protective gear: __ yes, __ no.
Clean stethoscope: __ yes, __ no. Oral care: __ yes, __ no. Suctioned: __ yes, __ no.
Repositioned: ___ yes, ___ no. Turned to: ___ left, ___ right, ___ backside ___.
Head of bed at: ______ degrees. Incontinence/skin breakdown: ____ yes, ____ no.
Linens wet or soiled: ____ yes, ____ no. Linens changed: ____ yes, _____ no.
Dressing changed: ____ yes, ____ no. Location: ____________________.
IV site checked: _____ yes, _____ no. IV tubing labeled: _____ yes, _____no.
IV fluids at: ____.
Pain level (0-10 scale.0-no pain, 10 intolerable): ________________.
Location of pain: ______________. Medicated for pain: ____ yes, ____ no.
Patient is alert/oriented: ____ yes, ____ no. New confusion: ___ yes, ____ no.
Vital signs: temp ____, pulse _____, resp _____, b/p _____, 02 _____ %, ____ liters.
Glucose level: _____. Insulin: ___ yes, ___ no. Type: ____________ # of units ____.

Nurse ____________, CNA ____________, in at _____ am/pm. Left at ______ am/pm.
Wash hands and wear gloves before touching patient: ______ yes, ______ no.
Wash hands before leaving room: ___ yes, ___ no. Wear protective gear: __ yes, __ no.
Clean stethoscope: __ yes, __ no. Oral care: __ yes, __ no. Suctioned: __ yes, __ no.
Repositioned: ___ yes, ___ no. Turned to: ___ left, ___ right, ___ backside ___.
Head of bed at: ______ degrees. Incontinence/skin breakdown: ____ yes, ____ no.
Linens wet or soiled: ____ yes, ____ no. Linens changed: ____ yes, _____ no.
Dressing changed: ____ yes, ____ no. Location: ____________________.
IV site checked: _____ yes, _____ no. IV tubing labeled: _____ yes, _____no.
IV fluids at: ____.
Pain level (0-10 scale.0-no pain, 10 intolerable): ________________.
Location of pain: ______________. Medicated for pain: ____ yes, ____ no.
Patient is alert/oriented: ____ yes, ____ no. New confusion: ___ yes, ____ no.
Vital signs: temp ____, pulse _____, resp _____, b/p _____, 02 _____ %, ____ liters.
Glucose level: _____. Insulin: ___ yes, ___ no. Type: ____________ # of units ____.

Nurse ____________, CNA ____________, in at _____ am/pm. Left at ______ am/pm.
Wash hands and wear gloves before touching patient: ______ yes, ______ no.
Wash hands before leaving room: ___ yes, ___ no. Wear protective gear: __ yes, __ no.
Clean stethoscope: __ yes, __ no. Oral care: __ yes, __ no. Suctioned: __ yes, __ no.
Repositioned: ___ yes, ___ no. Turned to: ___ left, ___ right, ___ backside ___.
Head of bed at: ______ degrees. Incontinence/skin breakdown: ____ yes, ____ no.
Linens wet or soiled: ____ yes, ____ no. Linens changed: ____ yes, _____ no.
Dressing changed: ____ yes, ____ no. Location: ____________________.
IV site checked: _____ yes, _____ no. IV tubing labeled: _____ yes, _____no.
IV fluids at: ____.
Pain level (0-10 scale.0-no pain, 10 intolerable): ________________.
Location of pain: ______________. Medicated for pain: ____ yes, ____ no.
Patient is alert/oriented: ____ yes, ____ no. New confusion: ___ yes, ____ no.
Vital signs: temp ____, pulse _____, resp _____, b/p _____, 02 _____ %, ____ liters.
Glucose level: _____. Insulin: ___ yes, ___ no. Type: ____________ # of units ____.

NURSING CARE FOR ______________________________

DATE ____________________, DAY NUMBER ____________________

INITIAL NIGHT SHIFT EXAM:

My nurse has _____ # of patients. CNA ___yes, ___no. Charge nurse ______________
Nurse ______________ RN/LPN came in at _________ am/pm. Left at _________ am/pm.
Did nurse wash hands and wear gloves before touching patient: _______ yes, _______ no.
Wash hands after touching patient and before leaving the room: _______ yes, _______ no.
Don't hesitate to request staff to wash their hands. This will help decrease the risk of spreading potentially lethal germs.
Did nurse wear protective gear (isolation precautions only): _______ yes, _______ no.
Did nurse provide oral care (to be done every two hours if unable to provide for self, also decreases risk of pneumonia, infections, and aspiration): _______ yes, _____ no.
If able to provide own oral care, then supplies at bedside: _______ yes, _______ no.
Was patient repositioned (every two hours if unable to turn self): _____ yes _____ no.
Head of bed at ________ degrees. This is important for patients on ventilators or on tube feedings. Anything less than thirty degrees places patients at risk for aspiration of stomach contents into the lungs causing aspiration pneumonia.
Checked for incontinence and skin breakdown: ____ yes, ____ no.
Patient's linens wet or soiled: ____ yes, ____ no. Linens changed: ____ yes, ____ no.
Time linens changed: ________ am/pm. Any skin redness or breakdown: ____ yes, ____ no.
If yes, what stage is pressure ulcer: ________. Acquired when: ______________.
List wounds not associated with pressure ulcers and how acquired: ______________
____.
Mattress type: ____.
Specialty mattresses are important to help prevent pressure ulcers)
If patient on ventilator or has tracheostomy, suction performed: _____ yes, _____ no.
Did nurse listen to lung sounds: _____ yes, _____ no.
Does patient have chest tubes: ____ yes, ____ no. Functioning _____ yes, _____ no.
Bowel sounds: ______ yes, ______ no. Bowel sounds active: ______ yes, ______ no.
Neurological exam: _____ yes, _____ no. Follow commands: _______ yes, ______ no.
Is patient alert and oriented to person, place, time, and events: ____ yes, ____ no.
If confused, patient is not oriented to: ___ person, ___ place, ___ time, ___ event.
Confusion began (time and date): ____.
Glasgow coma scale (checks conscious scale of patient): ________________________.
Intracranial pressure monitoring: ____ yes, ____ no.
If yes, pressure is at ________ mm mercury. (Normal is one to fifteen).
Moves extremities: ___ yes, ___ no.
Paralysis: (inability to move extremities) _______ yes, _______ no.
If yes, extremities affected and when paralysis began: __________________________.
Is patient in pain: ____ yes, ____ no. Describe pain and location _______________.
Patient able to eat: ___ yes, ___ no. What type of diet? _________________________.
If patient on tube feedings list type: ____________ at ____________ cc/ml per hour.
Nausea ____, vomiting ____. If so, describe: ___________________________________.
Patient has: Nasal gastric tube ______, Dobhoff tube _____, Peg or gastric tube ____.
When was feeding tube placed and what site: _____________________________________.
Catheter for draining urine: ____ yes, ____ no. If so, when placed: ______________.
Find out policy for allowed time to remain in bladder. Too long may cause infections.)
IV site(s) where: ______________________ when placed: __________________________.
IV fluids (types and rates): _____________________, _______________, ____________,
_____________________, _____________________, ___________________, ____________.
Is patient on oxygen: _____ yes, _____ no. If so, how much and route delivered (see oxygen routes): ____.
If patient on ventilator, list settings (see list on ventilator settings): _________
____.
Vital signs: temp ______, pulse ______, resp ______, b/p ______, o2 ______%,
current weight ______ pounds, ______ kg. Glucose level: ______
Insulin coverage: ____ yes, ____ no. Insulin type: ____________, # of units: ______.

NURSING CARE CONTINUED FOR ____________________
DATE ____________________, DAY NUMBER ____________________

FOLLOWING EXAMINATIONS FOR NIGHT SHIFT:

Nurse ____________, CNA ____________, in at ______ am/pm. Left at ______ am/pm.
Wash hands and wear gloves before touching patient: ______ yes, ______ no.
Wash hands before leaving room: ___ yes, ___ no. Wear protective gear: __ yes, __ no.
Clean stethoscope: __ yes, __ no. Oral care: __ yes, __ no. Suctioned: __ yes, __ no.
Repositioned: ___ yes, ___ no. Turned to: ___ left, ___ right, ___ backside ___.
Head of bed at: ________ degrees. Incontinence/skin breakdown: ____ yes, ____ no.
Linens wet or soiled: _____ yes, _____ no. Linens changed: _____ yes, ______ no.
Dressing changed: ____ yes, ____ no. Location: ______________________________.
IV site checked: _____ yes, _____ no. IV tubing labeled: _____ yes, _____no.
IV fluids at: ____.
Pain level (0-10 scale.0-no pain, 10 intolerable): ____________________________.
Location of pain: ____________________. Medicated for pain: ____ yes, ____ no.
Patient is alert/oriented: ____ yes, ____ no. New confusion: ____ yes, ____ no.
Vital signs: temp ____, pulse _____, resp _____, b/p _____, 02 _____ %, ____ liters.
Glucose level: _____. Insulin: ___ yes, ___ no. Type: _____________ # of units ____.

Nurse ____________, CNA ____________, in at ______ am/pm. Left at ______ am/pm.
Wash hands and wear gloves before touching patient: ______ yes, ______ no.
Wash hands before leaving room: ___ yes, ___ no. Wear protective gear: __ yes, __ no.
Clean stethoscope: __ yes, __ no. Oral care: __ yes, __ no. Suctioned: __ yes, __ no.
Repositioned: ___ yes, ___ no. Turned to: ___ left, ___ right, ___ backside ___.
Head of bed at: ________ degrees. Incontinence/skin breakdown: ____ yes, ____ no.
Linens wet or soiled: _____ yes, _____ no. Linens changed: _____ yes, ______ no.
Dressing changed: ____ yes, ____ no. Location: ______________________________.
IV site checked: _____ yes, _____ no. IV tubing labeled: _____ yes, _____no.
IV fluids at: ____.
Pain level (0-10 scale.0-no pain, 10 intolerable): ____________________________.
Location of pain: ____________________. Medicated for pain: ____ yes, ____ no.
Patient is alert/oriented: ____ yes, ____ no. New confusion: ____ yes, ____ no.
Vital signs: temp ____, pulse _____, resp _____, b/p _____, 02 _____ %, ____ liters.
Glucose level: _____. Insulin: ___ yes, ___ no. Type: _____________ # of units ____.

Nurse ____________, CNA ____________, in at ______ am/pm. Left at ______ am/pm.
Wash hands and wear gloves before touching patient: ______ yes, ______ no.
Wash hands before leaving room: ___ yes, ___ no. Wear protective gear: __ yes, __ no.
Clean stethoscope: __ yes, __ no. Oral care: __ yes, __ no. Suctioned: __ yes, __ no.
Repositioned: ___ yes, ___ no. Turned to: ___ left, ___ right, ___ backside ___.
Head of bed at: ________ degrees. Incontinence/skin breakdown: ____ yes, ____ no.
Linens wet or soiled: _____ yes, _____ no. Linens changed: _____ yes, ______ no.
Dressing changed: ____ yes, ____ no. Location: ______________________________.
IV site checked: _____ yes, _____ no. IV tubing labeled: _____ yes, _____no.
IV fluids at: ____.
Pain level (0-10 scale.0-no pain, 10 intolerable): ____________________________.
Location of pain: ____________________. Medicated for pain: ____ yes, ____ no.
Patient is alert/oriented: ____ yes, ____ no. New confusion: ____ yes, ____ no.
Vital signs: temp ____, pulse _____, resp _____, b/p _____, 02 _____ %, ____ liters.
Glucose level: _____. Insulin: ___ yes, ___ no. Type: _____________ # of units ____.

NURSING CARE CONTINUED FOR ____________________
DATE ____________________, DAY NUMBER ____________________

FOLLOWING EXAMINATIONS FOR NIGHT SHIFT:

Nurse ______________, CNA ______________, in at _____ am/pm. Left at ______ am/pm.
Wash hands and wear gloves before touching patient: ______ yes, ______ no.
Wash hands before leaving room: ___ yes, ___ no. Wear protective gear: __ yes, __ no.
Clean stethoscope: __ yes, __ no. Oral care: __ yes, __ no. Suctioned: __ yes, __ no.
Repositioned: ___ yes, ___ no. Turned to: ___ left, ___ right, ___ backside ___.
Head of bed at: ________ degrees. Incontinence/skin breakdown: ____ yes, ____ no.
Linens wet or soiled: _____ yes, _____ no. Linens changed: _____ yes, _____ no.
Dressing changed: ____ yes, ____ no. Location: ______________________.
IV site checked: _____ yes, _____ no. IV tubing labeled: _____ yes, _____no.
IV fluids at: ____.
Pain level (0-10 scale.0-no pain, 10 intolerable): ______________________.
Location of pain: ______________. Medicated for pain: _____ yes, ____ no.
Patient is alert/oriented: ____ yes, ____ no. New confusion: ____ yes, ____ no.
Vital signs: temp ____, pulse _____, resp ______, b/p ______, 02 _____ %, ____ liters.
Glucose level: _____. Insulin: ___ yes, ___ no. Type: ______________ # of units ____.

Nurse ______________, CNA ______________, in at _____ am/pm. Left at ______ am/pm.
Wash hands and wear gloves before touching patient: ______ yes, ______ no.
Wash hands before leaving room: ___ yes, ___ no. Wear protective gear: __ yes, __ no.
Clean stethoscope: __ yes, __ no. Oral care: __ yes, __ no. Suctioned: __ yes, __ no.
Repositioned: ___ yes, ___ no. Turned to: ___ left, ___ right, ___ backside ___.
Head of bed at: ________ degrees. Incontinence/skin breakdown: ____ yes, ____ no.
Linens wet or soiled: _____ yes, _____ no. Linens changed: _____ yes, _____ no.
Dressing changed: ____ yes, ____ no. Location: ______________________.
IV site checked: _____ yes, _____ no. IV tubing labeled: _____ yes, _____no.
IV fluids at: ____.
Pain level (0-10 scale.0-no pain, 10 intolerable): ______________________.
Location of pain: ______________. Medicated for pain: _____ yes, ____ no.
Patient is alert/oriented: ____ yes, ____ no. New confusion: ____ yes, ____ no.
Vital signs: temp ____, pulse _____, resp ______, b/p ______, 02 _____ %, ____ liters.
Glucose level: _____. Insulin: ___ yes, ___ no. Type: ______________ # of units ____.

Nurse ______________, CNA ______________, in at _____ am/pm. Left at ______ am/pm.
Wash hands and wear gloves before touching patient: ______ yes, ______ no.
Wash hands before leaving room: ___ yes, ___ no. Wear protective gear: __ yes, __ no.
Clean stethoscope: __ yes, __ no. Oral care: __ yes, __ no. Suctioned: __ yes, __ no.
Repositioned: ___ yes, ___ no. Turned to: ___ left, ___ right, ___ backside ___.
Head of bed at: ________ degrees. Incontinence/skin breakdown: ____ yes, ____ no.
Linens wet or soiled: _____ yes, _____ no. Linens changed: _____ yes, _____ no.
Dressing changed: ____ yes, ____ no. Location: ______________________.
IV site checked: _____ yes, _____ no. IV tubing labeled: _____ yes, _____no.
IV fluids at: ____.
Pain level (0-10 scale.0-no pain, 10 intolerable): ______________________.
Location of pain: ______________. Medicated for pain: _____ yes, ____ no.
Patient is alert/oriented: ____ yes, ____ no. New confusion: ____ yes, ____ no.
Vital signs: temp ____, pulse _____, resp ______, b/p ______, 02 _____ %, ____ liters.
Glucose level: _____. Insulin: ___ yes, ___ no. Type: ______________ # of units ____.

MEDICATION ADMINISTRATION LIST FOR ____________________
DATE ______________ DAY NUMBER ____________________

List the medication for each day. Routes of administration: oral, thru feeding tube, intravenous (IV), intramuscular (IM), subcutaneous (SQ), epidural or a catheter in your spinal column, rectal, topical, eye drops, and ear drops.

Medication: ______________ Route: ______________ Time: __________
Medication: ______________ Route: ______________ Time: __________
Medication: ______________ Route: ______________ Time: __________
Medication: ______________ Route: ______________ Time: __________
Medication: ______________ Route: ______________ Time: __________
Medication: ______________ Route: ______________ Time: __________
Medication: ______________ Route: ______________ Time: __________
Medication: ______________ Route: ______________ Time: __________
Medication: ______________ Route: ______________ Time: __________
Medication: ______________ Route: ______________ Time: __________
Medication: ______________ Route: ______________ Time: __________
Medication: ______________ Route: ______________ Time: __________
Medication: ______________ Route: ______________ Time: __________
Medication: ______________ Route: ______________ Time: __________
Medication: ______________ Route: ______________ Time: __________
Medication: ______________ Route: ______________ Time: __________
Medication: ______________ Route: ______________ Time: __________
Medication: ______________ Route: ______________ Time: __________
Medication: ______________ Route: ______________ Time: __________
Medication: ______________ Route: ______________ Time: __________
Medication: ______________ Route: ______________ Time: __________
Medication: ______________ Route: ______________ Time: __________
Medication: ______________ Route: ______________ Time: __________
Medication: ______________ Route: ______________ Time: __________
Medication: ______________ Route: ______________ Time: __________
Medication: ______________ Route: ______________ Time: __________
Medication: ______________ Route: ______________ Time: __________
Medication: ______________ Route: ______________ Time: __________
Medication: ______________ Route: ______________ Time: __________
Medication: ______________ Route: ______________ Time: __________
Medication: ______________ Route: ______________ Time: __________
Medication: ______________ Route: ______________ Time: __________
Medication: ______________ Route: ______________ Time: __________
Medication: ______________ Route: ______________ Time: __________
Medication: ______________ Route: ______________ Time: __________
Medication: ______________ Route: ______________ Time: __________
Medication: ______________ Route: ______________ Time: __________
Medication: ______________ Route: ______________ Time: __________
Medication: ______________ Route: ______________ Time: __________
Medication: ______________ Route: ______________ Time: __________
Medication: ______________ Route: ______________ Time: __________
Medication: ______________ Route: ______________ Time: __________
Medication: ______________ Route: ______________ Time: __________
Medication: ______________ Route: ______________ Time: __________
Medication: ______________ Route: ______________ Time: __________
Medication: ______________ Route: ______________ Time: __________
Medication: ______________ Route: ______________ Time: __________
Medication: ______________ Route: ______________ Time: __________
Medication: ______________ Route: ______________ Time: __________
Medication: ______________ Route: ______________ Time: __________
Medication: ______________ Route: ______________ Time: __________
Medication: ______________ Route: ______________ Time: __________
Medication: ______________ Route: ______________ Time: __________
Medication: ______________ Route: ______________ Time: __________

NOTES FOR DAY NUMBER ______________________________

DATE ______________________________

MEDICAL JOURNAL FOR ______________________________

DATE ____________________, DAY NUMBER ______________

VISITS FROM MY DOCTORS TODAY

Goals for today: ____

____

____.

Things to discuss with my doctor(s): ______________________________

____

____

Dr.__________ came in at ____ am/pm. Left at ____ am/pm.
We discussed ____.
Did doctor examine patient: ____ yes, ____ no.
Wash hands before touching patient: ____ yes, ____ no.
Wear gloves: ____ yes, ___ no. Clean stethoscope: ____ yes, ____ no.
Wear gown and mask (precautions only):____ yes, ____ no.
Wash hands before leaving the room: ____ yes, ____ no.

Dr.__________ came in at ____ am/pm. Left at ____ am/pm.
We discussed ____.
Did doctor examine patient: ____ yes, ____ no.
Wash hands before touching patient: ____ yes, ____ no.
Wear gloves: ____ yes, ___ no. Clean stethoscope: ____ yes, ____ no.
Wear gown and mask (precautions only):____ yes, ____ no.
Wash hands before leaving the room: ____ yes, ____ no.

Dr.__________ came in at ____ am/pm. Left at ____ am/pm.
We discussed ____.
Did doctor examine patient: ____ yes, ____ no.
Wash hands before touching patient: ____ yes, ____ no.
Wear gloves: ____ yes, ___ no. Clean stethoscope: ____ yes, ____ no.
Wear gown and mask (precautions only):____ yes, ____ no.
Wash hands before leaving the room: ____ yes, ____ no.

Dr.__________ came in at ____ am/pm. Left at ____ am/pm.
We discussed ____.
Did doctor examine patient: ____ yes, ____ no.
Wash hands before touching patient: ____ yes, ____ no.
Wear gloves: ____ yes, ___ no. Clean stethoscope: ____ yes, ____ no.
Wear gown and mask (precautions only):____ yes, ____ no.
Wash hands before leaving the room: ____ yes, ____ no.

Dr.__________ came in at ____ am/pm. Left at ____ am/pm.
We discussed ____.
Did doctor examine patient: ____ yes, ____ no.
Wash hands before touching patient: ____ yes, ____ no.
Wear gloves: ____ yes, ___ no. Clean stethoscope: ____ yes, ____ no.
Wear gown and mask (precautions only):____ yes, ____ no.
Wash hands before leaving the room: ____ yes, ____ no.

NURSING CARE FOR ______________________________

DATE ____________________, DAY NUMBER ____________________

INITIAL DAY SHIFT EXAM:

My nurse has ______ # of patients. CNA ___yes, ___no. Charge nurse ______________
Nurse ____________ RN/LPN came in at ________ am/pm. Left at ________ am/pm.
Did nurse wash hands and wear gloves before touching patient: _______ yes, _______ no.
Wash hands after touching patient and before leaving the room: _______ yes, _______ no.
Don't hesitate to request staff to wash their hands. This will help decrease the risk of spreading potentially lethal germs.
Did nurse wear protective gear (isolation precautions only): _______ yes, _______ no.
Did nurse provide oral care (to be done every two hours if unable to provide for self, also decreases risk of pneumonia, infections, and aspiration): _______ yes, _______ no.
If able to provide own oral care, then supplies at bedside: _______ yes, _______ no.
Was patient repositioned (every two hours if unable to turn self): _____ yes _____ no.
Head of bed at ________ degrees. This is important for patients on ventilators or on tube feedings. Anything less than thirty degrees places patients at risk for aspiration of stomach contents into the lungs causing aspiration pneumonia.
Checked for incontinence and skin breakdown: ____ yes, _____ no.
Patient's linens wet or soiled: ____ yes, ____ no. Linens changed: ____ yes, ____ no.
Time linens changed: ________ am/pm. Any skin redness or breakdown: ____ yes, ____ no.
If yes, what stage is pressure ulcer: ________. Acquired when: ______________.
List wounds not associated with pressure ulcers and how acquired: ______________
____
Mattress type: ____
Specialty mattresses are important to help prevent pressure ulcers)
If patient on ventilator or has tracheostomy, suction performed: _____ yes, _____ no.
Did nurse listen to lung sounds: _____ yes, _____ no.
Does patient have chest tubes: ____ yes, ____ no. Functioning _____ yes, _____ no.
Bowel sounds: _______ yes, _______ no. Bowel sounds active: _______ yes, _______ no.
Neurological exam: ______ yes, ______ no. Follow commands: _______ yes, _______ no.
Is patient alert and oriented to person, place, time, and events: _____ yes, _____ no.
If confused, patient is not oriented to: ___ person, ___ place, ___ time, ___ event.
Confusion began (time and date): ____
Glasgow coma scale (checks conscious scale of patient): _____________________
Intracranial pressure monitoring: _____ yes, _____ no.
If yes, pressure is at ________ mm mercury. (Normal is one to fifteen).
Moves extremities: ___ yes, ___ no.
Paralysis: (inability to move extremities) _______ yes, _______ no.
If yes, extremities affected and when paralysis began: ______________________.
Is patient in pain: ____ yes, ____ no. Describe pain and location ____________.
Patient able to eat: ____ yes, ____ no. What type of diet? ____________________.
If patient on tube feedings list type: __________ at __________ cc/ml per hour.
Nausea ____, vomiting ____. If so, describe: _________________________________.
Patient has: Nasal gastric tube _____, Dobhoff tube ____, Peg or gastric tube ____.
When was feeding tube placed and what site: _________________________________.
Catheter for draining urine: ____ yes, ____ no. If so, when placed: __________.
Find out policy for allowed time to remain in bladder. Too long may cause infections.)
IV site(s) where: ______________________ when placed: ________________________.
IV fluids (types and rates): __________________, __________________, __________,
______________________________, ______________________, _______________________.
Is patient on oxygen: _____ yes, _____ no. If so, how much and route delivered (see oxygen routes): ____.
If patient on ventilator, list settings (see list on ventilator settings): _________
____.
Vital signs: temp _____, pulse _____, resp _____, b/p _____, o2 _____%,
current weight _____ pounds, _____ kg. Glucose level: _____
Insulin coverage: ____ yes, ____ no. Insulin type: ____________, # of units: _____.

NURSING CARE CONTINUED FOR ______________________________
DATE ____________________, DAY NUMBER ____________________

FOLLOWING EXAMINATIONS FOR DAY SHIFT:

Nurse _____________, CNA _____________, in at _____ am/pm. Left at _____ am/pm.
Wash hands and wear gloves before touching patient: _____ yes, _____ no.
Wash hands before leaving room: ___ yes, ___ no. Wear protective gear: __ yes, __ no.
Clean stethoscope: __ yes, __ no. Oral care: __ yes, __ no. Suctioned: __ yes, __ no.
Repositioned: ___ yes, ___ no. Turned to: ___ left, ___ right, ___ backside ___.
Head of bed at: ______ degrees. Incontinence/skin breakdown: ____ yes, ____ no.
Linens wet or soiled: _____ yes, _____ no. Linens changed: _____ yes, _____ no.
Dressing changed: ____ yes, ____ no. Location: _____________________.
IV site checked: _____ yes, _____ no. IV tubing labeled: _____ yes, _____no.
IV fluids at: ____.
Pain level (0-10 scale.0-no pain, 10 intolerable): ____________________.
Location of pain: _____________. Medicated for pain: ____ yes, ____ no.
Patient is alert/oriented: ____ yes, ____ no. New confusion: ____ yes, ____ no.
Vital signs: temp ____, pulse _____, resp _____, b/p _____, 02 ____ %, ___ liters.
Glucose level: _____. Insulin: ___ yes, ___ no. Type: ___________ # of units ____.

Nurse _____________, CNA _____________, in at _____ am/pm. Left at _____ am/pm.
Wash hands and wear gloves before touching patient: _____ yes, _____ no.
Wash hands before leaving room: ___ yes, ___ no. Wear protective gear: __ yes, __ no.
Clean stethoscope: __ yes, __ no. Oral care: __ yes, __ no. Suctioned: __yes, __ no.
Repositioned: ___ yes, ___ no. Turned to: ___ left, ___right, ___ backside ___.
Head of bed at: ______ degrees. Incontinence/skin breakdown: ____ yes, ____ no.
Linens wet or soiled: _____ yes, _____ no. Linens changed: _____ yes, _____ no.
Dressing changed: ____ yes, ____ no. Location: _____________________.
IV site checked: _____ yes, _____ no. IV tubing labeled: _____ yes, _____no.
IV fluids at: ____.
Pain level (0-10 scale.0-no pain, 10 intolerable): ____________________.
Location of pain: _____________. Medicated for pain: ____ yes, ____ no.
Patient is alert/oriented: ____ yes, ____ no. New confusion: ____ yes, ____ no.
Vital signs: temp ____, pulse _____, resp _____, b/p _____, 02 ____ %, ___ liters.
Glucose level: _____. Insulin: ___ yes, ___ no. Type: ___________ # of units ____.

Nurse _____________, CNA _____________, in at _____ am/pm. Left at _____ am/pm.
Wash hands and wear gloves before touching patient: _____ yes, _____ no.
Wash hands before leaving room: ___ yes, ___ no. Wear protective gear: __ yes, __ no.
Clean stethoscope: __ yes, __ no. Oral care: __ yes, __ no. Suctioned: __ yes, __ no.
Repositioned: ___ yes, ___ no. Turned to: ___ left, ___ right, ___ backside ___.
Head of bed at: ______ degrees. Incontinence/skin breakdown: ____ yes, ____ no.
Linens wet or soiled: _____ yes, _____ no. Linens changed: _____ yes, _____ no.
Dressing changed: ____ yes, ____ no. Location: _____________________.
IV site checked: _____ yes, _____ no. IV tubing labeled: _____ yes, _____no.
IV fluids at: ____.
Pain level (0-10 scale.0-no pain, 10 intolerable): ____________________.
Location of pain: _____________. Medicated for pain: ____ yes, ____ no.
Patient is alert/oriented: ____ yes, ____ no. New confusion: ____ yes, ____ no.
Vital signs: temp ____, pulse _____, resp _____, b/p _____, 02 ____ %, ___ liters.
Glucose level: _____. Insulin: ___ yes, ___ no. Type: ___________ # of units ____.

NURSING CARE CONTINUED FOR ____________________
DATE ____________________, DAY NUMBER ____________________

FOLLOWING EXAMINATIONS FOR DAY SHIFT:

Nurse ______________, CNA ______________, in at _____ am/pm. Left at ______ am/pm.
Wash hands and wear gloves before touching patient: ______ yes, _____ no.
Wash hands before leaving room: ___ yes, ___ no. Wear protective gear: __ yes, __ no.
Clean stethoscope: __ yes, __ no. Oral care: __ yes, __ no. Suctioned: __ yes, __ no.
Repositioned: ___ yes, ___ no. Turned to: ___ left, ___ right, ___ backside ___.
Head of bed at: _______ degrees. Incontinence/skin breakdown: ___ yes, ___ no.
Linens wet or soiled: ____ yes, _____ no. Linens changed: ____ yes, ____ no.
Dressing changed: ____ yes, ____ no. Location: ______________________.
IV site checked: ____ yes, ____ no. IV tubing labeled: _____ yes, _____ no.
IV fluids at: ____.
Pain level (0-10 scale.0-no pain, 10 intolerable): ______________________.
Location of pain: ______________. Medicated for pain: ____ yes, ____ no.
Patient is alert/oriented: ____ yes, ____ no. New confusion: ____ yes, ____ no.
Vital signs: temp ____, pulse ____, resp _____, b/p _______, 02 ____%, ____ liters.
Glucose level: _____. Insulin: ___ yes, ___ no. Type: _________ # of units ____.

Nurse ______________, CNA ______________, in at _____ am/pm. Left at ______ am/pm.
Wash hands and wear gloves before touching patient: ______ yes, _____ no.
Wash hands before leaving room: ___ yes, ___ no. Wear protective gear: __ yes, __ no.
Clean stethoscope: __ yes, __ no. Oral care: __ yes, __ no. Suctioned: __ yes, __ no.
Repositioned: ___ yes, ___ no. Turned to: ___ left, ___ right, ___ backside ___.
Head of bed at: _______ degrees. Incontinence/skin breakdown: ___ yes, ___ no.
Linens wet or soiled: ____ yes, _____ no. Linens changed: ____ yes, ____ no.
Dressing changed: ____ yes, ____ no. Location: ______________________.
IV site checked: ____ yes, ____ no. IV tubing labeled: _____ yes, _____ no.
IV fluids at: ____.
Pain level (0-10 scale.0-no pain, 10 intolerable): ______________________.
Location of pain: ______________. Medicated for pain: ____ yes, ____ no.
Patient is alert/oriented: ____ yes, ____ no. New confusion: ____ yes, ____ no.
Vital signs: temp ____, pulse ____, resp _____, b/p _______, 02 ____%, ____ liters.
Glucose level: _____. Insulin: ___ yes, ___ no. Type: _________ # of units ____.

Nurse ______________, CNA ______________, in at _____ am/pm. Left at ______ am/pm.
Wash hands and wear gloves before touching patient: ______ yes, _____ no.
Wash hands before leaving room: ___ yes, ___ no. Wear protective gear: __ yes, __ no.
Clean stethoscope: __ yes, __ no. Oral care: __ yes, __ no. Suctioned: __ yes, __ no.
Repositioned: ___ yes, ___ no. Turned to: ___ left, ___ right, ___ backside ___.
Head of bed at: _______ degrees. Incontinence/skin breakdown: ___ yes, ___ no.
Linens wet or soiled: ____ yes, _____ no. Linens changed: ____ yes, ____ no.
Dressing changed: ____ yes, ____ no. Location: ______________________.
IV site checked: ____ yes, ____ no. IV tubing labeled: _____ yes, _____ no.
IV fluids at: ____.
Pain level (0-10 scale.0-no pain, 10 intolerable): ______________________.
Location of pain: ______________. Medicated for pain: ____ yes, ____ no.
Patient is alert/oriented: ____ yes, ____ no. New confusion: ____ yes, ____ no.
Vital signs: temp ____, pulse ____, resp _____, b/p _______, 02 ____%, ____ liters.
Glucose level: _____. Insulin: ___ yes, ___ no. Type: _________ # of units ____.

NURSING CARE FOR ______________________________

DATE ____________________, DAY NUMBER ______________________

INITIAL NIGHT SHIFT EXAM:

My nurse has _____ # of patients. CNA ___yes, ___no. Charge nurse _______________
Nurse ______________ RN/LPN came in at _________ am/pm. Left at _________ am/pm.
Did nurse wash hands and wear gloves before touching patient: ______ yes, ______ no.
Wash hands after touching patient and before leaving the room: ______ yes, ______ no.
Don't hesitate to request staff to wash their hands. This will help decrease the risk of spreading potentially lethal germs.
Did nurse wear protective gear (isolation precautions only): ______ yes, ______ no.
Did nurse provide oral care (to be done every two hours if unable to provide for self, also decreases risk of pneumonia, infections, and aspiration): ______ yes, _____ no.
If able to provide own oral care, then supplies at bedside: ______ yes, ______ no.
Was patient repositioned (every two hours if unable to turn self): _____ yes _____ no.
Head of bed at ________ degrees. This is important for patients on ventilators or on tube feedings. Anything less than thirty degrees places patients at risk for aspiration of stomach contents into the lungs causing aspiration pneumonia.
Checked for incontinence and skin breakdown: _____ yes, _____ no.
Patient's linens wet or soiled: ____ yes, ____ no. Linens changed: ____ yes, ____ no.
Time linens changed: _______ am/pm. Any skin redness or breakdown: ____ yes, ____ no.
If yes, what stage is pressure ulcer: ________. Acquired when: ________________.
List wounds not associated with pressure ulcers and how acquired: ____________
____.
Mattress type: ____.
Specialty mattresses are important to help prevent pressure ulcers)
If patient on ventilator or has tracheostomy, suction performed: _____ yes, _____ no.
Did nurse listen to lung sounds: _____ yes, _____ no.
Does patient have chest tubes: ____ yes, ____ no. Functioning _____ yes, _____ no.
Bowel sounds: ______ yes, ______ no. Bowel sounds active: ______ yes, ______ no.
Neurological exam: ______ yes, ______ no. Follow commands: ______ yes, ______ no.
Is patient alert and oriented to person, place, time, and events: _____ yes, _____ no.
If confused, patient is not oriented to: ___ person, ___ place, ___ time, ___ event.
Confusion began (time and date): ____.
Glasgow coma scale (checks conscious scale of patient): ______________________.
Intracranial pressure monitoring: ______ yes, ______ no.
If yes, pressure is at ________ mm mercury. (Normal is one to fifteen).
Moves extremities: ___ yes, ___ no.
Paralysis: (inability to move extremities) ________ yes, ________ no.
If yes, extremities affected and when paralysis began: ______________________.
Is patient in pain: ____ yes, ____ no. Describe pain and location ____________.
Patient able to eat: ____ yes, ____ no. What type of diet? ____________________.
If patient on tube feedings list type: ____________ at ___________ cc/ml per hour.
Nausea ____, vomiting ____. If so, describe: __________________________________.
Patient has: Nasal gastric tube _____, Dobhoff tube _____, Peg or gastric tube ____.
When was feeding tube placed and what site: __________________________________.
Catheter for draining urine: ____ yes, ____ no. If so, when placed: ___________.
Find out policy for allowed time to remain in bladder. Too long may cause infections.)
IV site(s) where: ________________ when placed: ______________________________.
IV fluids (types and rates): _______________________, ________________________,
_____________________, _____________________________, ________________________,
Is patient on oxygen: _____ yes, _____ no. If so, how much and route delivered (see oxygen routes): ____.
If patient on ventilator, list settings (see list on ventilator settings): ________
____.
Vital signs: temp ______, pulse ______, resp ______, b/p ______, o2 ______%,
current weight ______ pounds, ______ kg. Glucose level: ______
Insulin coverage: ____ yes, ____ no. Insulin type: ____________, # of units: ______.

NURSING CARE CONTINUED FOR ____________________
DATE ____________________, DAY NUMBER ____________________

FOLLOWING EXAMINATIONS FOR NIGHT SHIFT:

Nurse ____________, CNA ____________, in at ______ am/pm. Left at ______ am/pm.
Wash hands and wear gloves before touching patient: ______ yes, ___ no.
Wash hands before leaving room: ___ yes, ___ no. Wear protective gear: __ yes, __ no.
Clean stethoscope: __ yes, __ no. Oral care: __ yes, __ no. Suctioned: __ yes, __ no.
Repositioned: ___ yes, ___ no. Turned to: ___ left, ___ right, ___ backside ___.
Head of bed at: ______ degrees. Incontinence/skin breakdown: ____ yes, ___ no.
Linens wet or soiled: ____ yes, _____ no. Linens changed: ____ yes, ____ no.
Dressing changed: ____ yes, ____ no. Location: ____________________.
IV site checked: ____ yes, ____ no. IV tubing labeled: ____ yes, ____ no.
IV fluids at: ____.
Pain level (0-10 scale.0-no pain, 10 intolerable): ______________.
Location of pain: ____________. Medicated for pain: ____ yes, ___ no.
Patient is alert/oriented: ___ yes, __ no. New confusion: ___ yes, __ no.
Vital signs: temp ____, pulse ____, resp ____, b/p ____, 02 ____ %, ____ liters.
Glucose level: ____. Insulin: ___ yes, __ no. Type: ________ # of units ___.

Nurse ____________, CNA ____________, in at ______ am/pm. Left at ______ am/pm.
Wash hands and wear gloves before touching patient: ______ yes, ___ no.
Wash hands before leaving room: ___ yes, ___ no. Wear protective gear: __ yes, __ no.
Clean stethoscope: __ yes, __ no. Oral care: __ yes, __ no. Suctioned: __ yes, __ no.
Repositioned: ___ yes, ___ no. Turned to: ___ left, ___ right, ___ backside ___.
Head of bed at: ______ degrees. Incontinence/skin breakdown: ____ yes, ___ no.
Linens wet or soiled: ____ yes, _____ no. Linens changed: ____ yes, ____ no.
Dressing changed: ____ yes, ____ no. Location: ____________________.
IV site checked: ____ yes, ____ no. IV tubing labeled: ____ yes, ____ no.
IV fluids at: ____.
Pain level (0-10 scale.0-no pain, 10 intolerable): ______________.
Location of pain: ____________. Medicated for pain: ____ yes, ___ no.
Patient is alert/oriented: ___ yes, __ no. New confusion: ___ yes, __ no.
Vital signs: temp ____, pulse ____, resp ____, b/p ____, 02 ____ %, ____ liters.
Glucose level: ____. Insulin: ___ yes, __ no. Type: ________ # of units ___.

Nurse ____________, CNA ____________, in at ______ am/pm. Left at ______ am/pm.
Wash hands and wear gloves before touching patient: ______ yes, ___ no.
Wash hands before leaving room: ___ yes, ___ no. Wear protective gear: __ yes, __ no.
Clean stethoscope: __ yes, __ no. Oral care: __ yes, __ no. Suctioned: __ yes, __ no.
Repositioned: ___ yes, ___ no. Turned to: ___ left, ___ right, ___ backside ___.
Head of bed at: ______ degrees. Incontinence/skin breakdown: ____ yes, ___ no.
Linens wet or soiled: ____ yes, _____ no. Linens changed: ____ yes, ____ no.
Dressing changed: ____ yes, ____ no. Location: ____________________.
IV site checked: ____ yes, ____ no. IV tubing labeled: ____ yes, ____ no.
IV fluids at: ____.
Pain level (0-10 scale.0-no pain, 10 intolerable): ______________.
Location of pain: ____________. Medicated for pain: ____ yes, ___ no.
Patient is alert/oriented: ___ yes, __ no. New confusion: ___ yes, __ no.
Vital signs: temp ____, pulse ____, resp ____, b/p ____, 02 ____ %, ____ liters.
Glucose level: ____. Insulin: ___ yes, __ no. Type: ________ # of units ___.

NURSING CARE CONTINUED FOR ____________________
DATE ____________________, DAY NUMBER ____________________

FOLLOWING EXAMINATIONS FOR NIGHT SHIFT:

Nurse ______________, CNA ______________, in at _____ am/pm. Left at ______ am/pm.
Wash hands and wear gloves before touching patient: ________ yes, ________ no.
Wash hands before leaving room: ___ yes, ___ no. Wear protective gear: __ yes, __ no.
Clean stethoscope: __ yes, __ no. Oral care: __ yes, __ no. Suctioned: __ yes, __ no.
Repositioned: ___ yes, ___ no. Turned to: ___ left, ___ right, ___ backside ___.
Head of bed at: _______ degrees. Incontinence/skin breakdown: ____ yes, ____ no.
Linens wet or soiled: ____ yes, ____ no. Linens changed: ____ yes, _____ no.
Dressing changed: ____ yes, ____ no. Location: ______________________________.
IV site checked: _____ yes, _____ no. IV tubing labeled: _____ yes, _____no.
IV fluids at: ____.
Pain level (0-10 scale.0-no pain, 10 intolerable): _________________________.
Location of pain: _______________. Medicated for pain: _____ yes, ____ no.
Patient is alert/oriented: ____ yes, ____ no. New confusion: ____ yes, ____ no.
Vital signs: temp ____, pulse _____, resp _____, b/p _____, 02 _____ %, ____ liters.
Glucose level: _____. Insulin: ___ yes, ___ no. Type: ____________ # of units ____.

Nurse ______________, CNA ______________, in at _____ am/pm. Left at ______ am/pm.
Wash hands and wear gloves before touching patient: ________ yes, ________ no.
Wash hands before leaving room: ___ yes, ___ no. Wear protective gear: __ yes, __ no.
Clean stethoscope: __ yes, __ no. Oral care: __ yes, __ no. Suctioned: __ yes, __ no.
Repositioned: ___ yes, ___ no. Turned to: ___ left, ___ right, ___ backside ___.
Head of bed at: _______ degrees. Incontinence/skin breakdown: ____ yes, ____ no.
Linens wet or soiled: ____ yes, ____ no. Linens changed: ____ yes, _____ no.
Dressing changed: ____ yes, ____ no. Location: ______________________________.
IV site checked: _____ yes, _____ no. IV tubing labeled: _____ yes, _____no.
IV fluids at: ____.
Pain level (0-10 scale.0-no pain, 10 intolerable): _________________________.
Location of pain: _______________. Medicated for pain: _____ yes, ____ no.
Patient is alert/oriented: ____ yes, ____ no. New confusion: ____ yes, ____ no.
Vital signs: temp ____, pulse _____, resp _____, b/p _____, 02 _____ %, ____ liters.
Glucose level: _____. Insulin: ___ yes, ___ no. Type: ____________ # of units ____.

Nurse ______________, CNA ______________, in at _____ am/pm. Left at ______ am/pm.
Wash hands and wear gloves before touching patient: ________ yes, ________ no.
Wash hands before leaving room: ___ yes, ___ no. Wear protective gear: __ yes, __ no.
Clean stethoscope: __ yes, __ no. Oral care: __ yes, __ no. Suctioned: __ yes, __ no.
Repositioned: ___ yes, ___ no. Turned to: ___ left, ___ right, ___ backside ___.
Head of bed at: _______ degrees. Incontinence/skin breakdown: ____ yes, ____ no.
Linens wet or soiled: ____ yes, ____ no. Linens changed: ____ yes, _____ no.
Dressing changed: ____ yes, ____ no. Location: ______________________________.
IV site checked: _____ yes, _____ no. IV tubing labeled: _____ yes, _____no.
IV fluids at: ____.
Pain level (0-10 scale.0-no pain, 10 intolerable): _________________________.
Location of pain: _______________. Medicated for pain: _____ yes, ____ no.
Patient is alert/oriented: ____ yes, ____ no. New confusion: ____ yes, ____ no.
Vital signs: temp ____, pulse _____, resp _____, b/p _____, 02 _____ %, ____ liters.
Glucose level: _____. Insulin: ___ yes, ___ no. Type: ____________ # of units ____.

MEDICATION ADMINISTRATION LIST FOR ________________

DATE ____________ DAY NUMBER ________________

List the medication for each day. Routes of administration: oral, thru feeding tube, intravenous (IV), intramuscular (IM), subcutaneous (SQ), epidural or a catheter in your spinal column, rectal, topical, eye drops, and ear drops.

Medication: ____________ Route: ____________ Time: ____________
Medication: ____________ Route: ____________ Time: ____________
Medication: ____________ Route: ____________ Time: ____________
Medication: ____________ Route: ____________ Time: ____________
Medication: ____________ Route: ____________ Time: ____________
Medication: ____________ Route: ____________ Time: ____________
Medication: ____________ Route: ____________ Time: ____________
Medication: ____________ Route: ____________ Time: ____________
Medication: ____________ Route: ____________ Time: ____________
Medication: ____________ Route: ____________ Time: ____________
Medication: ____________ Route: ____________ Time: ____________
Medication: ____________ Route: ____________ Time: ____________
Medication: ____________ Route: ____________ Time: ____________
Medication: ____________ Route: ____________ Time: ____________
Medication: ____________ Route: ____________ Time: ____________
Medication: ____________ Route: ____________ Time: ____________
Medication: ____________ Route: ____________ Time: ____________
Medication: ____________ Route: ____________ Time: ____________
Medication: ____________ Route: ____________ Time: ____________
Medication: ____________ Route: ____________ Time: ____________
Medication: ____________ Route: ____________ Time: ____________
Medication: ____________ Route: ____________ Time: ____________
Medication: ____________ Route: ____________ Time: ____________
Medication: ____________ Route: ____________ Time: ____________
Medication: ____________ Route: ____________ Time: ____________
Medication: ____________ Route: ____________ Time: ____________
Medication: ____________ Route: ____________ Time: ____________
Medication: ____________ Route: ____________ Time: ____________
Medication: ____________ Route: ____________ Time: ____________
Medication: ____________ Route: ____________ Time: ____________
Medication: ____________ Route: ____________ Time: ____________
Medication: ____________ Route: ____________ Time: ____________
Medication: ____________ Route: ____________ Time: ____________
Medication: ____________ Route: ____________ Time: ____________
Medication: ____________ Route: ____________ Time: ____________
Medication: ____________ Route: ____________ Time: ____________
Medication: ____________ Route: ____________ Time: ____________
Medication: ____________ Route: ____________ Time: ____________
Medication: ____________ Route: ____________ Time: ____________
Medication: ____________ Route: ____________ Time: ____________
Medication: ____________ Route: ____________ Time: ____________
Medication: ____________ Route: ____________ Time: ____________
Medication: ____________ Route: ____________ Time: ____________
Medication: ____________ Route: ____________ Time: ____________
Medication: ____________ Route: ____________ Time: ____________
Medication: ____________ Route: ____________ Time: ____________
Medication: ____________ Route: ____________ Time: ____________
Medication: ____________ Route: ____________ Time: ____________
Medication: ____________ Route: ____________ Time: ____________
Medication: ____________ Route: ____________ Time: ____________
Medication: ____________ Route: ____________ Time: ____________
Medication: ____________ Route: ____________ Time: ____________
Medication: ____________ Route: ____________ Time: ____________
Medication: ____________ Route: ____________ Time: ____________

NOTES FOR DAY NUMBER ______________________

DATE ______________________

MY CANCER JOURNAL

This section of the journal is designed for those that have cancer. This is designed to assist you in recording your treatment schedule. If you need assistance regarding explaining and interpreting cancer and cancer research contact: Cancer Information Center at 1-800-4-CANCER or 1-800-422-6237 or instant live message on the internet at https://cissecure.nci.nih.gov/livehelp/welcome.asp

Date diagnosed: ____________________ Today's date: ____________________

My hematologist / oncologist: ____________________

Phone # ____________________ Fax # ____________________

Address: ____________________

I have ____________________

Stage: I / IA, IB, IC / II / IIA, IIB, IIC, IIE / III / IIIA, IIIB, IIIC, IIIE, IIIS, IIIE+S / IV / IVA, IVB, IVC.

Grade: 1 / 2 / 3 / IV

ABCD rating: A / B / C / D

Current trial phase: I / I/II / II / II/III / III / IV

Bone marrow transplant: ___ yes, ___ no. Reaction: ___ yes, ___ no, when: __________.

My protocol # ____________________ Today is day # _______ of my protocol.

Type of implanted access: ____________________ Date inserted: ____________________.

Huber needle size: ___________ White blood cell count: _________ Hemoglobin: _______

Hematocrit: _______________ Platelet count: ________________ My ANC: ________________.

My chemotherapy schedule: ____________________

____

____

____

Current chemotherapy medications: ____________________

____

____

____

____

MY CANCER JOURNAL

My current radiation schedule: ______________________

____

____

____

____

Complications associated with chemotherapy or radiation: ______________________

____

____

____

____

____

Adverse reactions: _______ yes, _______ no.

Type and treatment: ______________________

____

____

____

Notes: ______________________

____

____

____

____

____

____

____

____

____

____

____

MY CANCER JOURNAL

Day number: ____________________ of treatment. Date: ____________________

Day nurse: ______________ Night nurse: ______________ CNA: ______ yes, ______ no.

Visit from Hematologist / Oncologist: ____ yes, ____ no. Time of visit: ____________

My lab test done today: ____

WBC: ________ H&H: __________ PLT: __________ ANC: __________ Nadir: ________

Chemotherapy schedule: ____

____

Pretreatment given: ______ yes, ______ no. Type: ______________________________

Radiation: ______ yes, ______ no. Location: ______________________________

Type of radiation: ____

Other treatments or procedures: ____

____

Reactions: ______ yes, ______ no. Treatment: ______________________________

Day number: ____________________ of treatment. Date: ____________________

Day nurse: ______________ Night nurse: ______________ CNA: ______ yes, ______ no.

Visit from Hematologist / Oncologist: ____ yes, ____ no. Time of visit: ____________

Lab tests done today: ____

WBC: ________ H&H: __________ PLT: __________ ANC: __________ Nadir: ________

Chemotherapy schedule: ____

Pretreatment given: ______ yes, ______ no. Type: ______________________________

____

Radiation: ______ yes, ______ no. Location: ______________________________

Type of radiation: ____

Other treatments or procedures: ____

____

Reactions: ______ yes, ______ no. Treatment: ______________________________

MY CANCER JOURNAL

Day number: ______________________ of treatment. Date: ______________________________

Day nurse: ________________ Night nurse: _______________ CNA: _____ yes, _____ no.

Visit from Hematologist / Oncologist: ____ yes, ____ no. Time of visit: __________

My lab test done today: ____

WBC: __________ H&H: __________ PLT: ___________ ANC: ___________ Nadir: _________

Chemotherapy schedule: ____

____

Pretreatment given: ______ yes, ______ no. Type: ____________________________________

Radiation: ______ yes, ______ no. Location: ____

Type of radiation: ____

Other treatments or procedures: ____

____

Reactions: ______ yes, ______ no. Treatment: ____

Day number: ______________________ of treatment. Date: ______________________________

Day nurse: ________________ Night nurse: _______________ CNA: _____ yes, _____ no.

Visit from Hematologist / Oncologist: ____ yes, ____ no. Time of visit: __________

Lab tests done today: ____

WBC: __________ H&H: __________ PLT: ___________ ANC: ___________ Nadir: _________

Chemotherapy schedule: ____

Pretreatment given: ______ yes, ______ no. Type: ____________________________________

____

Radiation: ______ yes, ______ no. Location: ____

Type of radiation: ____

Other treatments or procedures: ____

____

Reactions: ______ yes, ______ no. Treatment: ____

MY CANCER JOURNAL

Day number: ____________________ of treatment. Date: ____________________

Day nurse: ______________ Night nurse: ______________ CNA: ______ yes, ______ no.

Visit from Hematologist / Oncologist: ____ yes, ____ no. Time of visit: ____________

My lab test done today: ____

WBC: __________ H&H: __________ PLT: __________ ANC: __________ Nadir: ________

Chemotherapy schedule: ____

____

Pretreatment given: ______ yes, ______ no. Type: ______________________________

Radiation: ______ yes, ______ no. Location: ______________________________

Type of radiation: ____

Other treatments or procedures: ____

____

Reactions: ______ yes, ______ no. Treatment: ______________________________

Day number: ____________________ of treatment. Date: ____________________

Day nurse: ______________ Night nurse: ______________ CNA: ______ yes, ______ no.

Visit from Hematologist / Oncologist: ____ yes, ____ no. Time of visit: ____________

Lab tests done today: ____

WBC: __________ H&H: __________ PLT: __________ ANC: __________ Nadir: ________

Chemotherapy schedule: ____

Pretreatment given: ______ yes, ______ no. Type: ______________________________

____

Radiation: ______ yes, ______ no. Location: ______________________________

Type of radiation: ____

Other treatments or procedures: ____

____

Reactions: ______ yes, ______ no. Treatment: ______________________________

MY CANCER JOURNAL

Day number: ______________________ of treatment. Date: ______________________

Day nurse: ________________ Night nurse: ______________ CNA: ______ yes, ______ no.

Visit from Hematologist / Oncologist: ____ yes, ____ no. Time of visit: __________

My lab test done today: ____

WBC: __________ H&H: __________ PLT: ____________ ANC: ____________ Nadir: ________

Chemotherapy schedule: ____

____

Pretreatment given: _______ yes, _______ no. Type: ____________________________

Radiation: _______ yes, _______ no. Location: ______________________________

Type of radiation: ____

Other treatments or procedures: ______________________________________

____

Reactions: _______ yes, _______ no. Treatment: ______________________________

Day number: ______________________ of treatment. Date: ______________________

Day nurse: ________________ Night nurse: ______________ CNA: ______ yes, ______ no.

Visit from Hematologist / Oncologist: ____ yes, ____ no. Time of visit: __________

Lab tests done today: ____

WBC: __________ H&H: __________ PLT: ____________ ANC: ____________ Nadir: ________

Chemotherapy schedule: ____

Pretreatment given: _______ yes, _______ no. Type: ____________________________

____

Radiation: _______ yes, _______ no. Location: ______________________________

Type of radiation: ____

Other treatments or procedures: ______________________________________

____

Reactions: _______ yes, _______ no. Treatment: ______________________________

MY CANCER JOURNAL

Day number: ______________________ of treatment. Date: ______________________

Day nurse: ________________ Night nurse: ______________ CNA: ______ yes, ______ no.

Visit from Hematologist / Oncologist: ____ yes, ____ no. Time of visit: __________

My lab test done today: ____

WBC: __________ H&H: __________ PLT: ___________ ANC: ___________ Nadir: _______

Chemotherapy schedule: ____

____

Pretreatment given: _______ yes, _______ no. Type: ___________________________

Radiation: _______ yes, _______ no. Location: ______________________________

Type of radiation: ____

Other treatments or procedures: ____________________________________

____

Reactions: _______ yes, _______ no. Treatment: _____________________________

Day number: ______________________ of treatment. Date: ______________________

Day nurse: ________________ Night nurse: ______________ CNA: ______ yes, ______ no.

Visit from Hematologist / Oncologist: ____ yes, ____ no. Time of visit: __________

Lab tests done today: ____

WBC: __________ H&H: __________ PLT: ___________ ANC: ___________ Nadir: _______

Chemotherapy schedule: ____

Pretreatment given: _______ yes, _______ no. Type: ___________________________

____

Radiation: _______ yes, _______ no. Location: ______________________________

Type of radiation: ____

Other treatments or procedures: ____________________________________

____

Reactions: _______ yes, _______ no. Treatment: _____________________________

MY CANCER JOURNAL

Day number: ____________________ of treatment. Date: ____________________________

Day nurse: _______________ Night nurse: ______________ CNA: _____ yes, _____ no.

Visit from Hematologist / Oncologist: ___ yes, ___ no. Time of visit: _________

My lab test done today: ____

WBC: __________ H&H: __________ PLT: _________ ANC: __________ Nadir: ________

Chemotherapy schedule: ____

____

Pretreatment given: ______ yes, ______ no. Type: ________________________________

Radiation: ______ yes, ______ no. Location: _____________________________________

Type of radiation: ____

Other treatments or procedures: ____

____

Reactions: ______ yes, ______ no. Treatment: ____________________________________

Day number: ____________________ of treatment. Date: ____________________________

Day nurse: _______________ Night nurse: ______________ CNA: _____ yes, _____ no.

Visit from Hematologist / Oncologist: ___ yes, ___ no. Time of visit: _________

Lab tests done today: ____

WBC: __________ H&H: __________ PLT: _________ ANC: __________ Nadir: ________

Chemotherapy schedule: ____

Pretreatment given: ______ yes, ______ no. Type: ________________________________

____

Radiation: ______ yes, ______ no. Location: _____________________________________

Type of radiation: ____

Other treatments or procedures: ____

____

Reactions: ______ yes, ______ no. Treatment: ____________________________________

MY CANCER JOURNAL

Day number: ______________________ of treatment. Date: ______________________

Day nurse: _________________ Night nurse: _____________ CNA: ______ yes, ______ no.

Visit from Hematologist / Oncologist: ____ yes, ____ no. Time of visit: ________________

My lab test done today: ____

WBC: __________ H&H: ___________ PLT: ____________ ANC: ____________ Nadir: _______

Chemotherapy schedule: ____

____

Pretreatment given: _______ yes, _______ no. Type: ____________________

Radiation: _______ yes, _______ no. Location: ____________________

Type of radiation: ____

Other treatments or procedures: ____________________________________

____

Reactions: _______ yes, _______ no. Treatment: ____________________

Day number: ______________________ of treatment. Date: ______________________

Day nurse: _________________ Night nurse: _____________ CNA: ______ yes, ______ no.

Visit from Hematologist / Oncologist: ____ yes, ____ no. Time of visit: ________________

Lab tests done today: ____

WBC: __________ H&H: ___________ PLT: ____________ ANC: ____________ Nadir: _______

Chemotherapy schedule: ____

Pretreatment given: _______ yes, _______ no. Type: ____________________

____

Radiation: _______ yes, _______ no. Location: ____________________

Type of radiation: ____

Other treatments or procedures: ____________________________________

____

Reactions: _______ yes, _______ no. Treatment: ____________________

MY CANCER JOURNAL

Day number: ______________________ of treatment. Date: ______________________

Day nurse: ________________ Night nurse: ________________ CNA: ______ yes, ______ no.

Visit from Hematologist / Oncologist: ____ yes, ____ no. Time of visit: __________

My lab test done today: ____

WBC: __________ H&H: __________ PLT: ____________ ANC: __________ Nadir: ________

Chemotherapy schedule: ____

____

Pretreatment given: _______ yes, _______ no. Type: ______________________________

Radiation: _______ yes, _______ no. Location: ______________________________

Type of radiation: ____

Other treatments or procedures: ____

____

Reactions: _______ yes, _______ no. Treatment: ______________________________

Day number: ______________________ of treatment. Date: ______________________

Day nurse: ________________ Night nurse: ________________ CNA: ______ yes, ______ no.

Visit from Hematologist / Oncologist: ____ yes, ____ no. Time of visit: __________

Lab tests done today: ____

WBC: __________ H&H: __________ PLT: ____________ ANC: __________ Nadir: ________

Chemotherapy schedule: ____

Pretreatment given: _______ yes, _______ no. Type: ______________________________

____

Radiation: _______ yes, _______ no. Location: ______________________________

Type of radiation: ____

Other treatments or procedures: ____

____

Reactions: _______ yes, _______ no. Treatment: ______________________________

MY CANCER JOURNAL

Day number: ____________________ of treatment. Date: ____________________

Day nurse: ______________ Night nurse: ______________ CNA: _____ yes, _____ no.

Visit from Hematologist / Oncologist: ___ yes, ___ no. Time of visit: ________

My lab test done today: ____

WBC: ________ H&H: ________ PLT: ________ ANC: ________ Nadir: ______

Chemotherapy schedule: ____

____

Pretreatment given: ______ yes, _____ no. Type: ______________________

Radiation: ______ yes, ______ no. Location: __________________________

Type of radiation: ____

Other treatments or procedures: ______________________________________

____

Reactions: ______ yes, ______ no. Treatment: _________________________

Day number: ____________________ of treatment. Date: ____________________

Day nurse: ______________ Night nurse: ______________ CNA: _____ yes, _____ no.

Visit from Hematologist / Oncologist: ___ yes, ___ no. Time of visit: ________

Lab tests done today: ____

WBC: ________ H&H: ________ PLT: ________ ANC: ________ Nadir: ______

Chemotherapy schedule: ____

Pretreatment given: ______ yes, _____ no. Type: ______________________

____

Radiation: ______ yes, ______ no. Location: __________________________

Type of radiation: ____

Other treatments or procedures: ______________________________________

____

Reactions: ______ yes, ______ no. Treatment: _________________________

MY CANCER JOURNAL

Day number: ________________________ of treatment. Date: ________________________

Day nurse: __________________ Night nurse: ______________ CNA: ______ yes, ______ no.

Visit from Hematologist / Oncologist: ____ yes, ____ no. Time of visit: __________

My lab test done today: ____

WBC: __________ H&H: __________ PLT: __________ ANC: __________ Nadir: ________

Chemotherapy schedule: ____

____

Pretreatment given: ______ yes, ______ no. Type: ______________________________

Radiation: ______ yes, ______ no. Location: ____________________________________

Type of radiation: ____

Other treatments or procedures: ____

____

Reactions: ______ yes, ______ no. Treatment: ____________________________________

Day number: ________________________ of treatment. Date: ________________________

Day nurse: __________________ Night nurse: ______________ CNA: ______ yes, ______ no.

Visit from Hematologist / Oncologist: ____ yes, ____ no. Time of visit: __________

Lab tests done today: ____

WBC: __________ H&H: __________ PLT: __________ ANC: __________ Nadir: ________

Chemotherapy schedule: ____

Pretreatment given: ______ yes, ______ no. Type: ______________________________

____

Radiation: ______ yes, ______ no. Location: ____________________________________

Type of radiation: ____

Other treatments or procedures: ____

____

Reactions: ______ yes, ______ no. Treatment: ____________________________________

MY CANCER JOURNAL

Day number: ____________________ of treatment. Date: ____________________

Day nurse: ______________ Night nurse: ____________ CNA: _____ yes, _____ no.

Visit from Hematologist / Oncologist: ___ yes, ___ no. Time of visit: ________

My lab test done today: ____

WBC: ________ H&H: __________ PLT: ___________ ANC: __________ Nadir: ______

Chemotherapy schedule: ____

____

Pretreatment given: ______ yes, ______ no. Type: ______________________

Radiation: ______ yes, ______ no. Location: ____________________________

Type of radiation: ____

Other treatments or procedures: ________________________________

____

Reactions: ______ yes, ______ no. Treatment: ___________________________

Day number: ____________________ of treatment. Date: ____________________

Day nurse: ______________ Night nurse: ____________ CNA: _____ yes, _____ no.

Visit from Hematologist / Oncologist: ___ yes, ___ no. Time of visit: ________

Lab tests done today: ____

WBC: ________ H&H: __________ PLT: ___________ ANC: __________ Nadir: ______

Chemotherapy schedule: ____

Pretreatment given: ______ yes, ______ no. Type: ______________________

____

Radiation: ______ yes, ______ no. Location: ____________________________

Type of radiation: ____

Other treatments or procedures: ________________________________

____

Reactions: ______ yes, ______ no. Treatment: ___________________________

MY CANCER JOURNAL

Day number: ____________________ of treatment. Date: ____________________

Day nurse: ______________ Night nurse: ______________ CNA: _____ yes, _____ no.

Visit from Hematologist / Oncologist: ____ yes, ____ no. Time of visit: ____________

My lab test done today: ____

WBC: __________ H&H: __________ PLT: __________ ANC: __________ Nadir: ________

Chemotherapy schedule: ____

____

Pretreatment given: ______ yes, ______ no. Type: ____________________________

Radiation: ______ yes, ______ no. Location: ____________________________

Type of radiation: ____

Other treatments or procedures: ____________________________________

____

Reactions: ______ yes, ______ no. Treatment: ____________________________

Day number: ____________________ of treatment. Date: ____________________

Day nurse: ______________ Night nurse: ______________ CNA: _____ yes, _____ no.

Visit from Hematologist / Oncologist: ____ yes, ____ no. Time of visit: ____________

Lab tests done today: ____

WBC: __________ H&H: __________ PLT: __________ ANC: __________ Nadir: ________

Chemotherapy schedule: ____

Pretreatment given: ______ yes, ______ no. Type: ____________________________

____

Radiation: ______ yes, ______ no. Location: ____________________________

Type of radiation: ____

Other treatments or procedures: ____________________________________

____

Reactions: ______ yes, ______ no. Treatment: ____________________________

MY CANCER JOURNAL

Day number: ____________________ of treatment. Date: ____________________

Day nurse: ______________ Night nurse: ______________ CNA: _____ yes, _____ no.

Visit from Hematologist / Oncologist: ___ yes, ___ no. Time of visit: __________

My lab test done today: ____

WBC: ________ H&H: ________ PLT: ________ ANC: ________ Nadir: ________

Chemotherapy schedule: ____

____

Pretreatment given: ______ yes, ______ no. Type: ____________________

Radiation: ______ yes, ______ no. Location: ____________________

Type of radiation: ____

Other treatments or procedures: ______________________________

____

Reactions: ______ yes, ______ no. Treatment: ____________________

Day number: ____________________ of treatment. Date: ____________________

Day nurse: ______________ Night nurse: ______________ CNA: _____ yes, _____ no.

Visit from Hematologist / Oncologist: ___ yes, ___ no. Time of visit: __________

Lab tests done today: ____

WBC: ________ H&H: ________ PLT: ________ ANC: ________ Nadir: ________

Chemotherapy schedule: ____

Pretreatment given: ______ yes, ______ no. Type: ____________________

____

Radiation: ______ yes, ______ no. Location: ____________________

Type of radiation: ____

Other treatments or procedures: ______________________________

____

Reactions: ______ yes, ______ no. Treatment: ____________________

MY CANCER JOURNAL

Day number: ______________________ of treatment. Date: ______________________

Day nurse: ________________ Night nurse: ________________ CNA: ______ yes, ______ no.

Visit from Hematologist / Oncologist: ____ yes, ____ no. Time of visit: ____________

My lab test done today: ____

WBC: __________ H&H: __________ PLT: ____________ ANC: ____________ Nadir: ________

Chemotherapy schedule: ____

____

Pretreatment given: _______ yes, _______ no. Type: ______________________

Radiation: _______ yes, _______ no. Location: ______________________________

Type of radiation: ____

Other treatments or procedures: ______________________________________

____

Reactions: _______ yes, _______ no. Treatment: ______________________________

Day number: ______________________ of treatment. Date: ______________________

Day nurse: ________________ Night nurse: ________________ CNA: ______ yes, ______ no.

Visit from Hematologist / Oncologist: ____ yes, ____ no. Time of visit: ____________

Lab tests done today: ____

WBC: __________ H&H: __________ PLT: ____________ ANC: ____________ Nadir: ________

Chemotherapy schedule: ____

Pretreatment given: _______ yes, _______ no. Type: ______________________

____

Radiation: _______ yes, _______ no. Location: ______________________________

Type of radiation: ____

Other treatments or procedures: ______________________________________

____

Reactions: _______ yes, _______ no. Treatment: ______________________________

MY CANCER JOURNAL

Day number: ____________ of treatment. Date: ____________

Day nurse: ____________ Night nurse: ____________ CNA: ______ yes, ______ no.

Visit from Hematologist / Oncologist: ____ yes, ____ no. Time of visit: ________

My lab test done today: ____________________________

WBC: ________ H&H: ________ PLT: ________ ANC: ________ Nadir: ________

Chemotherapy schedule: ____________________________

____

Pretreatment given: ______ yes, ______ no. Type: ____________

Radiation: ______ yes, ______ no. Location: ____________

Type of radiation: ____________________________

Other treatments or procedures: ____________________________

____

Reactions: ______ yes, ______ no. Treatment: ____________

Day number: ____________ of treatment. Date: ____________

Day nurse: ____________ Night nurse: ____________ CNA: ______ yes, ______ no.

Visit from Hematologist / Oncologist: ____ yes, ____ no. Time of visit: ________

Lab tests done today: ____________________________

WBC: ________ H&H: ________ PLT: ________ ANC: ________ Nadir: ________

Chemotherapy schedule: ____________________________

Pretreatment given: ______ yes, ______ no. Type: ____________

____

Radiation: ______ yes, ______ no. Location: ____________

Type of radiation: ____________________________

Other treatments or procedures: ____________________________

____

Reactions: ______ yes, ______ no. Treatment: ____________

SPECIAL DELIVERY

I entered the hospital at ______ am/pm. I was admitted to room # _____ at ____ am/pm.

My physicians name: ______________________________

Physician(s) delivering my baby: ______________________________

Nurse name(s): ______________________________

Type of delivery planned: ______________ Type performed: ______________

Epidural: _____ yes, _____ no. Side Effects: _____ yes, _____ no,

Side effects: ______________________________

Medications administered: ______________________________

____

Time: __________ am/pm. Dilated upon first examination: __________ centimeters.

Effacement upon first examination: ________ %. Station: minus ______ plus ______

Fetal heart rate: ______________ Fetal movement: ________ yes, ______ no.

Person performing examination: ______________________________.

Examiner wash hands/wear gloves: ________ yes, ________ no.

Time: __________ am/pm. Dilated: ________ centimeters. Effacement: ________ %.

Effacement ________ %. Station: minus ____ plus ____.

Fetal heart rate: _____. Fetal movement: ___yes, ___no.

Person performing examination: ______________________________

Examiner wash hands/wear gloves: _______ yes, _______ no.

Time: __________ am/pm. Dilated: ________ centimeters. Effacement: ________ %.

Effacement ________ %. Station: minus ____ plus ____.

Fetal heart rate: _____. Fetal movement: ___yes, ___no.

Person performing examination: ______________________________

Examiner washed hands/wear gloves: ______________________________

Time: __________ am/pm. Dilated: ________ centimeters. Effacement: ________ %.

Effacement ________ %. Station: minus ____ plus ____.

Fetal heart rate: _____. Fetal movement: ___yes, ___no.

Person performing examination: ______________________________

Examiner washed hands/wear gloves: ______________________________

SPECIAL DELIVERY

Time: ____________ am/pm. Dilated: __________ centimeters. Effacement: _________ %.

Effacement _________ %. Station: minus ___ plus ___.

Fetal heart rate: _____. Fetal movement: ___yes, ___no.

Person performing examination: ______________________________________

Examiner wash hands/wear gloves: ______ yes, ______ no.

Time: ____________ am/pm. Dilated: __________ centimeters. Effacement: _________ %.

Effacement _________ %. Station: minus ___ plus ___.

Fetal heart rate: _____. Fetal movement: ___yes, ___no.

Person performing examination: ______________________________________

Examiner wash hands/wear gloves: ______ yes, ______ no.

Time: ____________ am/pm. Dilated: __________ centimeters. Effacement: _________ %.

Effacement _________ %. Station: minus ___ plus ___.

Fetal heart rate: _____. Fetal movement: ___yes, ___no.

Person performing examination: ______________________________________

Examiner wash hands/wear gloves: ______ yes, ______ no.

Time: ____________ am/pm. Dilated: __________ centimeters. Effacement: _________ %.

Effacement _________ %. Station: minus ___ plus ___.

Fetal heart rate: _____. Fetal movement: ___yes, ___no.

Person performing examination: ______________________________________

Examiner wash hands/wear gloves: ______ yes, ______ no.

Time: ____________ am/pm. Dilated: __________ centimeters. Effacement: _________ %.

Effacement _________ %. Station: minus ___ plus ___.

Fetal heart rate: _____. Fetal movement: ___yes, ___no.

Person performing examination: ______________________________________

Examiner wash hands/wear gloves: ______ yes, ______ no.

Time: ____________ am/pm. Dilated: __________ centimeters. Effacement: _________ %.

Effacement _________ %. Station: minus ___ plus ___.

Fetal heart rate: _____. Fetal movement: ___yes, ___no.

Person performing examination: ______________________________________

Examiner wash hands/wear gloves: ______ yes, ______ no.

SPECIAL DELIVERY

Time: ____________ am/pm. Dilated: __________ centimeters. Effacement: _________ %.

Effacement _________ %. Station: minus ___ plus ___.

Fetal heart rate: ____. Fetal movement: ___yes, ___no.

Person performing examination: ____

Examiner wash hands/wear gloves: ______ yes, ______ no.

Time: ____________ am/pm. Dilated: __________ centimeters. Effacement: _________ %.

Effacement _________ %. Station: minus ___ plus ___.

Fetal heart rate: ____. Fetal movement: ___yes, ___no.

Person performing examination: ____

Examiner wash hands/wear gloves: ______ yes, ______ no.

Time: ____________ am/pm. Dilated: __________ centimeters. Effacement: _________ %.

Effacement _________ %. Station: minus ___ plus ___.

Fetal heart rate: ____. Fetal movement: ___yes, ___no.

Person performing examination: ____

Examiner wash hands/wear gloves: ______ yes, ______ no.

Time: ____________ am/pm. Dilated: __________ centimeters. Effacement: _________ %.

Effacement _________ %. Station: minus ___ plus ___.

Fetal heart rate: ____. Fetal movement: ___yes, ___no.

Person performing examination: ____

Examiner wash hands/wear gloves: ______ yes, ______ no.

Time: ____________ am/pm. Dilated: __________ centimeters. Effacement: _________ %.

Effacement _________ %. Station: minus ___ plus ___.

Fetal heart rate: ____. Fetal movement: ___yes, ___no.

Person performing examination: ____

Examiner wash hands/wear gloves: ______ yes, ______ no.

Time: ____________ am/pm. Dilated: __________ centimeters. Effacement: _________ %.

Effacement _________ %. Station: minus ___ plus ___.

Fetal heart rate: ____. Fetal movement: ___yes, ___no.

Person performing examination: ____

Examiner wash hands/wear gloves: ______ yes, ______ no.

SPECIAL DELIVERY

Length of labor: ____________ Hours, ______ Minutes.

Uncomplicated Delivery: _______ Yes, _______ No.

List complications: ______________________________

Baby #1 Name: ______________________________

Weight: __________ Pounds __________ Ounces. Length: ______________ Inches.

Male: ________ Female: ________ Apgar score: ______________

Baby #2 Name: ______________________________

Weight: __________ Pounds __________ Ounces. Length: ______________ Inches.

Male: ________ Female: ________ Apgar score: ______________

Baby #3 Name: ______________________________

Weight: __________ Pounds __________ Ounces. Length: ______________ Inches.

Male: ________ Female: ________ Apgar score: ______________

Baby #4 Name: ______________________________

Weight: __________ Pounds __________ Ounces. Length: ______________ Inches.

Male: ________ Female: ________ Apgar score: ______________

Baby #5 Name: ______________________________

Weight: __________ Pounds __________ Ounces. Length: ______________ Inches.

Male: ________ Female: ________ Apgar score: ______________

MEDICAL SUPPLY LIST FOR ____________________
DATES ____________________ TO ____________________

List the type of supplies that were provided to assist in your care. The types of materials used for bathing, blood pressure cuffs and oxygen probes, bandages and tape for wounds, IV start kits and tubing, all types of oxygen tubing and masks, materials used for bedside procedures, etc. Although the list is almost endless this will give you a better idea of what to list. You may want to keep a list of supplies left in the room not used upon discharge from the facility. Compare your list to your itemized bill. Bring your own toiletries if you have the opportunity. The charge for these items can be very costly.

Note: There is a daily charge if you are on a specialty bed to reduce the risk of pressure ulcers. Ask to be informed of the daily rate charge. Make sure you are sitting down when you receive this information.

DAY 1: ____________________

DAY 2: ____________________

DAY 3: ____________________

DAY 4: ____________________

DAY 5: ____________________

DAY 6: ____________________

DAY 7: ____________________

MEDICAL SUPPLY LIST FOR ____________________

DATES ____________________ TO ____________________

DAY 8: ____________________

DAY 9: ____________________

DAY 10: ____________________

DAY 11: ____________________

DAY 12: ____________________

DAY 13: ____________________

DAY 14: ____________________

DAY 15: ____________________

DAY 16: ____________________

MEDICAL SUPPLY LIST FOR ______________________________

DATES __________________ TO __________________________

DAY 17: ____

____

____

DAY 18: ____

____

____

DAY 19: ____

____

____

DAY 20: ____

____

____

DAY 21: ____

____

____

DAY 22: ____

____

____

DAY 23: ____

____

____

DAY 24: ____

____

____

DAY 25: ____

____

____

MEDICAL SUPPLY LIST FOR ______________________________

DATES __________________ TO __________________________

DAY 26: ____

____

____

DAY 27: ____

____

____

DAY 28: ____

____

____

DAY 29: ____

____

____

DAY 30: ____

____

____

SUPPLIES LEFT UNOPENED UPON DISCHARGE FROM FACILITY: ____________

____

____

____

____

____

____

QUESTIONS REGARDING SUPPLIES: __________________________

____

____

____

Index

C

D

E

F

G

H

I

J

K

L

M

N

O

P

Q

R

S

T

U

V

W